An Atlas of

Oxygen-cardiorespirograms in Newborn Infants

Renate Huch, MD
Professor, Department of Obstetrics & Gynaecology
University Hospital,
Zurich, Switzerland

Albert Huch, MD
Professor, Department of Obstetrics & Gynaecology
University Hospital,
Zurich, Switzerland

Gösta Rooth, MD
Professor, Perinatal Research Unit, Department of Paediatrics
University Hospital
Uppsala, Sweden

in collaboration with

Falk Fallenstein, MSc
Department of Obstetrics & Gynaecology
University Hospital,
Zurich, Switzerland

Harald Schachinger, MD
Department of Paediatrics
University Hospital,
Berlin, West Germany

Wolfe Medical Publications Ltd

Published by Wolfe Medical Publications Ltd, 1983
Printed by Royal Smeets Offset b.v., Weert, Netherlands
ISBN 0 7234 0770 3

This book is one of the titles in the series of Wolfe Medical Atlases, a series which brings together probably the world's largest systematic published collection of diagnostic photographs.
For a full list of Atlases in the series, plus forthcoming titles and details of our surgical, dental and veterinary Atlases, please write to Wolfe Medical Publications Ltd, Wolfe House, 3 Conway Street, London W1P 6HE.

General Editor, Wolfe Medical Atlases:
G. Barry Carruthers, MD(Lond)

Foreword

Over the past decade, physicians and nurses who care for newborn infants have had access to ever more equipment designed to provide continuous information about vital signs. The monitors now widely used in intensive care settings allow prompt intervention when apnoea occurs, for example. The ability to follow transcutaneous oxygen tensions and see changes with usual nursing procedures such as feeding and suctioning provides valuable information to nurses who sometimes alter their actions to lessen wide swings in oxygenation. Those of us who have used continuous monitors would not like to return to the era of sporadic sampling of information.

Even though we are convinced of the value of monitoring vital signs, we are at the same time aware of deficiencies in our knowledge of natural variation. We have come to depend on information about extensive changes before we knew the limits of normal. Little notice has been taken of patterns of change as they may appear when simultaneous recordings of heart rate, respiration, transcutaneous oxygen tension and activity are considered together.

The first step in defining normal variations is presented in this Atlas, compiled by three of the world's authorities in the field. The combined experience of the Huchs and Gösta Rooth, and their meticulous attention to detail, makes them ideally qualified to provide these most welcome data. The observations on 3000 term infants in the first week of life, carefully analysed, provide new information of value to students of postnatal adaptations, and to all who should be alert to departures from normal.

Mary Ellen Avery, MD
Thomas Morgan Rotch Professor of Pediatrics
Department of Pediatrics
Harvard Medical School
Children's Hospital Medical Center
Boston, Massachusetts, U.S.A.

Contents

1 Introduction

In the last 10 years we have seen an increased use of non-invasive, biophysical diagnostic methods in perinatal medicine. The main reason for this is their easy handling and the availability of new methods. Once a transducer is suitably placed there is a continuous flow of information which can be collected without major requirements in equipment or personnel.

One by one the electrocardiogram, heart rate monitors, and equipment to monitor respiration and transcutaneous oxygen tension measurements (tc$P\text{O}_2$) have come to be used in the intensive care units of perinatal medicine. There have so far been only a few consistent efforts to evaluate synchronously the continuous recording of several parameters.

This is not surprising as doctors in training are taught to evaluate individual measurements and to compare them with given mean values and confidence limits. Far less attention has been paid to dynamic changes of continuous parameters and the significance of interactions for recognition of pathophysiological patterns.

Compared with single measurements, the continuous monitoring of any single parameter is incomparably accurate because the information must, at each instant, relate to the information obtained before and later. Thus, a logical sequence of information is obtained. This may form recognizable patterns which may be related to physiological or pathophysiological processes, something that can never be achieved with single measurements.

The oxygen-cardiorespirograms to be discussed represent such combinations of biophysical, non-invasive and continuous recordings of several variables. Before we can be certain that a pattern in the oxygen-cardiorespirogram represents the onset of a disturbance or a manifest one we must know the range of the normal picture; in other words we must ascertain how much the pattern varies in healthy newborn infants. It is the aim of the present Atlas to describe and statistically to define the oxygen-cardiorespirogram in the first week of life from our experience with 3000 healthy newborn infants.

2 Methods

2.1 The oxygen-cardiorespirogram

The term oxygen-cardiorespirogram was introduced by us some 10 years ago in the course of our studies on neonatal adaptation and diagnosis of neonatal cardiorespiratory disorders. The term signifies simultaneous, polygraphic recordings of the non-invasive, continuous monitoring of transcutaneous *oxygen* tension, heart rate *(cardio)* and *respir*ation. The *gram* implies the recording.

The oxygen-cardiorespirogram is obtained by the use of four electrodes, the transcutaneous Po_2 electrode and the three ECG electrodes positioned on the chest of the infant as illustrated in Fig. 2.1.1.

Fig. 2.1.2 shows an oxygen-cardiorespirogram. Although the curves may be displayed in any order we have found it convenient to show, read from top to bottom, respiratory rate in the first channel which is obtained tachyometrically from the chest wall movements. The latter are recorded as changes in the transthoracic impedance in the channel below. The third channel is the beat-to-beat heart rate obtained from the electrocardiograph. Channel four is transcutaneous Po_2 and the bottom channel is called 'flow'. It gives the amount of energy needed to maintain the oxygen electrode at a constant temperature. One of the factors cooling the system is the blood entering the heated area. The channel therefore indicates relative changes in blood flow.

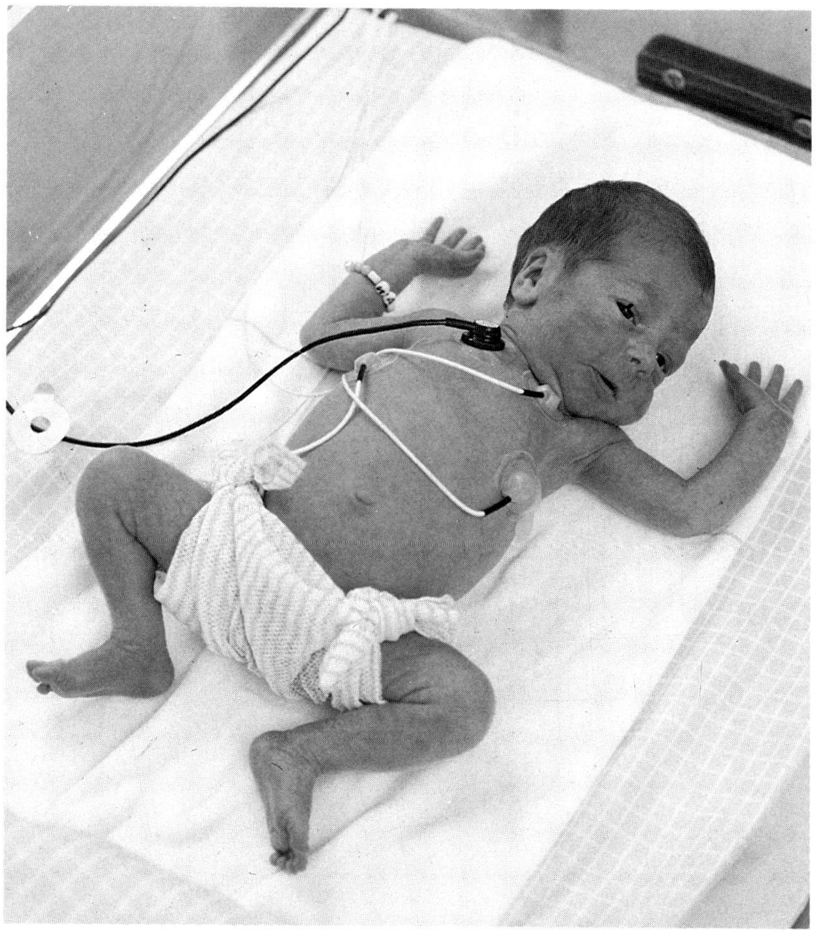

Fig. 2.1.1 Newborn infant with the electrodes for the oxygen-cardiorespirogram
(reproduced with the permission of the parents).

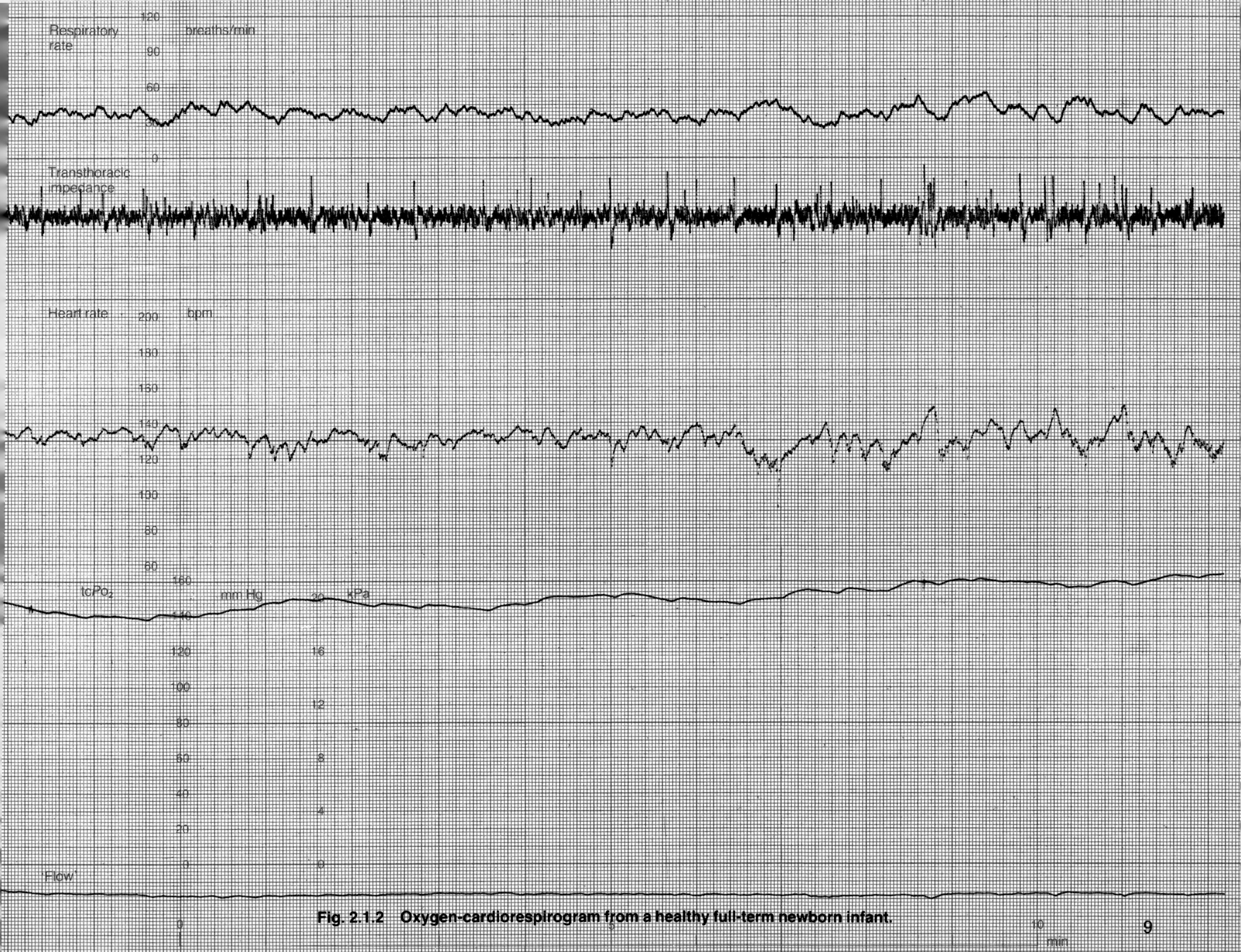

Fig. 2.1.2 Oxygen-cardiorespirogram from a healthy full-term newborn infant.

2.2 The individual measurements

2.2.1 Respiration

Respiration is monitored as variation in the impedance between two electrodes between which a high frequency current is applied. During chest wall movements there are changes in the air/fluid ratio of the lung and thereby also of the transthoracic impedance. Using a frequency of 100 kHz the impedance changes are in the range 0–3 kΩ. Fig. 2.2.1 shows schematically the principle of these measurements.

The transthoracic impedance changes in the oxygen-cardiorespirogram are, as mentioned, displayed in the second channel from the top. Respiratory rate is derived from this primary signal. Respiratory rate may be shown as breath-to-breath rate or some average value may be used. Most recordings in this Atlas have a mean over 3 seconds which gives a picture resembling that obtained by breath-to-breath displays. Sometimes Monitor II was used which averages over 20 seconds. The curve then shown is damped and will not reveal rapid changes.

Respiratory rate is expressed in breaths/min. The transthoracic impedance will mainly be referred to as large or small excursions. The transthoracic impedance changes depend upon many, partly variable factors such as the position of the electrodes, boundary resistance between the electrode and the skin, the size and the properties of the electrode, skin humidity etc, and may therefore not be used quantitatively to estimate tidal volume.

By choosing an optimal sensitivity it is usually possible to detect also minor variations in respiration as well as apnoea. The limitation of the technique lies in the fact that chest movements and consequently changes in the air/fluid ratio and the impedance may occur without corresponding alveolar gas exchange. This limitation is minimized in the oxygen-cardiorespirogram as tcP_{O_2} indicates the efficacy of the ventilation.

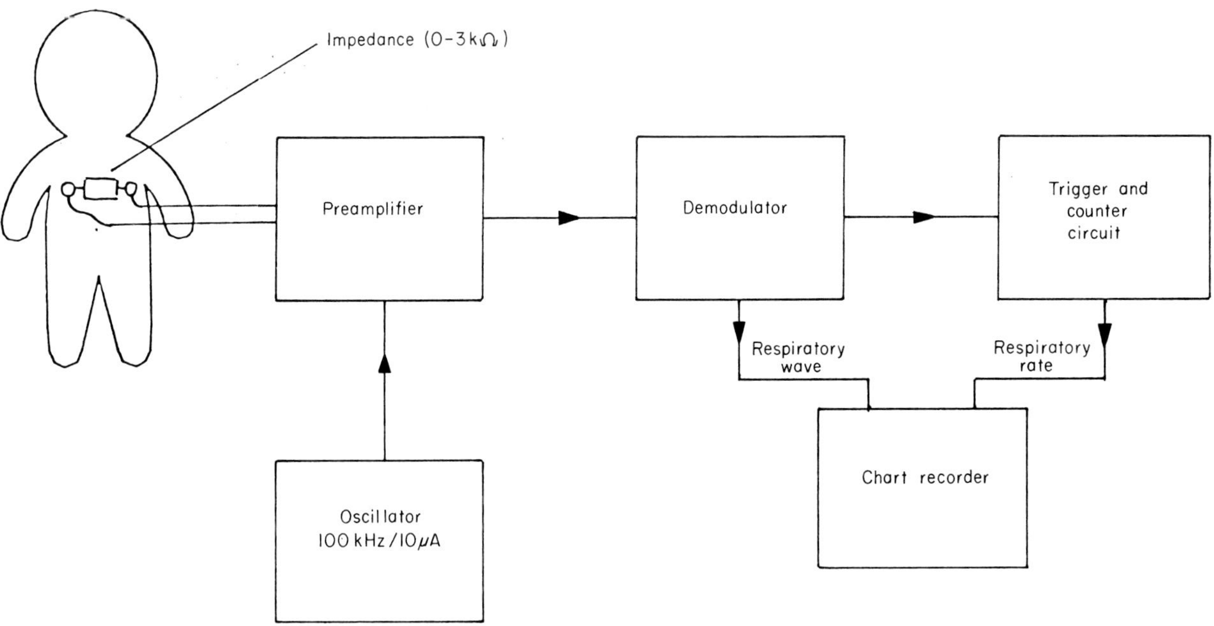

Fig. 2.2.1 Measurement of transthoracic impedance changes.

2.2.2 Heart rate

ECG monitoring has been in use as long as neonatal intensive care units have been operating and either from the ECG or by auscultation a mean heart rate has been obtained. Surprisingly enough beat-to-beat heart rate registration was first introduced in obstetrics. Thus distinct patterns of decelerations, accelerations, amplitude and frequency of long-term variability were described and related to the condition of the fetus. Beat-to-beat registration, which includes recording of the heart rate, is necessary for this pattern recognition. In obstetrics empirical clinical experience has substantiated the present classifications of patterns as innocuous or pathological. In neonatal medicine the clinical use of beat-to-beat heart rate is just beginning to emerge.

As Fig. 2.2.2 shows the basic signal utilized is the R wave of the ECG. This signal is transformed into another, standardized electrical signal. This is called triggering. The quality of the final information depends upon the temporal fit of the raw signal to the trigger impulse.

As the figure illustrates, beat-to-beat heart rate is calculated from the time interval (t) between two consecutive R waves using the formula: heart rate = 1/t.

The display of the beat-to-beat heart rate between 50 and 210 bpm on an 8 cm chart allows for the recognition of patterns. It should be remembered that the finest structure, i.e. the real beat-to-beat heart rate differences, the so-called short-term variability, cannot be seen in detail with the usual chart speeds of 1–3 cm/min. With the naked eye we can only see larger waves, called long-term variability. To allow for international comparability the scales of the *x* and the *y* axis in the heart rate display must be uniform and this is taken into account in the oxygen-cardiorespirogram.

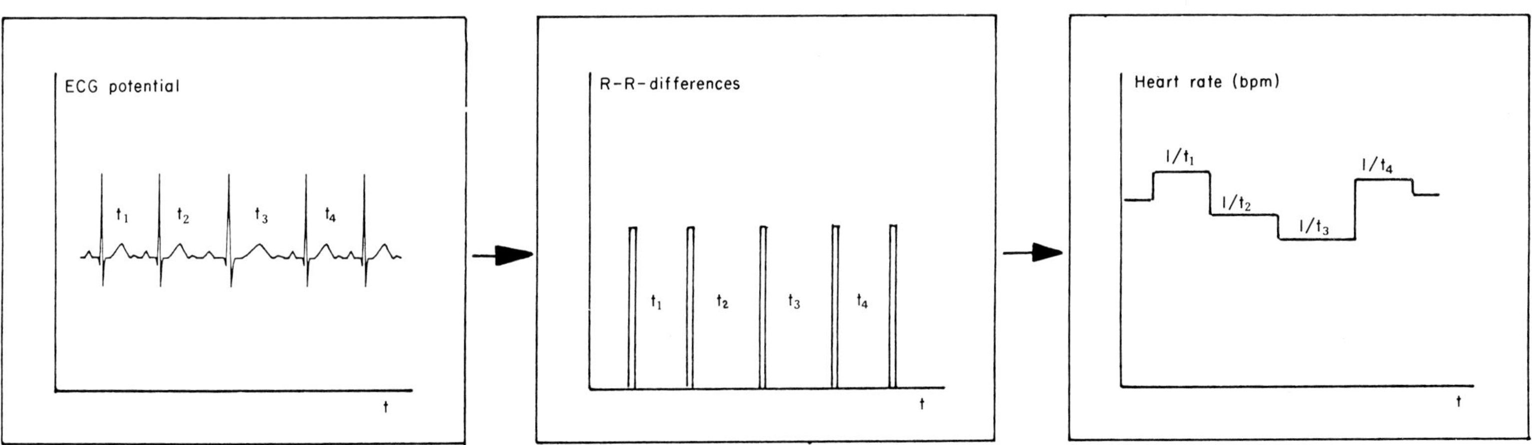

Fig. 2.2.2 Computation of beat-to-beat heart rate.

2.2.3 Transcutaneous oxygen tension (tcP_{O_2})

It is possible to monitor the partial pressure of oxygen by a suitable electrode placed on the skin because oxygen molecules diffuse through intact skin. The oxygen gradient from the capillaries of the skin to its surface is normally zero or a few mm Hg (< 0.5 kPa). It requires a maximal, or close to maximal hyperaemia to achieve a P_{O_2} on the skin surface which is of the same order of magnitude as that of the arterial blood.

Experience has shown that an adequate arterialization can only be reached by the use of heat, either direct heating via the electrode or by diathermy. The hyperthermia, regulated within narrow limits, may also be used to monitor the relative local blood flow under the electrode, as already indicated above.

All modern P_{O_2} methods are polarographic using the Clark type electrode (Clark, 1956).

By polarography oxygen is reduced at the platinum or gold cathode using an applied voltage of about 0.8 V. The resulting current is proportional to the number of oxygen molecules and therefore also proportional to the oxygen pressure. The heating needed for the transcutaneous use of the P_{O_2} electrode is usually applied directly to the silver reference electrode. The complex physiological and technical aspects of the system: electrode-heating-skin have recently been discussed in detail (Huch, Huch and Lübbers, 1981).

Fig. 2.2.3.1 schematically illustrates some of the basic features to take into account in this measuring system. The arrows indicate the factors which increase or decrease the final P_{O_2} level.

The temperature of the heating, the site of measurement, the properties of the membrane, and the diameter of the platinum cathode have all been empirically chosen so that tcP_{O_2} will be very similar to PaO_2.

Heated tc P_{O_2} electrode
45°C
Membranes
43°C
O_2 diffusion through avascular epidermis
40-41°C
Subepidermal capillary network

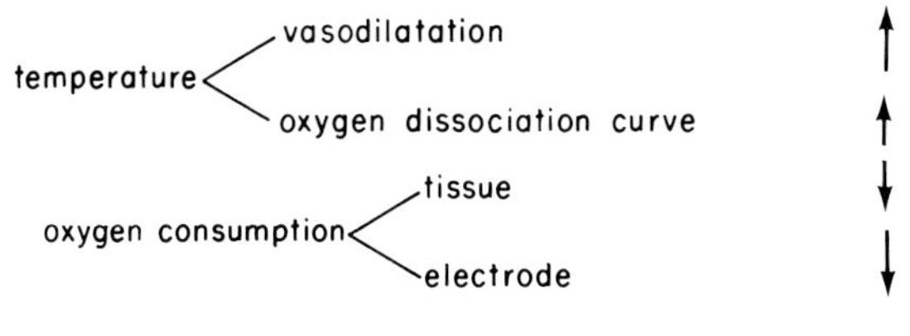

Fig. 2.2.3.1 Principle of transcutaneous measurement of blood P_{O_2}.

The 95 per cent response time of the electrode itself is about 10 seconds and shows almost immediate response to changes in $P\text{O}_2$. However the tc$P\text{O}_2$ electrode on the skin shows changes with a delay of 10–15 seconds. The delay after variation in inspired FiO_2 is due to mixing time in the lung, circulation time, and diffusion time from the capillaries through the skin to the electrode membrane and to the cathode. This must be taken into account when comparing tc$P\text{O}_2$ in the oxygen-cardiorespirogram to the instantaneous changes in heart rate and in respiration.

As indicated above a series of factors affect tc$P\text{O}_2$ in relation to $P\text{aO}_2$ in both directions and tc$P\text{O}_2$ is therefore never the same as, but similar to $P\text{aO}_2$. Several studies have shown the good agreement between $P\text{aO}_2$ and tc$P\text{O}_2$ in neonatal studies.

There may be a good agreement between arterial and transcutaneous $P\text{O}_2$ even in dying children, but any time the circulation is seriously impaired the blood flow under the electrode may be insufficient to raise tc$P\text{O}_2$ to the $P\text{aO}_2$ level. Therefore if infants are in shock or suspected shock the tc$P\text{O}_2$ values should always be compared with arterial values before a similarity is assumed.

For a recent review see Huch, Huch and Lübbers (1981).

Fig. 2.2.3.2 shows the correlation between arterial and transcutaneous $P\text{O}_2$ in 325 blood samples during the first day of life (Schachinger, 1980). His cases are also part of the material presented in this Atlas. The correlation coefficient is 0.99. As may be seen from the lowest $P\text{O}_2$ values, some of his infants had cardiac or respiratory diseases, although, as in this Atlas, the majority were healthy newborn infants.

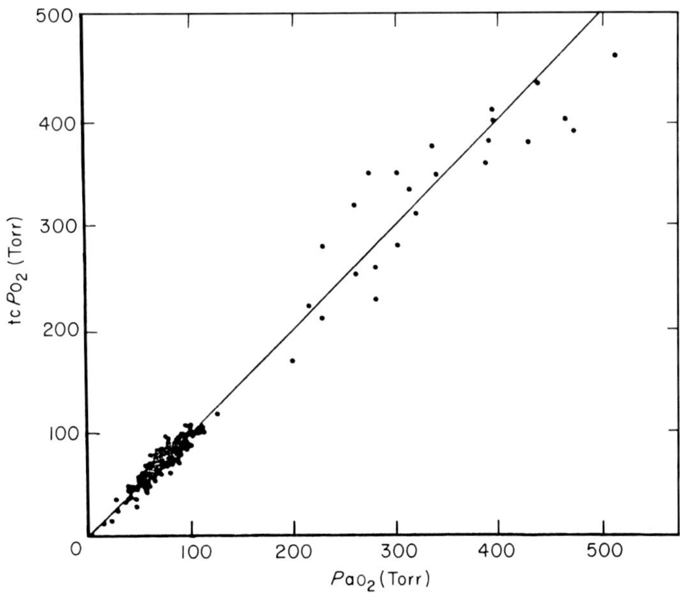

Fig. 2.2.3.2 Correlation between arterial $P\text{O}_2$ ($P\text{aO}_2$) and transcutaneous $P\text{O}_2$ (tc$P\text{O}_2$) (n = 325) in newborn infants during the first week of life. (From Schachinger, 1980.) (SI conversion 7.5 mm Hg (Torr) = 1 kPa.)

Peabody, Gregory, Willis and Tooley (1978) studied sick preterm newborn infants and found a correlation coefficient of 0.98 (Fig. 2.2.3.3) and confirmed that only under grave pathological conditions is there a risk that tc$P\text{O}_2$ will underestimate $P\text{aO}_2$ in neonates.

The point of this short review and the following data is to emphasize that the transcutaneous $P\text{O}_2$ values shown in the oxygen-cardiorespirograms are well correlated to $P\text{aO}_2$ and give representative information both about $P\text{aO}_2$ levels and changes. In 14 cases arterial blood sampling was performed at the same time as the oxygen-cardiorespirograms illustrated in this Atlas. Fig. 2.2.3.4 shows the good agreement between $P\text{aO}_2$ and tc$P\text{O}_2$ in this small series also. The correlation coefficient is 0.98.

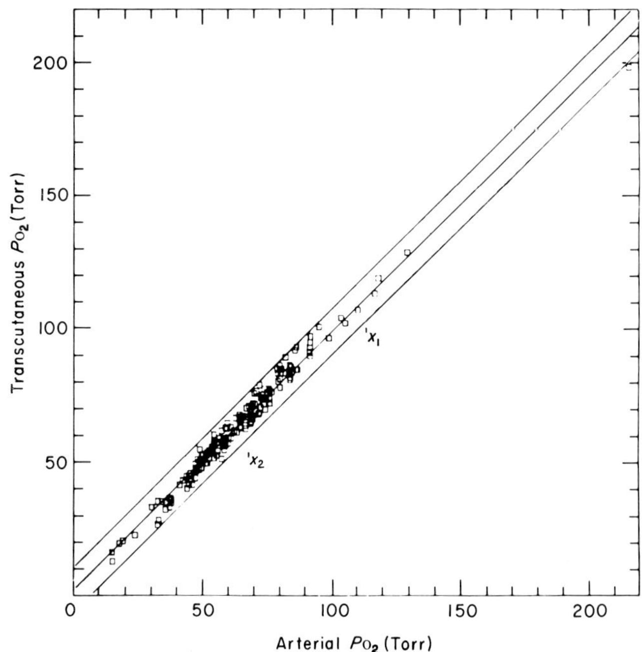

Fig. 2.2.3.3 Correlation between arterial $P\text{O}_2$ ($P\text{aO}_2$) and transcutaneous $P\text{O}_2$ (tc$P\text{O}_2$) in 30 sick infants.

By permission from Peabody, Gregory, Willis and Tooley (1978). (SI conversion: 7.5 mm Hg (Torr) = 1 kPa.)

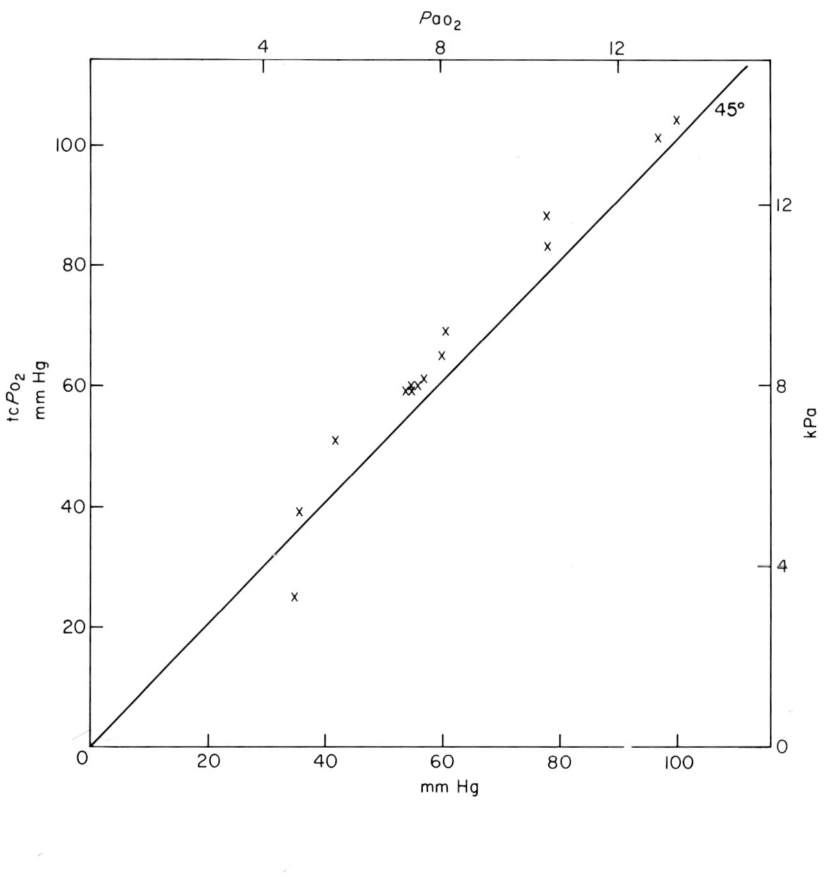

Fig. 2.2.3.4 Correlation between arterial $P\text{O}_2$ ($P\text{aO}_2$) and transcutaneous $P\text{O}_2$ (tc$P\text{O}_2$). The 14 simultaneous measurements referred to in Chapters 4–9 are shown. $y = 0.44 + 1.08x$, $r = 0.98$.

2.2.4 'Flow'

Several methods have been devised to measure blood flow by the use of heat. The transcutaneous Po_2 electrode uses heat, as indicated, by monitoring the amount of energy needed to maintain the core of the electrode at a constant, preset temperature. When blood with a temperature of 37°C enters the heated area with a core temperature of the electrode at 45°C the energy output is increased. This increase is proportional to the blood flow provided other influences are eliminated. Such factors are the heat conduction by the tissues and heat loss through the skin.

It follows that the absolute value of the energy requirement for the heating is influenced by many factors other than blood flow and actually they account for over 95 per cent of the energy output. The electronic equipment therefore needs some compensation so that the signal may be sufficiently amplified to indicate blood flow changes (see Fig. 2.5.4). The electrode should preferably be isolated in order to reduce the influence of variations in the surrounding temperature.

In the Atlas 'flow' is only shown in a few instances, i.e. those in which significant flow changes were observed. These will be discussed in relation to simultaneous changes in other channels.

2.3 The oxycardiorespirograph

Fig. 2.3 shows the combination equipment which Hellige, Freiburg, FRG, supplies for the recording of oxygen-cardiorespirograms, and which has been used for all the oxygen-cardiorespirograms presented in this Atlas. The instrument has:

- two channel oscilloscope for display of the signals
- beat-to-beat heart rate and ECG monitor
- transthoracic impedance meter (Apnoea monitor) for recording respiratory excursions and respiratory rate
- unit for transcutaneous Po_2 and 'flow' using the Transoxode (Dräger, Lübeck, FRG)
- six channel recorder with variable chart speeds.

This compact unit is advantageous in the nursery. However, oxygen-cardiorespirograms may be obtained using a combination of available equipment for transcutaneous Po_2, beat-to-beat heart rate and transthoracic impedance and by displaying the output for all the instruments on one common recorder.

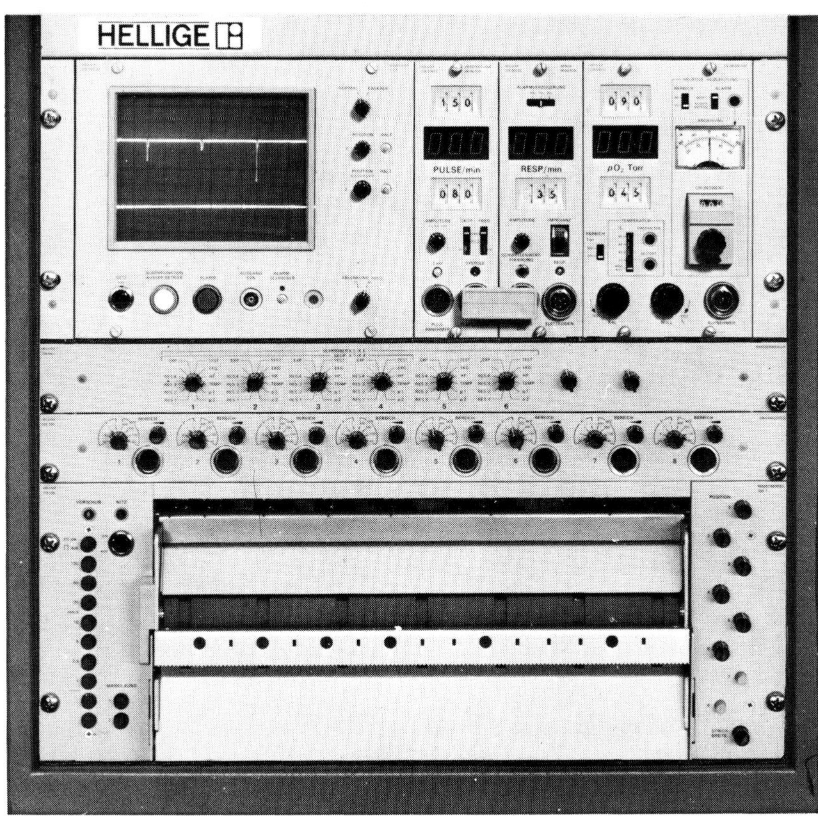

Fig. 2.3 The oxycardiorespirograph.

2.4 How to obtain the oxygen-cardiorespirogram

2.4.1 Position and calibration of the electrodes for the respiration and heart rate

For the recording of the transthoracic impedance changes, indicating the chest wall excursions, two silver-silverchloride electrodes covered with a commercially available contact jelly are placed as far as possible from each other laterally on the lower rib cage on each side. They are affixed with self-adhesive rings.

The monitor gives the number of inspirations per minute. In order to trigger the counter the inspirations must be over a certain threshold level. Therefore, for each infant a suitable sensitivity must be tried out in order to prevent trigger errors such as illustrated in Fig. 2.6.1. If the sensitivity is wrong either inspirations will not be counted or the respiratory excursions will be cut off when they are large as during crying.

The electrocardiogram is also obtained from these two electrodes. A third, indifferent one serves to eliminate AC disturbances. The trigger impulse needed for heart rate is automatically regulated. The calibration of both respiratory rate and heart rate is automatic and part of the electronic equipment.

2.4.2 Position and calibration of the tcP_{O_2} electrode

Whenever possible the tcP_{O_2} electrode should be placed on the trunk of a patient as it is more likely to find there an adequate concentration of capillaries in the subcutaneous tissues than on the extremities. With preterm or full-term newborn infants it is also necessary to measure over areas supplied by large, praeductal arteries. Therefore the right upper part of the thorax is particularly suitable.

Fig. 2.4.2 shows an oxygen-cardiorespirogram recorded with two tcP_{O_2} electrodes. One was positioned, as advocated, on the right upper part of the chest, and the other electrode was placed on the lower abdomen. The effect of the right-to-left shunt in the ductus is seen in the lower tcP_{O_2} level recorded by the electrode below the ductus.

Like the ECG electrode, the tcP_{O_2} electrode is affixed to the skin with a self-adhesive ring. Vacuum may also be used and is recommended for immediate monitoring after birth if the skin is still moist.

As the calibration curve for the oxygen electrode is linear it suffices to calibrate at two points with known P_{O_2} values. For the higher point it is best to use air, which depending upon the barometric pressure has a P_{O_2} of about 160 mm Hg (21.3 kPa). The lower calibration point should be zero, preferably using pure nitrogen or, as a second alternative, a so called zero-solution commercially available.

The core temperature of the electrode must be the same during calibration as during the measurements. Studying newborn full-term infants as well as adults we use 45°C. For monitoring preterm infants or fetuses the temperature should be set at 44°C.

After about two hours of recording the tcP_{O_2} electrode should be repositioned in order to reduce the risk of thermal skin lesions. The air calibration should be checked at the same time.

As mentioned in Chapter 2.3, only the relative energy requirements for maintaining a constant temperature are recorded and called ‘flow’. Using the oxycardiorespirograph the energy needed for the heating of the tcP_{O_2} electrode is displayed on an analog scale. When, after 10 to 20 minutes, adequate hyperaemia is attained the output of the basal heating energy is compensated to zero and only heating energy changes (‘flow’ changes) are shown.

Fig. 2.4.2 Oxygen-cardiorespirogram from a full-term infant with normal Apgar score. A second tcP_{O_2} electrode was positioned below the ductus. Both in air and during the oxygen test the electrode below the ductus showed lower values indicating a right – left shunt in the ductus. See also Fig. 4.7.4.2.

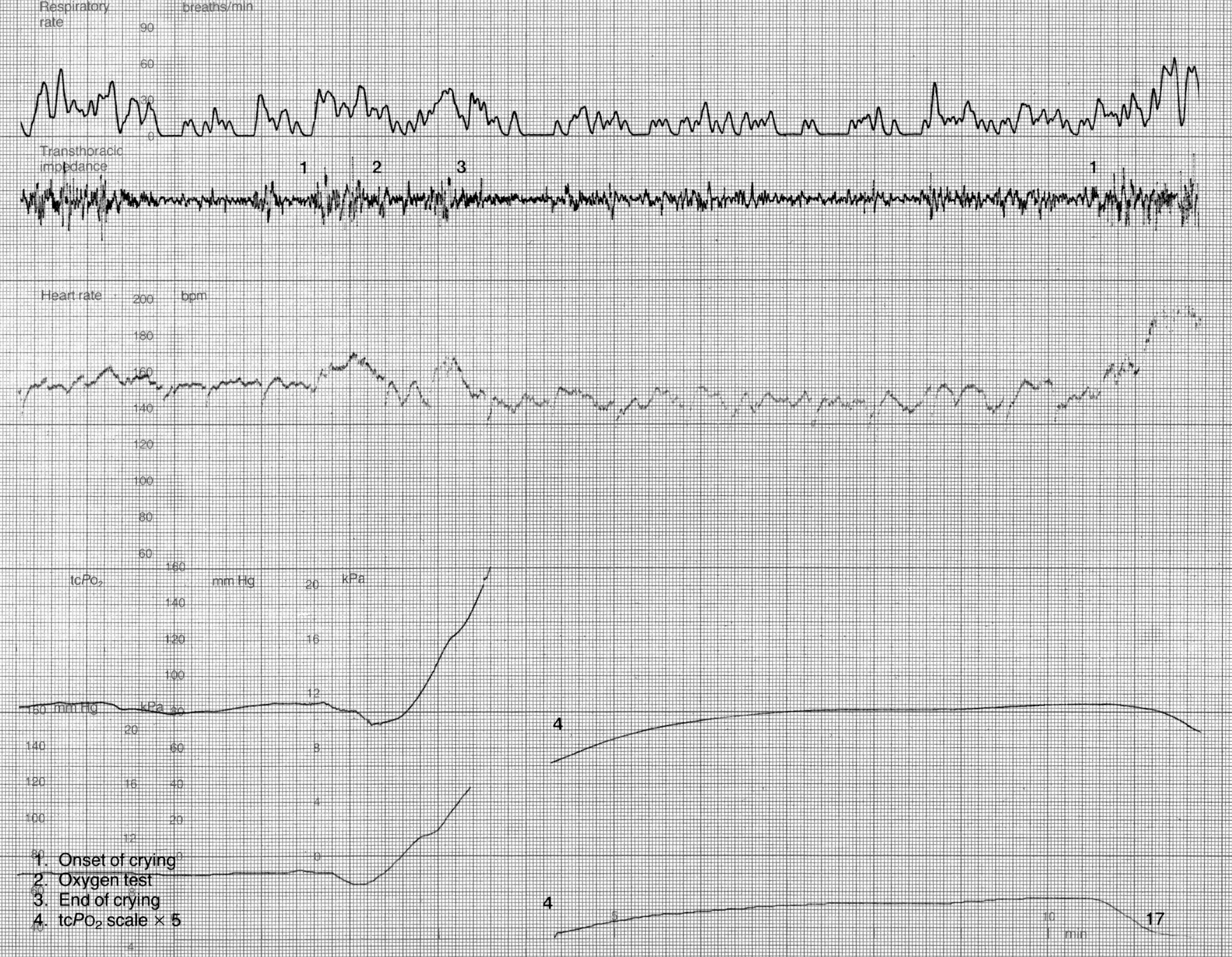

Respiratory rate
breaths/min
90
60
30
0
Transthoracic impedance
1
2
3
1
Heart rate
bpm
200
180
160
140
120
100
80
60
tcPo_2
mm Hg
kPa
160
140
120
100
80
60
40
20
0
20
16
12
8
4
0
4
4
5
10
min
17
1. Onset of crying
2. Oxygen test
3. End of crying
4. tcPo_2 scale × 5

2.4.3 Chart speed

A prerequisite for recognizing and comparing patterns in the oxygen-cardiorespirogram is that a standardized chart speed is used. In clinical fetal monitoring chart speeds between 1 and 3 cm/min are used. In this Atlas the chart speed has consistently been 2 cm/min. Fig. 2.4.3 shows how different the oxygen-cardiorespirograms look at different chart speeds.

Fig. 2.4.3 Oxygen-cardiorespirogram at three chart speeds.
a 0.5 cm/min.
b 2 cm/min (standard).
c 6 cm/min.

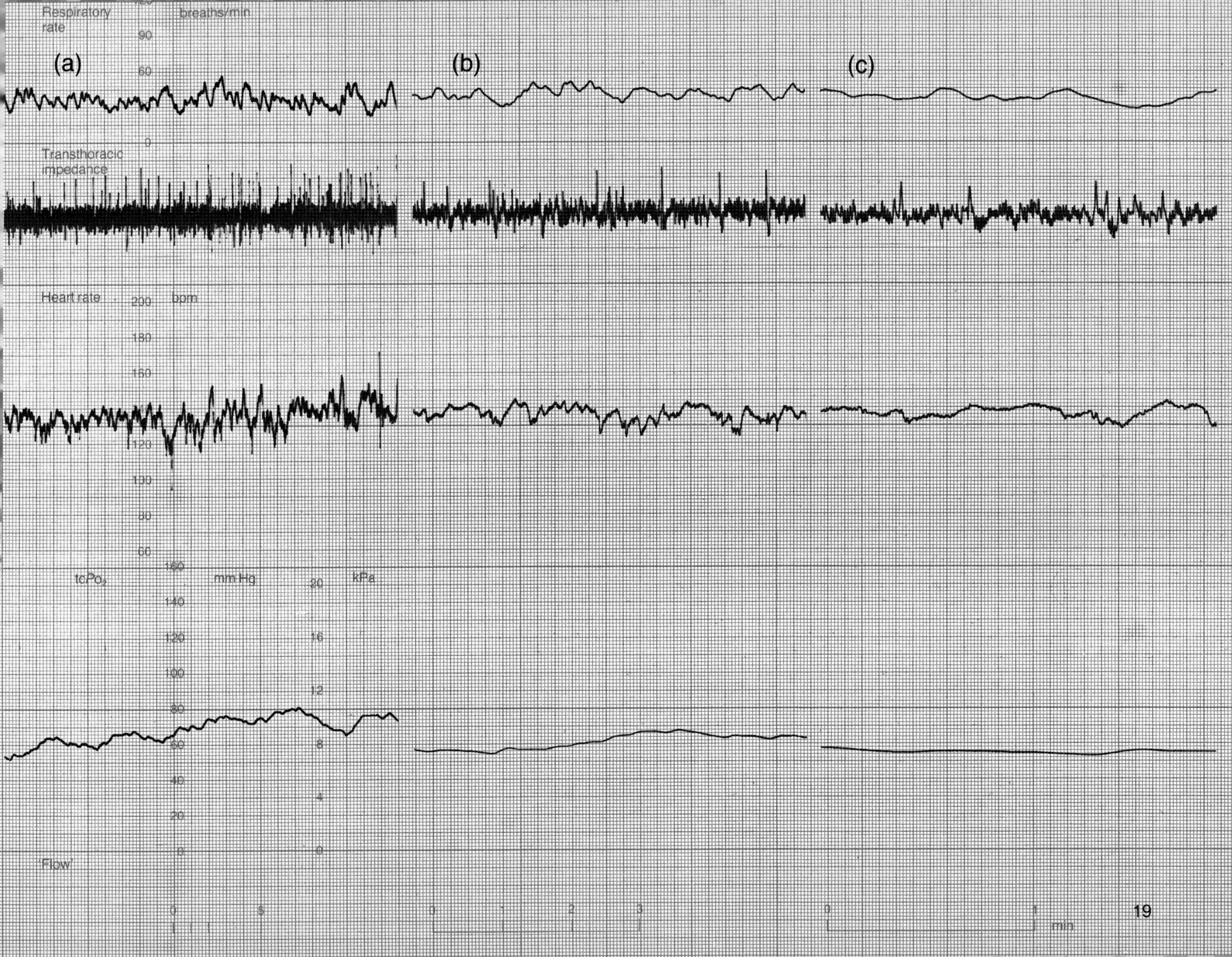
Respiratory rate
breaths/min
90
60
0
(a)
(b)
(c)
Transthoracic impedance
Heart rate
200
bpm
180
160
120
100
80
60
tcPo_2
160
mm Hg
20
kPa
140
120
16
100
12
80
60
8
40
4
20
0
0
'Flow'
0
5
0
1
2
3
0
1
min
19

2.5 Evaluation of the oxygen-cardiorespirogram – definitions

In describing the individual oxygen-cardiorespirograms in Chapters 4 – 9 and in the statistical analyses in Chapter 10 standardized definitions and terms have been used. The curves were evaluated by inspection and/or by computer and we describe whether the level is constant, variable, rhythmic, or if there is periodicity. One single mean baseline value for the whole time of recording was estimated disregarding the unquiet periods.

2.5.1 Respiration

(a) Respiratory rate breaths/min — visual; computer: arithmetic mean of the breath-to-breath rate over the quiet periods

(b) Transthoracic impedance, apnoea, small or large, regular or irregular excursions — visual

2.5.2 Heart rate

(a) Baseline heart rate beats/min (bpm) — visual; computer: arithmetic mean of the beat-to-beat heart rate over the quiet periods

(b) Variability

1. Short-term variability. This cannot be adequately evaluated visually and is therefore not referred to as the Atlas describes what is *seen* in the oxygen-cardiorespirograms. However, a phasic unidirectional short-term variability is the basis for the long-term variability.

2. Long-term variability. Amplitude beats/min — visual: (I) The distance between the highest and the lowest heart rate during one minute disregarding spikes and artifacts. (II) The estimation of the mean of these values over the quiet observation periods.
computer: See Fig. 2.5.2. (I) Using a moving window over 30 s the individual beat-to-beat heart rates were found. (II) The frequency distribution of these heart beats was generated. (III) The distance between the 90 and the 10 percentiles of this distribution was calculated. (IV) Multiplying this by 1.2 the long-term variability was obtained. (V) The mean over the quiet observation periods was calculated.

This computer approach allows for the calculation of the amplitude of the long-term variability in a manner which largely eliminates spikes and artifacts.

The frequency of long-term variability is not commented upon, being difficult to evaluate objectively both visually and by computer.

(c) 1. Spikes. Fast positive or negative changes in heart rate lasting < 3 s with return to initial level — visual

2. Decelerations. Temporary decrease in heart rate lasting > 3 s — visual

3. Accelerations. Temporary increase in heart rate lasting > 3 s — visual

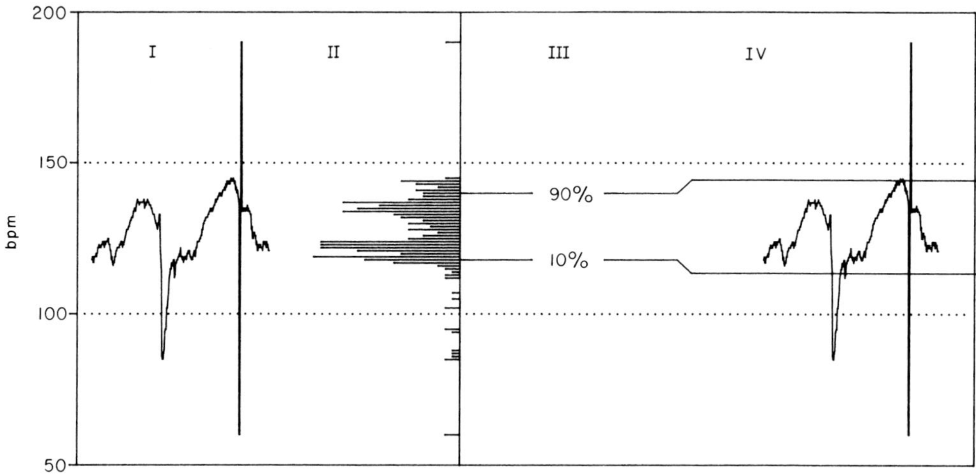

Fig. 2.5.2 The principle of the computer calculation of the amplitude of heart rate long-term variability.
I, Beat-to-beat heart rate registration. II, Frequency distribution of the heart rate values in I. III, 90 and 10 percentiles of this distribution. IV, The distance between the 90 and the 10 percentiles multiplied by 1.2 gives the amplitude of the long-term variability in beats/min.

2.5.3 tcP_{O_2}

(a) Level mm Hg (kPa)	visual computer: arithmetic mean of all levels over the quiet observation periods.
(b) Variability mm Hg (kPa)	visual: (I) Estimation of the interval between the highest and the lowest value in 1 min. (II) The estimated mean over all the quiet observation periods. computer: (I) Obtaining the interval between the highest and the lowest value in 1 min. (II) The arithmetic mean of this over all the quiet observation periods.
(c) Rate of increase mm Hg (kPa) Only evaluated during the oxygen test	visual: Description if a peak value comes fast or slow. computer: The highest rate of the tcP_{O_2} increase.

2.5.4 'Flow'

As already commented upon no units are given for 'flow'. Only visual descriptions are made in relation to covariability in some of the other variables. Fig. 2.5.4 illustrates the influence of different amplifications on the 'flow' signal.

Fig. 2.5.4 The influence of different amplification on the 'flow' curve.
(a) Simultaneous registration of neonatal heart rate and 'flow' with the standard sensitivity of the 'flow' channel.
(b) The same with twice the usual sensitivity of the flow channel.
The covariability between heart rate and 'flow' is more distinctly displayed in (b).

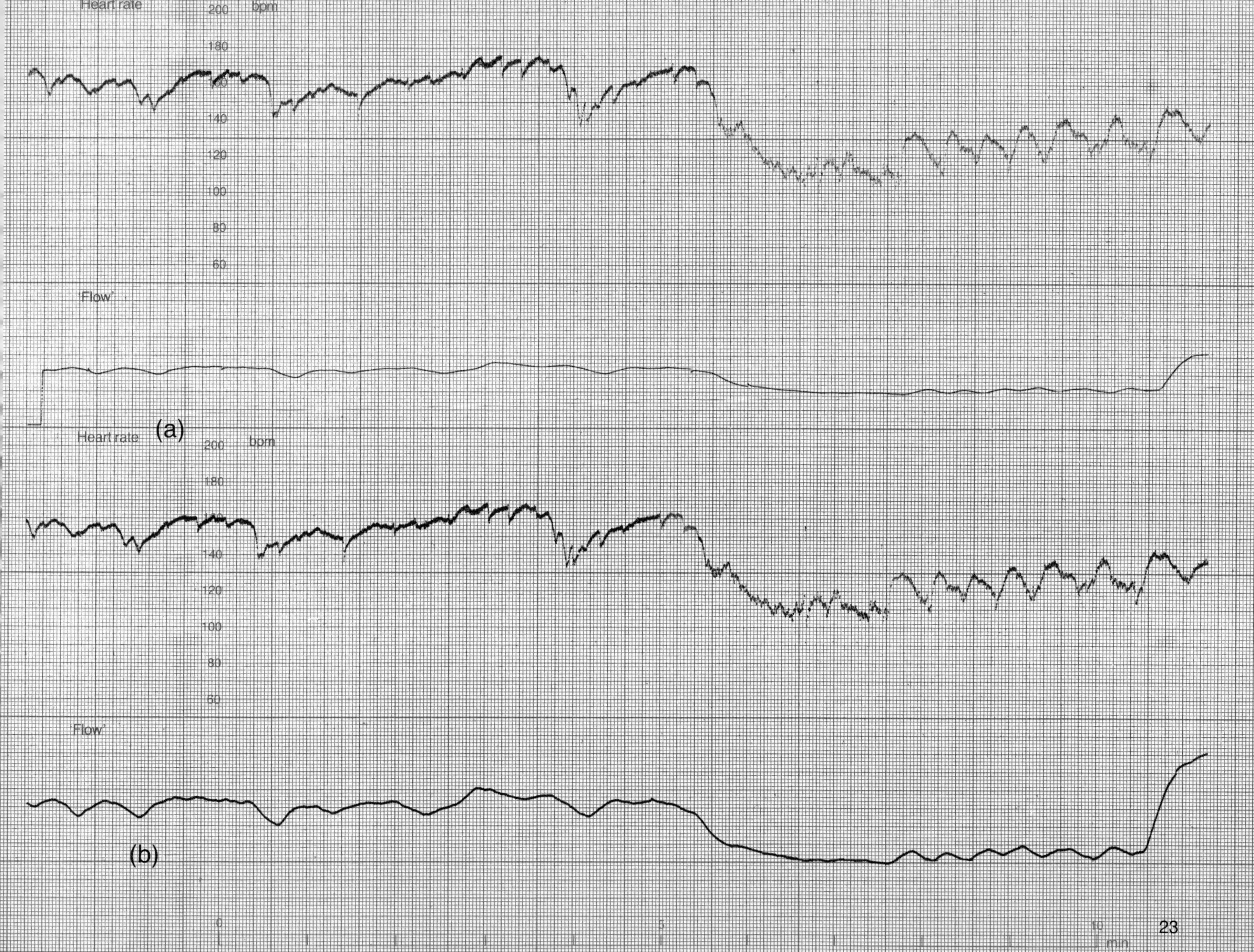
Heart rate
200
bpm
180
160
140
120
100
80
60
'Flow'
(a)
Heart rate
200
bpm
180
160
140
120
100
80
60
'Flow'
(b)
0
5
10
min

2.6 Artifacts and errors

2.6.1 Transthoracic impedance and respiratory rate

1. When the infants move, impedance changes may occur simulating respiratory excursions.
2. The impedance changes resulting from the heart action, although usually small, may simulate respiratory movements thereby masking apneoa.
3. With too high sensitivity the respiratory excursions are cut off.
4. With too low sensitivity, as mentioned, the impedance changes may not reach the threshold level for triggering the respiratory rate meter. Fig. 2.6.1 illustrates such errors.

Fig. 2.6.1 Artifacts in the respiratory rate curve.
Three examples of loss of respiratory rate recording due to trigger error.

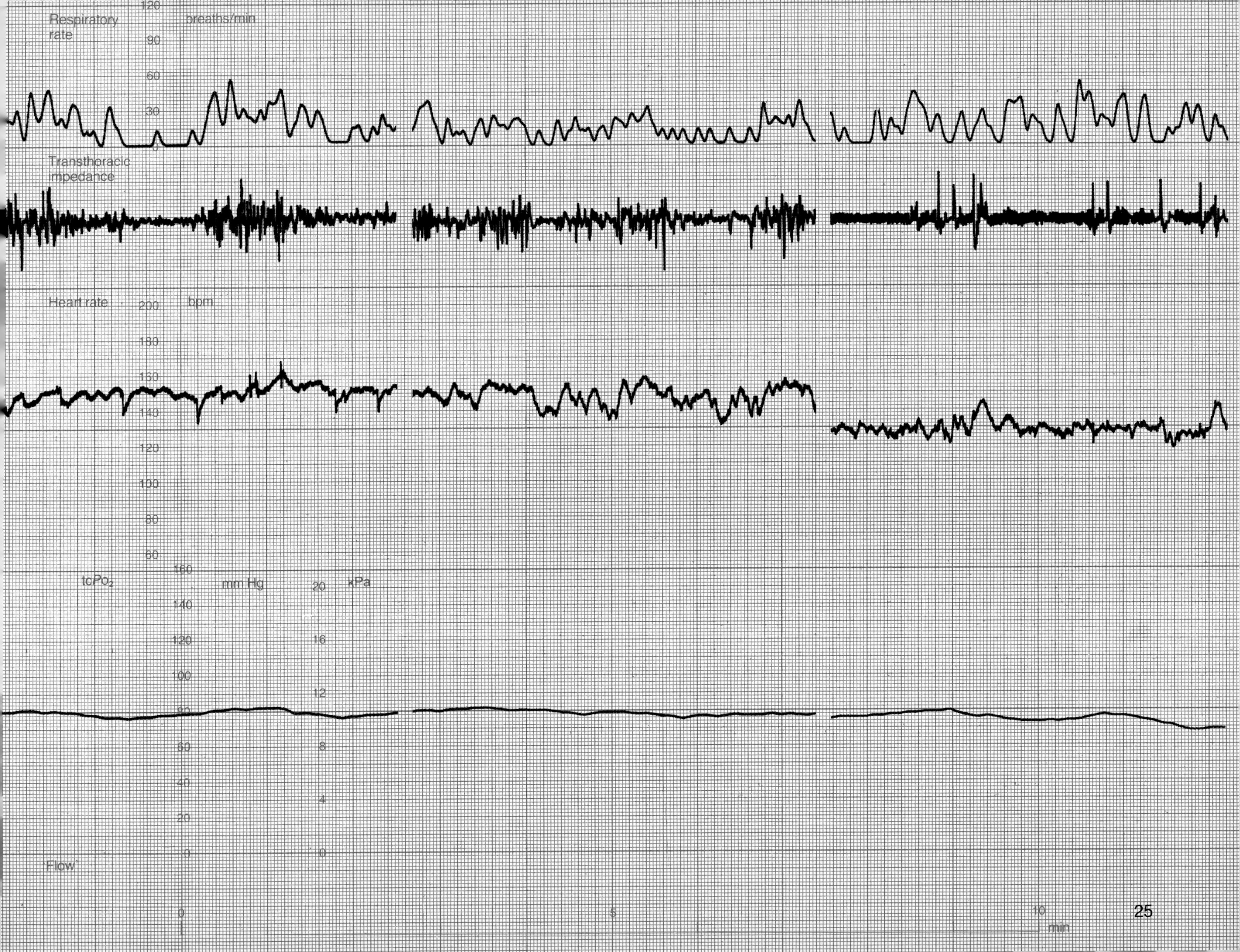
Respiratory rate
breaths/min
120
90
60
30
0
Transthoracic impedance
Heart rate
bpm
200
180
160
140
120
100
80
60
tcPo2
mm Hg
kPa
160
140
120
100
80
60
40
20
0
20
16
12
8
4
0
'Flow'
0
5
10
min

2.6.2 Heart rate

1. The transthoracic impedance changes may be superimposed on the heart rate simulating a large amplitude of the long-term variability. See Fig. 2.6.2.1.
2. Faulty skin contact with the electrodes or moving the cables may produce spikes. See Fig. 2.6.2.1.
3. Extrasystole produces artifacts which cannot be visually differentiated from spikes. If spikes occur frequently an ECG check for extrasystole must be made. See Fig. 2.6.2.2.

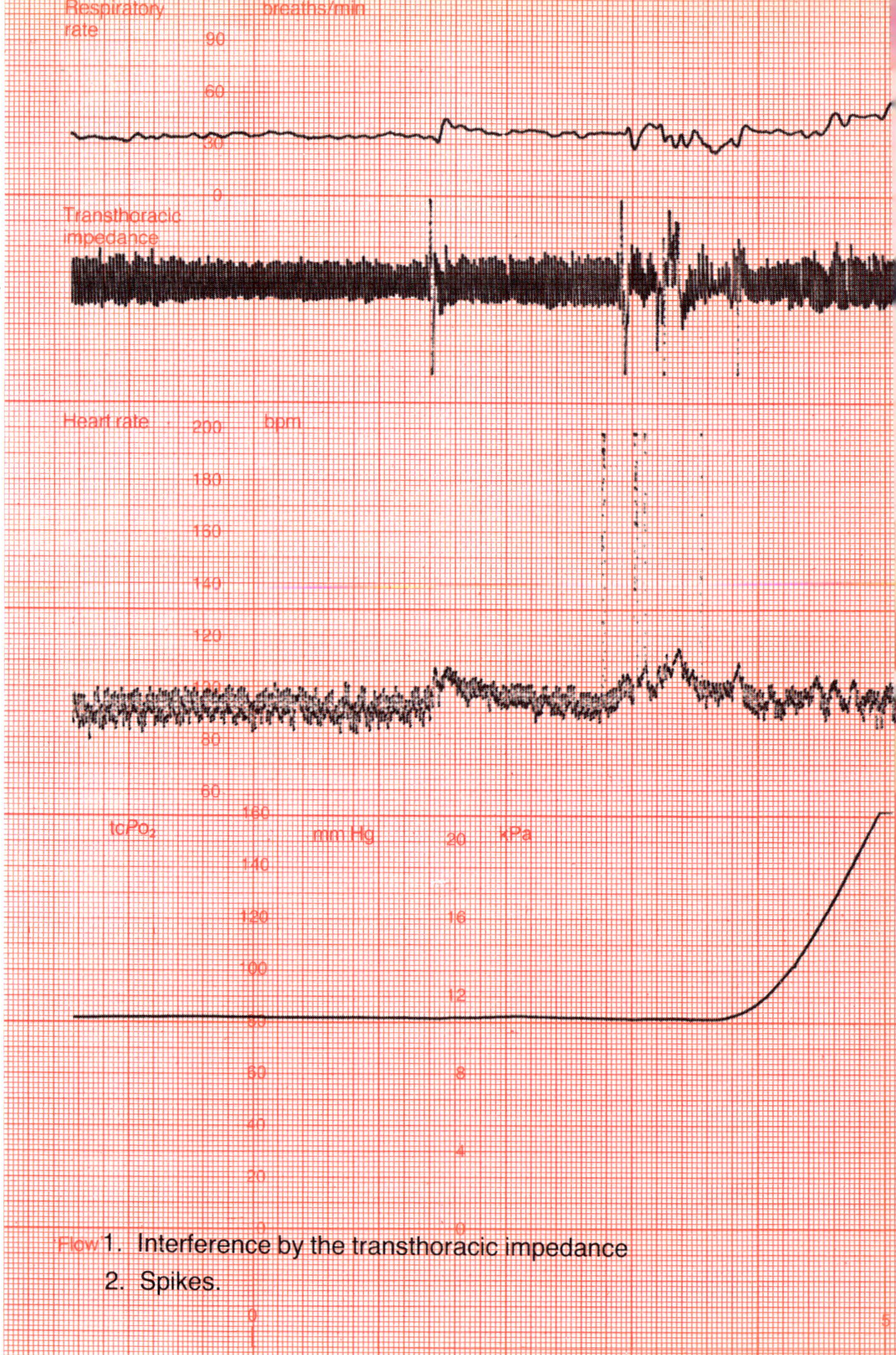

Fig. 2.6.2.1 Artifacts in the heart rate curve.

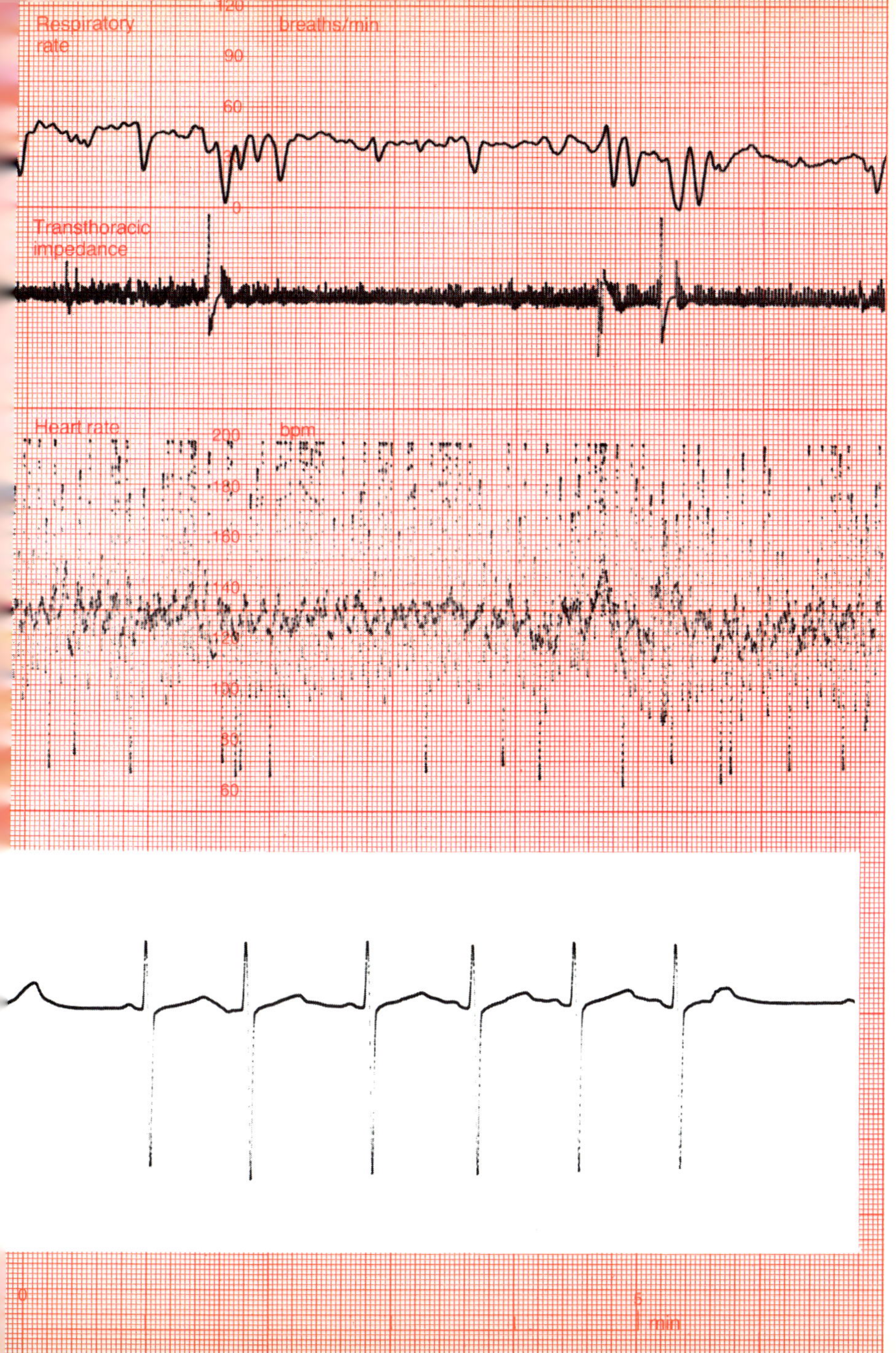

Fig. 2.6.2.2 Artifacts in the heart rate recording because of supraventricular and ventricular extrasystole as shown in the electrocardiogram (lower curve).

2.6.3 tcPO_2

1. If the tcPO_2 electrode is not well fixed to the skin the electrode may temporarily be disconnected. As PO_2 is higher in air than in the blood sharp increases occur as illustrated in Fig. 2.6.3. Physiologically such rapid increases do not occur.
2. As mentioned in 2.4.2, the temperature of the electrode must be set at the same reading during calibration as during the actual measurements. If this is not done, the level of the tcPO_2 values is erroneous but the direction of the changes is correct.

Fig. 2.6.3 Artifacts in the tcPO_2 curve because of intermittent disconnection of the electrode. At the same time spikes appear in the heart rate recording. Both these disturbances are due to movements.

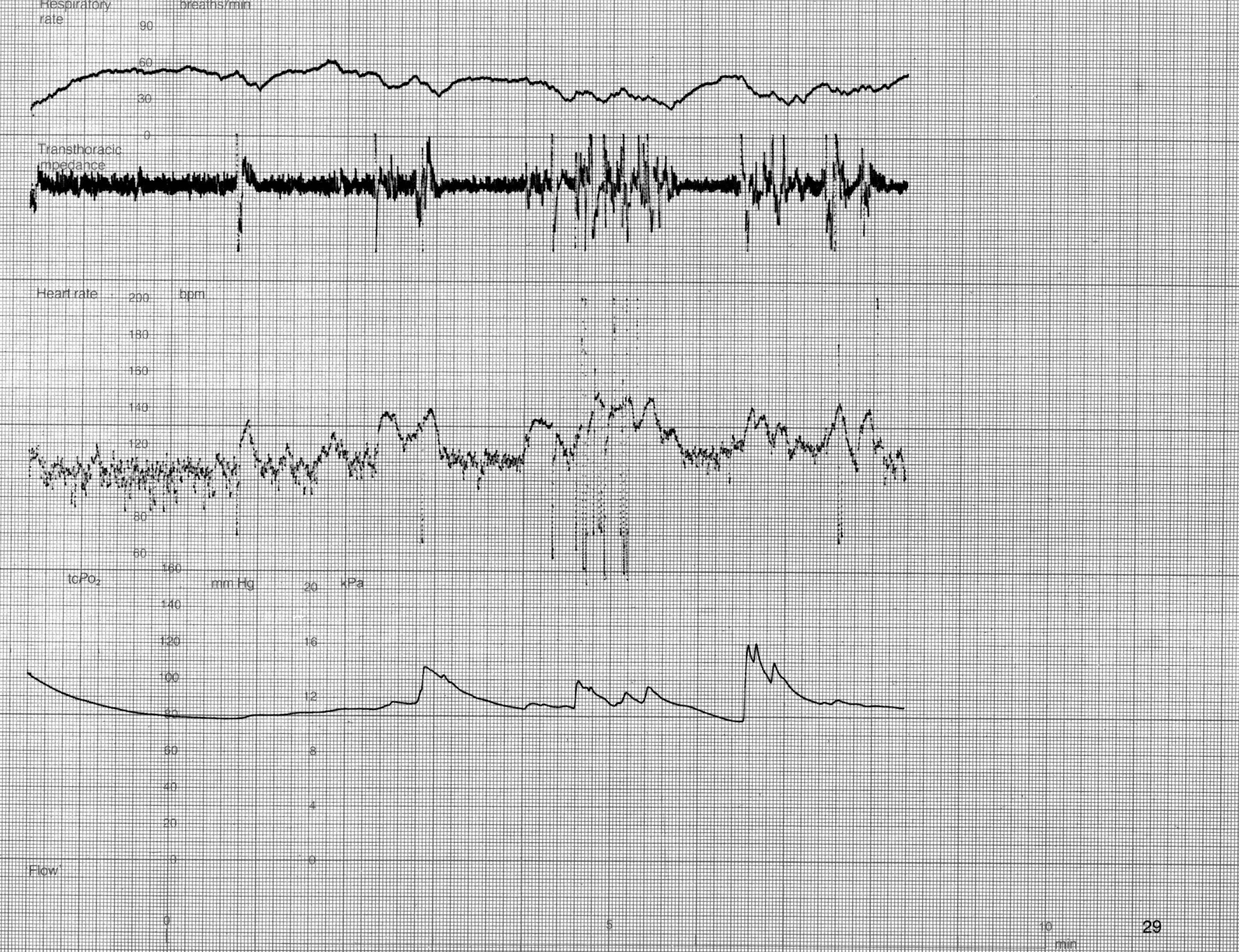
Respiratory rate
breaths/min
120
90
60
30
0
Transthoracic impedance
Heart rate
bpm
200
180
160
140
120
80
60
$tcPo_2$
mm Hg
kPa
160
140
120
100
80
60
40
20
0
20
16
12
8
4
0
Flow
0
5
10
min

3 The material

In the years 1976 to 1978, 3000 newborn infants in the Department of Obstetrics and Gynaecology, University of Marburg*, FRG were studied using oxygen-cardiorespirograms for at least one hour. Gradually the primarily scientific study became a routine check-up on all the newborn infants. For practical reasons the time interval between birth and recording varied.

The oxygen-cardiorespirograms were obtained using the oxycardiorespirograph (Hellige, Freiburg, FRG) and the tcP_{O_2} electrode manufactured by Dräger, Lübeck, FRG. See also Chapter 2.

Early clamping of the cord was done as a clinical routine. When monitoring was performed within the first hour of life the infants were without clothes in an incubator. Otherwise they were dressed and in standard cribs.

During the monitoring, the activity state of the infants was continuously observed and recorded. The following activity states were noted:

- Sleep (quiet sleep, active sleep, undetermined sleep).
- Awake quiet (i.e. no gross body movements).
- Awake unquiet (i.e. gross body movements, sobbing).
- Crying.
- Sucking and suckling.

Furthermore all interventions with the infants were noted such as arterial puncture, oxygen test (onset and end), bottle feeding as well as other clinical and diagnostic procedures.

For the oxygen test pure oxygen was warmed and humidified and applied to the infant through a plastic box placed over the head. The test was continued until a plateau was reached in tcP_{O_2} but never for more than 15 minutes.

Arterial blood was drawn from the right radial artery after puncture. The acid – base and blood gases were determined using the automatic bloodgas analyser IL 613 from Instrumentation Laboratories Lexington, Mass., USA.

The studies were made with the informed consent of the mothers who moreover were usually present during the whole recording.

All the oxygen-cardiorespirograms were used to illustrate, in Chapters 4 – 9, the influence of the activity states, age, Apgar score, type of birth, anaesthesia and analgesia etc. However, the statistical analyses in Chapter 10 only refer to infants who were clinically well at the time of study and who had a birthweight $\geq$ 2500 g. Only when studying the influence of birthweight were healthy infants with a birthweight down to 2000 g included.

The oxygen-cardiorespirograms of all the healthy infants were visually evaluated as described in Chapter 2. All the observations were made when the infants were quiet with the exception of the tcP_{O_2} decrease during crying. For each infant and each variable only one mean value was noted derived from variable time spans. The unequal numbers in the statistical analysis is due to technical difficulties in the clinical recording. All the data noted were stored and analysed with Hewlett Packard desk computer HP 9825 A and HP 9845 B.

*Before R.H. and A.H. moved to the University of Zurich/Switzerland.

The oxygen-cardiorespirograms of 500 of the newborn infants were in addition computer stored for subsequent analysis. A special unit was built utilizing commercially available tape cassettes. The unit has the following characteristics:

No. of channels	6
Sampling rate per channel	33.3 Hz
Resolution per channel	11 bit (about 2000 amplitude steps)
Storage capacity	120 min (with C-120 cassettes)

By the subsequent transfer to the computer, data reduction was made taking into account the natural structure of the individual variables of the oxygen-cardiorespirogram.

Channel	data frequency (Hz)	Resolution (bit)
1. Respiratory rate	1	8
2. Transthoracic impedance	8	8
3. Heart rate	4	8
4. tcP_{O_2}	1	8
5. 'Flow'	1	8

The sixth channel was used for recording the activity states. The data thus reduced, were stored on mini floppy discs using a Commodore CBM 3032 for subsequent calculations.

In some of the infants whose oxygen-cardiorespirograms were stored on tape it was possible to do repeated recordings thus allowing a study of the evolution of the oxygen-cardiorespirogram during the first week of life. Chapter 5.2 gives some individual examples and statistical studies are presented in Chapter 10.

4 Oxygen-cardiorespirograms

Fig. 4.1.1

Birthweight: 3300 g

Apgar score: 9/10

Age (in hours) at recording:	7

Delivery: vaginal

Cord blood acid – base and blood gases						
	pH	$P\text{CO}_2$ mm Hg	kPa	$P\text{O}_2$ mm Hg	kPa	Base deficit mmol/l
Umbilical vein	7.33	38	5.1	26	3.5	4.4

Activity state	Awake, quiet.
Respiratory rate	Mainly between 30 and 40 breaths/min (Monitor II).
Transthoracic impedance	Mainly regular excursions with occasional deeper breaths.
Heart rate	Between 90 and 120 bpm with such marked variation that no basal heart rate can be identified. Occasional short decelerations concomitant with the deep inspirations.
tc$P\text{O}_2$	Between 74 and 85 mm Hg (9.9 and 11.3 kPa).

Comments Variable respiration, heart rate and tc$P\text{O}_2$ is found in the quiet but awake infant.

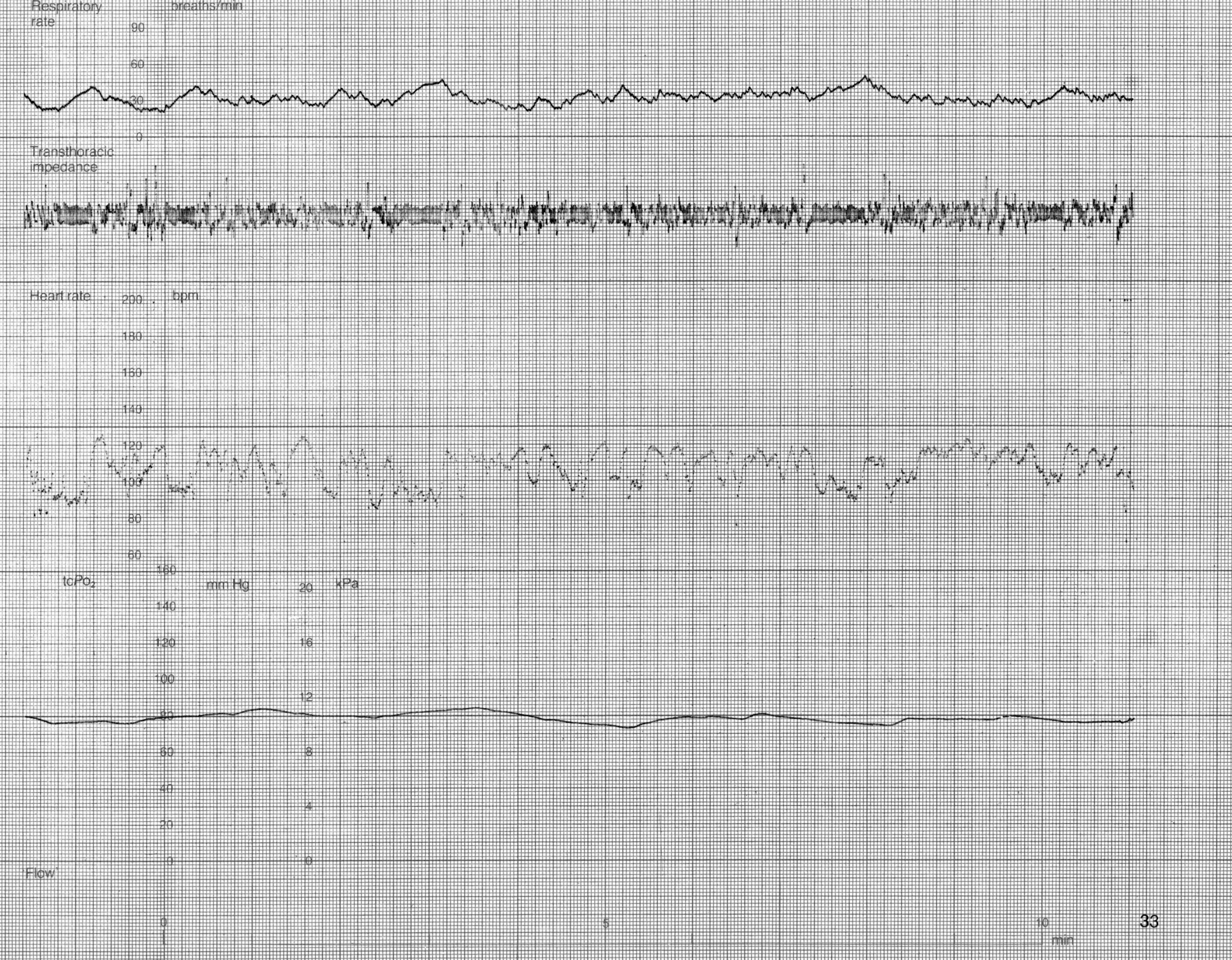
Respiratory rate
breaths/min
120
90
60
30
0
Transthoracic impedance
Heart rate
bpm
200
180
160
140
120
100
80
60
tcPo$_2$
mm Hg
kPa
160
140
120
100
80
60
40
20
0
20
16
12
8
4
0
Flow
0
5
10
min

Fig. 4.1.2

Birthweight: 3500 g

Apgar score: 10

Age (in hours) at recording: ½

Delivery: vaginal

Activity state	First unquiet then quiet and awake.
Respiratory rate	Between 0 and 40 breaths/min (probably incorrect triggering).
Transthoracic impedance	The excursions were irregular all the time and of larger amplitude during the unquiet periods.
Heart rate	Baseline heart rate about 150 bpm with an amplitude of long-term variability $\leq$ 20 bpm.
tc$P$O$_2$	About 73 mm Hg (9.7 kPa) in the unquiet period and 80 mm Hg (10.7 kPa) in the quiet phase.

Comments A typical oxygen-cardiorespirogram of the awake infant. The tc$P$O$_2$ is higher when the infant is quiet. The small tc$P$O$_2$ waves reflect the variations in the breathing.

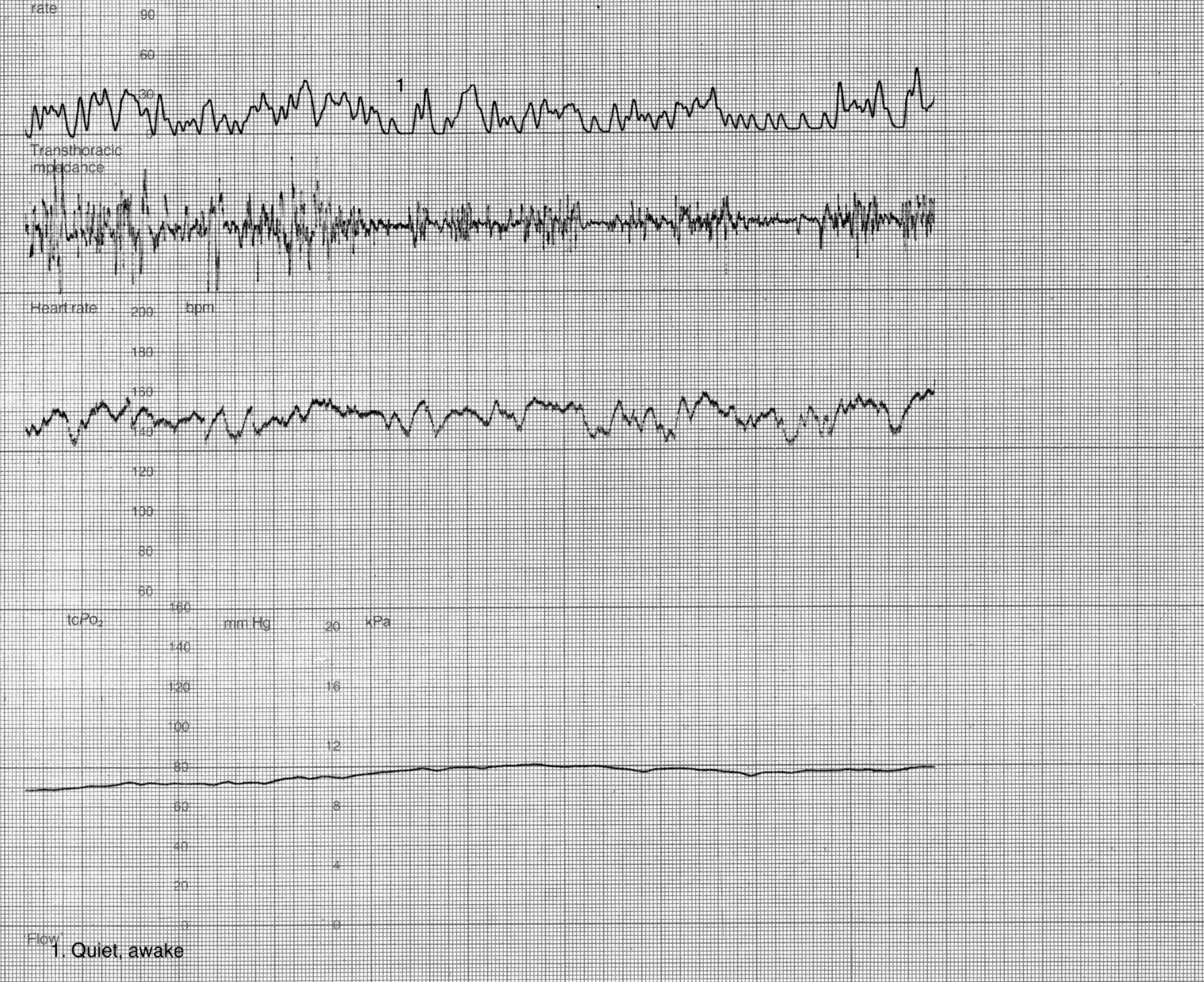

1. Quiet, awake

Fig. 4.2.1

Birthweight: 3640 g

Apgar score: 8/10/10

Age (in hours) at recording: 1

Delivery: vaginal

Activity state	Awake, unquiet.
Respiratory rate	Very undulating between 25 and 110 breaths/min.
Transthoracic impedance	Distinct rhythm changes in the amplitude synchronous to the changes in respiratory rate.
Heart rate	Baseline heart rate about 130 bpm with an amplitude of long-term variability $\leq$ 15 bpm. There are occasional very short decelerations but without distinct association with the breathing pattern.
tcP_{O_2}	Between 70 and 78 mm Hg (9.3 and 10.4 kPa) with small changes.

Comments In this case the infant was unquiet all the time and both respiratory rate and transthoracic impedance showed marked variations. The heart rate variability, although less pronounced than in the two previous figures is still marked. As in Fig. 4.1.2 the tcP_{O_2} changes are small.

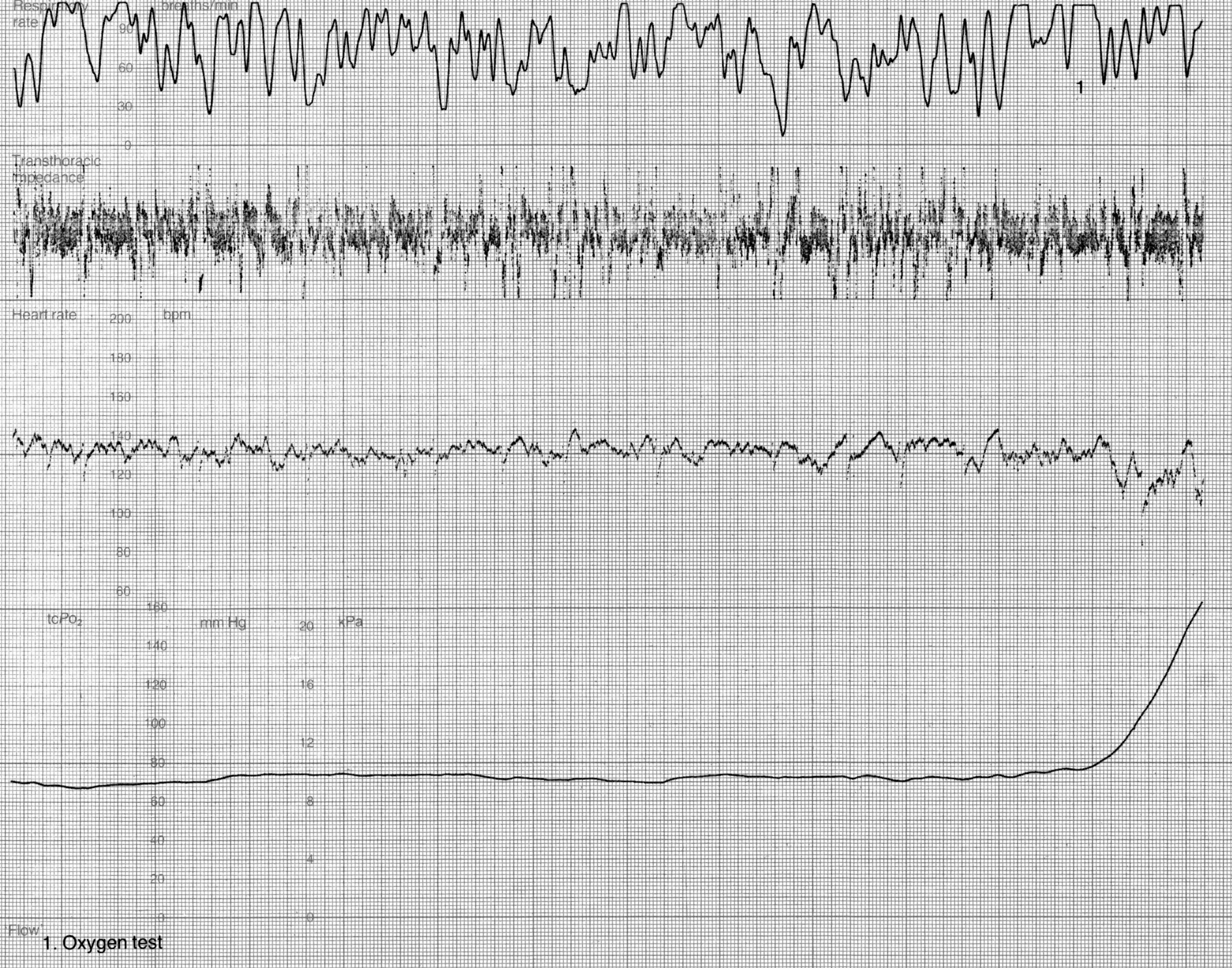
Respiratory rate
breaths/min
120
90
60
30
0
1
Transthoracic impedance
Heart rate
bpm
200
180
160
140
120
100
80
60
tcPo_2
mm Hg
kPa
160
140
120
100
80
60
40
20
0
20
16
12
8
4
0
'Flow'
1. Oxygen test
0
5
10
min

Fig. 4.2.2

Birthweight: 2950 g

Apgar score: 9/10

Age (in hours) at recording:	3

Delivery: vaginal

Activity state	Awake and unquiet. Early, in the middle, and late in the recording more quiet phases.
Respiratory rate	Usually between 30 and 45 breaths/min, occasionally slower.
Transthoracic impedance	Large irregular excursions during the unquiet phases and more regular ones in the quieter parts.
Heart rate	Baseline heart rate about 110 bpm when quiet with an amplitude of long-term variability $\leqslant$ 20 bpm and occasional short decelerations, not related to any of the other parameters except that they are more pronounced in the most unquiet period.
tc$P\text{O}_2$	The level of tc$P\text{O}_2$ fell to 68 mm Hg (9.1 kPa) during the most unquiet phase and increased to 81 mm Hg (10.8 kPa) when more quiet.

Comments This figure is more varied than Fig. 4.2.1 and heart rate is distinctly affected by changes in the intensity of the activity.

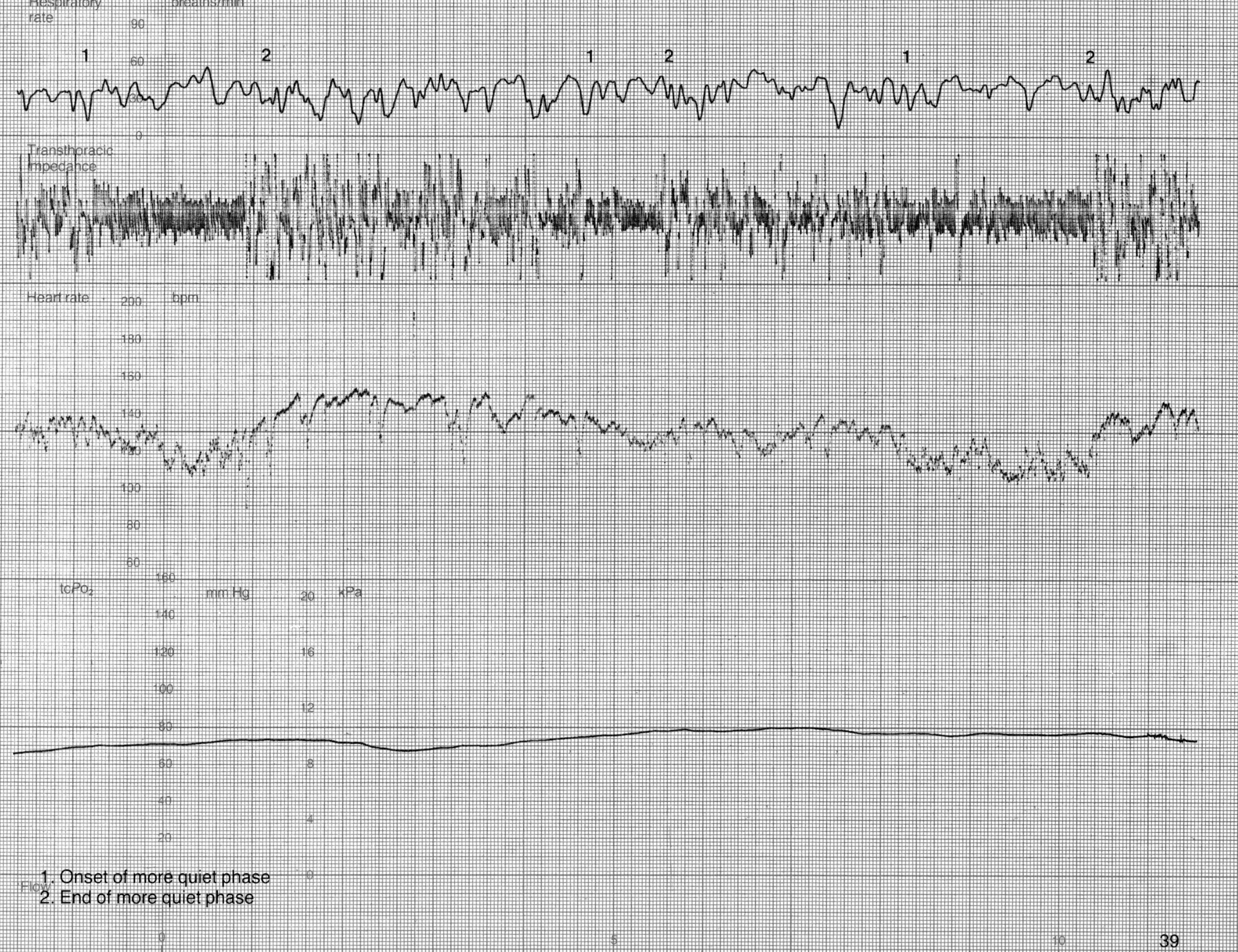
Respiratory rate
breaths/min
120
90
60
30
0
1
2
1
2
1
2
Transthoracic impedance
Heart rate
bpm
200
180
160
140
120
100
80
60
tcP_{O_2}
mm Hg
kPa
160
140
120
100
80
60
40
20
20
16
12
8
4
0
Flow
0
5
10
min
1. Onset of more quiet phase
2. End of more quiet phase

Fig. 4.3.1.a

Birthweight: 2710 g

Apgar score: 9/10/10

Age (in hours) at recording:	12

Delivery: vaginal

Activity state	Quiet sleep.
Respiratory rate	Between 35 and 40 breaths/min.
Transthoracic impedance	Very regular except for occasional deeper breaths.
Heart rate	Baseline heart rate was 100–110 bpm with accelerations synchronous to the deep breaths. The variability was only just discernible ($\leq$ 5 bpm).
tcP_{O_2}	About 95 mm Hg (12.7 kPa).
'Flow'	Constant 'flow' except for the increases during the deep breaths.

Comments See Fig. 4.3.1.c.

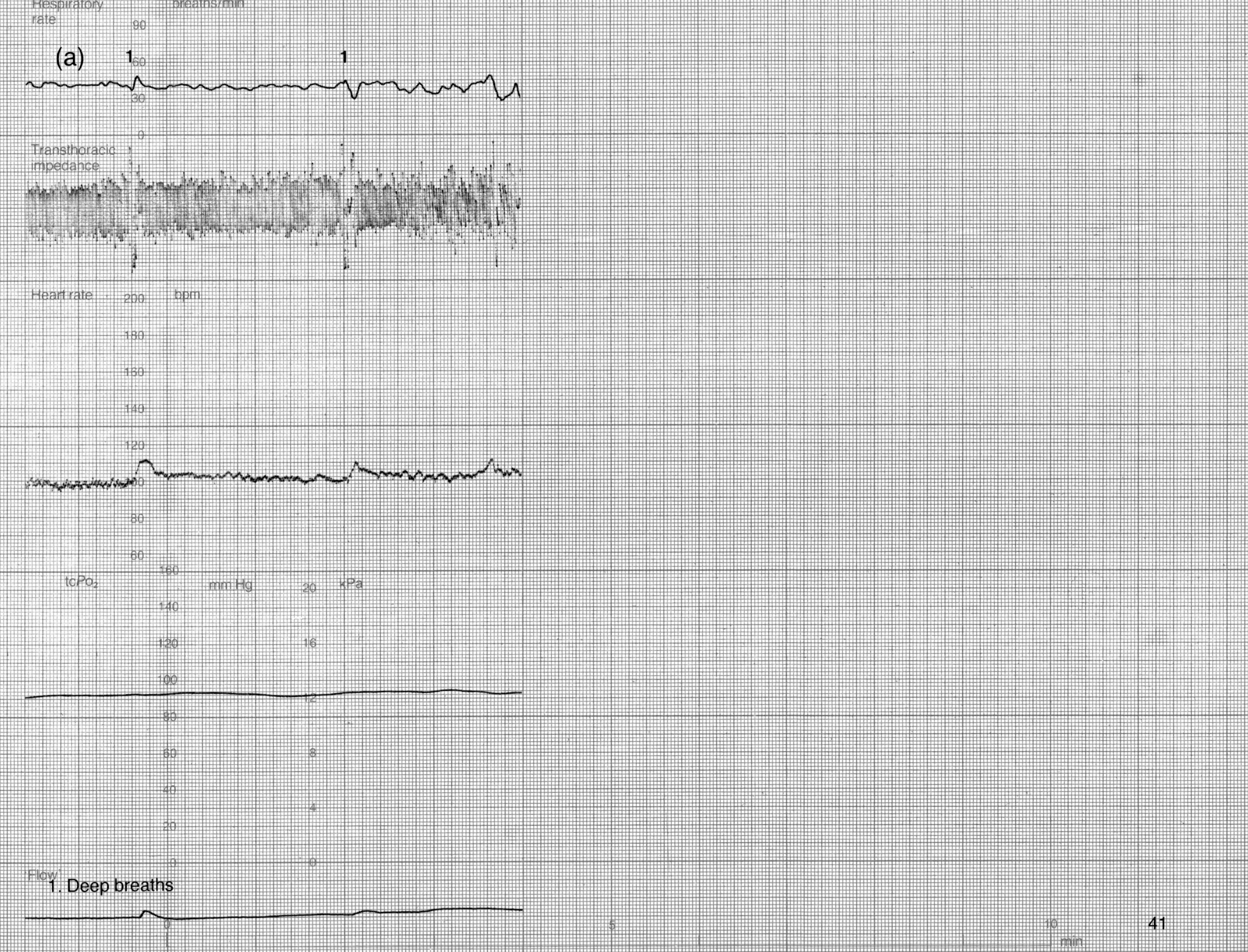

Respiratory rate
breaths/min
120
90
60
30
0
(a)
1
1
Transthoracic impedance
Heart rate
bpm
200
180
160
140
120
100
80
60
tcPo$_2$
mm Hg
kPa
160
140
120
100
80
60
40
20
0
20
16
12
8
4
0
Flow
1. Deep breaths
0
5
10
min

Fig. 4.3.1.b

Birthweight: 3900 g

Apgar score: 9/10/10

Age (in hours) at recording: 4

Delivery: vaginal

Cord blood acid – base and blood gases							
	pH	PCO_2 mm Hg	kPa	PO_2 mm Hg	kPa	Base deficit* mmol/l
Umbilical artery	7.37	39	5.2	13	1.7	2.4
Umbilical vein	7.43	30	4.0	22	2.9	4.1

Activity state	Quiet sleep.
Respiratory rate	Between 35 and 40 breaths/min.
Transthoracic impedance	Very regular with occasional deeper inspirations and apnoea.
Heart rate	Baseline heart rate was about 120 bpm. Long-term variability: about 10 bpm but difficult to evaluate because of artifacts. Decelerations parallel to the deep breaths.
tcPO_2	About 75 mm Hg (10 kPa) with small changes.
'Flow'	Small fluctuations without relation to the other variables.

*Base deficit (= –Base excess) was calculated as base deficit of the extracellular fluid according to Siggaard-Andersen, O. (1967) Therapeutic aspects of acid – base disorders. In *Modern Trends in Anaesthesia*, vol III, Evans, F. and Gray, T. C. Ed. Butterworth & Co, London and Rooth, G. (1974) *Acid – Base and Electrolyte Balance*, Wolfe, London and Year Book Publishers, Chicago.

It will be seen that in the majority of the cases base deficit was more pronounced in the umbilical vein blood than in blood from the umbilical artery. This is in contrast to most data in the literature. This discrepancy cannot be accounted for by methodological errors, as repeated and different tests have confirmed our measurements.

Comments See Fig. 4.3.1.c.

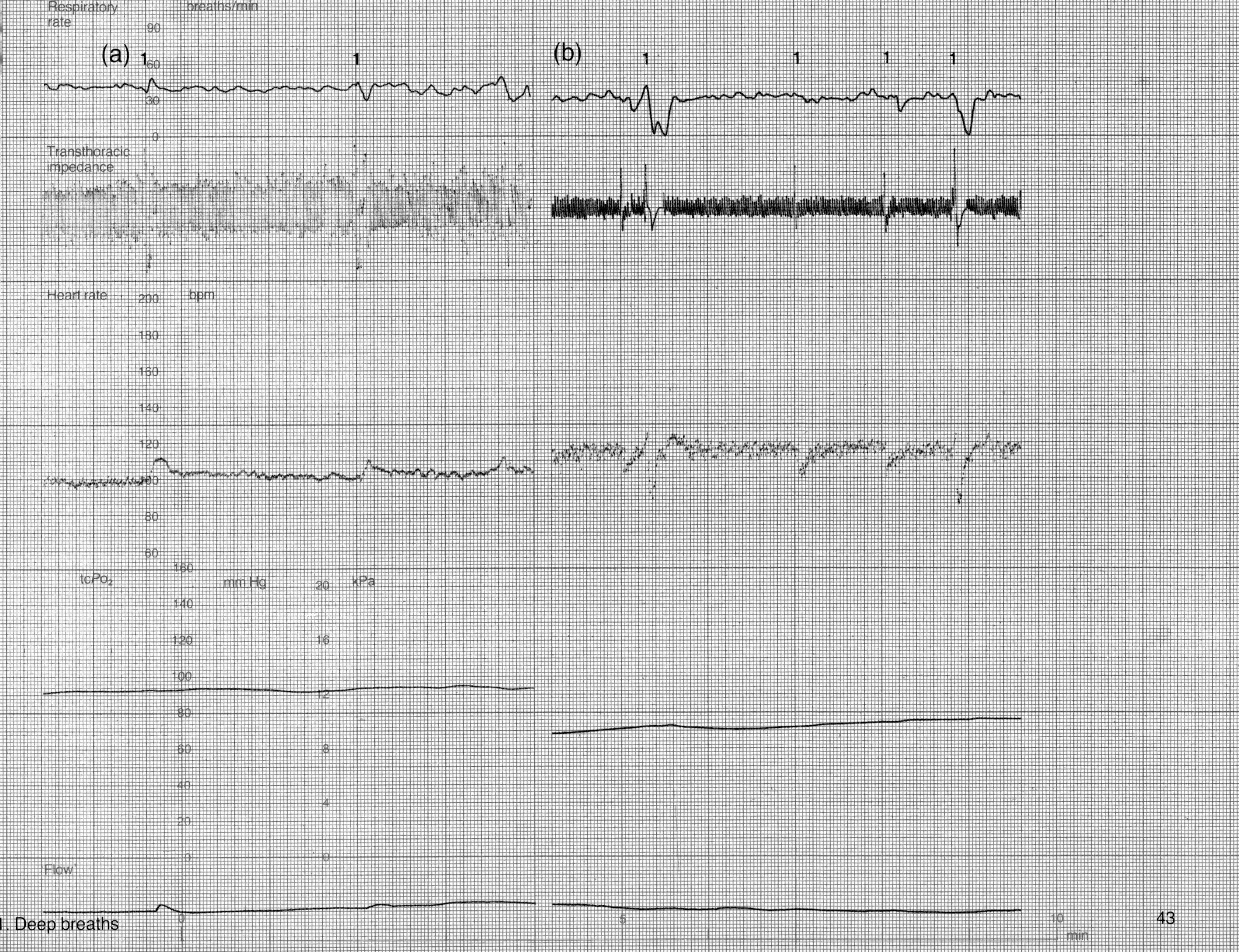

Respiratory rate
breaths/min
120
90
60
30
0
(a)
(b)
1
Transthoracic impedance
Heart rate
bpm
200
180
160
140
120
100
80
60
tcPo₂
mm Hg
kPa
160
140
120
100
80
60
40
20
0
20
16
12
8
4
0
Flow
0
5
10
min
1. Deep breaths

Fig. 4.3.1.c

Birthweight: 3480 g

Apgar score: 8/10/10

Age (in hours) at recording: 7

Delivery: vaginal

Activity state	Quiet sleep.
Respiratory rate	Very constant at 30 breaths/min except during the spells of deep breaths.
Transthoracic impedance	No changes in amplitude or level of excursions except during some deep breaths.
Heart rate	Baseline heart rate was about 120 bpm with an amplitude of long-term variability $\leq$ 5 bpm.
tc$P$O$_2$	A gradual increase from 72 to 80 mm Hg (9.6 to 10.7 kPa).

Comments (a–c) In quiet sleep very similar pictures are seen from case to case. All the parameters show small changes particularly the heart rate variability. During quiet sleep occasional deep breaths occur and this is revealed in the transthoracic impedance and in the heart rate, and sometimes also in 'flow'. In quiet sleep tc$P$O$_2$ usually is stable as illustrated in **a** and **b** but occasionally tc$P$O$_2$ increases as in **c**.

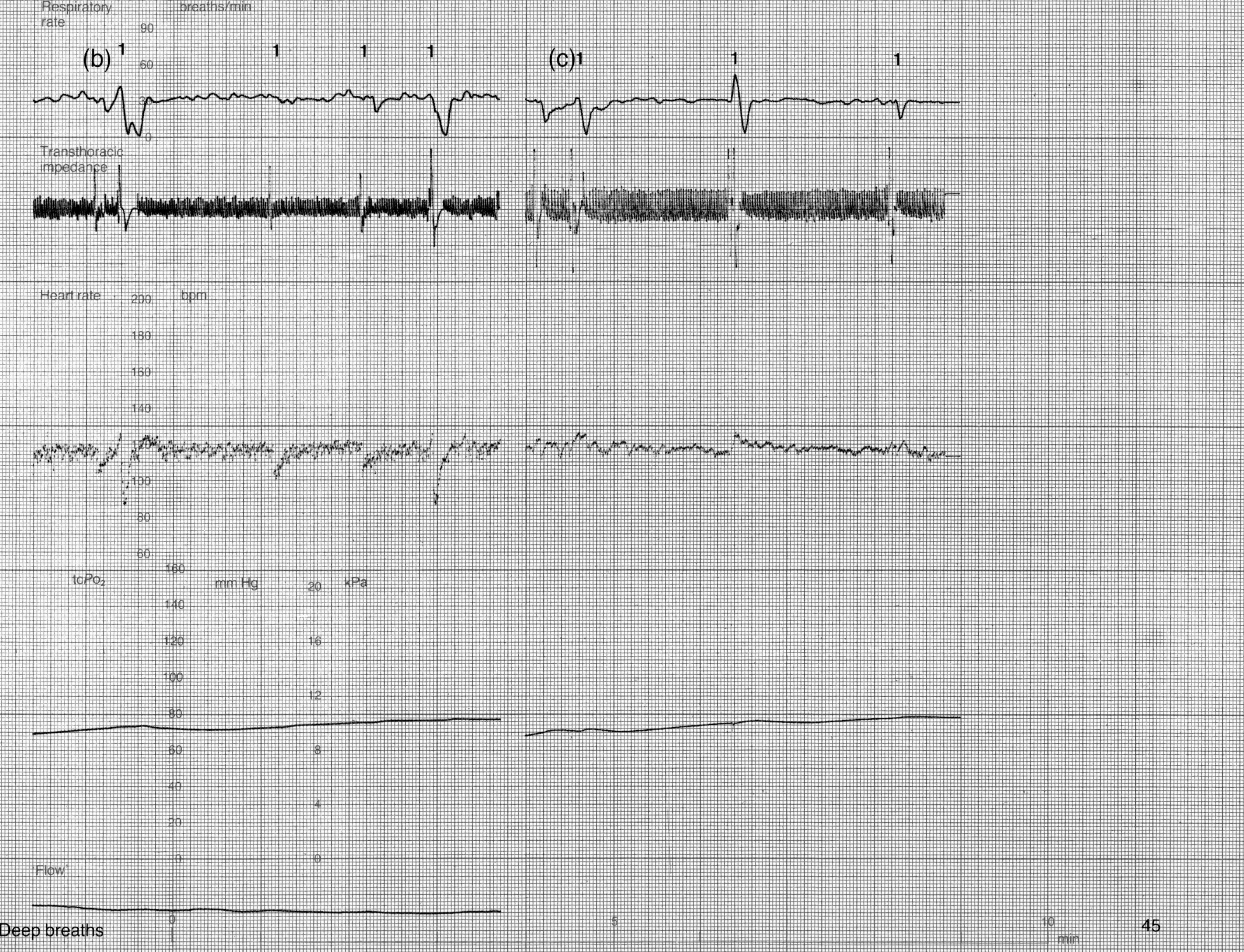

. Deep breaths

Fig. 4.3.2

Birthweight: 3480 g

Apgar score: 8/10/10

Age (in hours) at recording:	12

Delivery: vaginal

Activity state	Active sleep – quiet sleep.
Respiratory rate	During active sleep respiratory rate varied cyclically between 5 and 70 breaths/min. During quiet sleep it was between 60 and 65 breaths/min.
Transthoracic impedance	Periodic changes in the amplitude of the excursions during active sleep, but almost no changes during quiet sleep except for the occasional deep breath.
Heart rate	Initially baseline heart rate was about 100 bpm with marked long-term ($\geq$ 20 bpm) variability. During quiet sleep heart rate was almost constant at 115 bpm and the amplitude of the long-term variability was $\leq$ 5 bpm.
tc$P\text{O}_2$	Gradual fall from > 100 mm Hg (13.3 kPa) to 72 mm Hg (9.6 kPa) and a subsequent increase during quiet sleep to 113 mm Hg (15.1 kPa) not included in the figure.

Comments This registration illustrates the gradual transition from active to quiet sleep. During active sleep tc$P\text{O}_2$ gradually fell and increased during quiet sleep as also seen in Fig. 4.3.1.c.

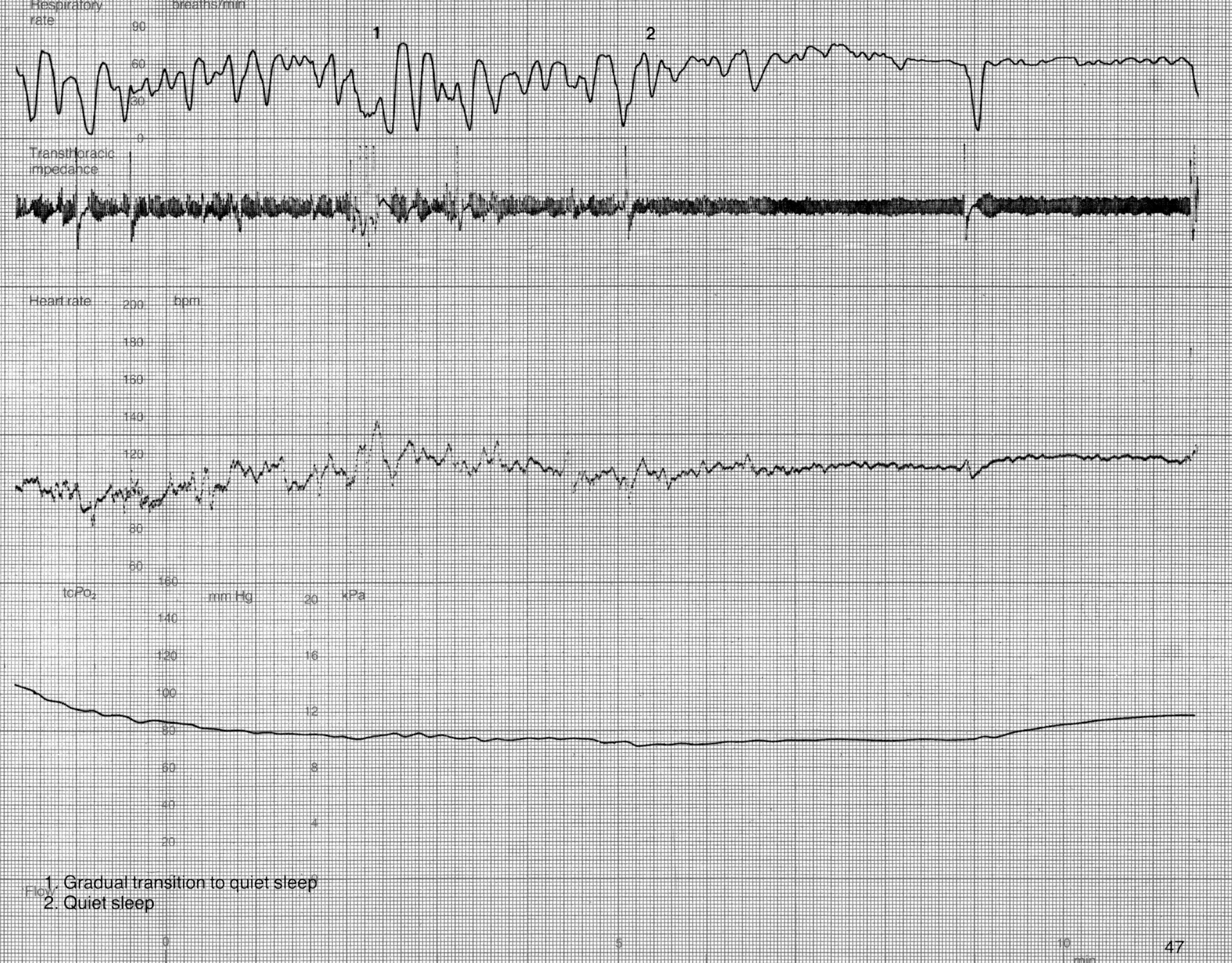
Respiratory rate
breaths/min
120
90
60
30
0
1
2
Transthoracic impedance
Heart rate
bpm
200
180
160
140
120
80
60
tcPo2
mm Hg
kPa
160
140
120
100
80
60
40
20
20
16
12
8
4
0
Flow
1. Gradual transition to quiet sleep
2. Quiet sleep
0
5
10
min

Fig. 4.3.3

Birthweight: 3120 g

Apgar score: 9/10/10

Age (in hours) at recording: 1

Delivery: Caesarean section

Activity state	Awake, unquiet, crying and quiet sleep.
Respiratory rate	Cyclic changes between 15 and 90 breaths/min which were much reduced in amplitude during quiet sleep.
Transthoracic impedance	Marked changes in magnitude and level of the excursions during the active phase. Occasional deep inspirations occur during quiet sleep.
Heart rate	Baseline heart rate was about 130 bpm with distinct long-term amplitude $\leqslant$ 20 bpm in the awake, unquiet period. In quiet sleep long-term variability was distinct with an amplitude $\leqslant$ 15 bpm.
tcP_{O_2}	A maximal level of 84 mm Hg (11.2 kPa) was seen during active phase and increased to 90 mm Hg (12.0 kPa) during the quiet phase.

Comments This oxygen-cardiorespirogram is an example of transition from awake, unquiet to quiet sleep.

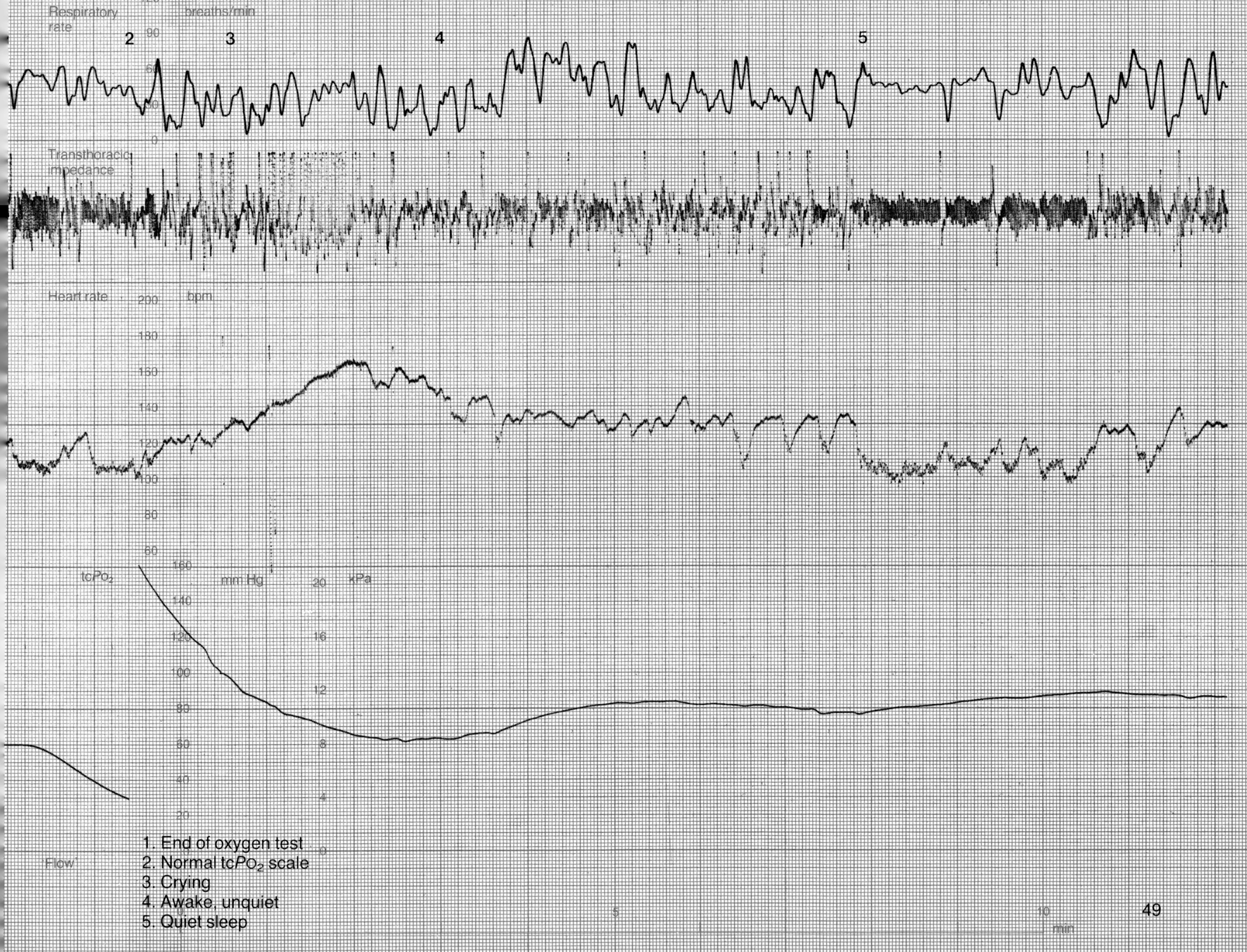
Respiratory rate
breaths/min
2
3
4
5
Transthoracic impedance
Heart rate
bpm
tcPo2
mm Hg
kPa
Flow
1. End of oxygen test
2. Normal tcPo2 scale
3. Crying
4. Awake, unquiet
5. Quiet sleep
min

Fig. 4.4.1.a

Birthweight: 3140 g

Apgar score: 7/8/10

Age (in hours) at recording: 4

Delivery: Caesarean section

Activity state	Active sleep.
Respiratory rate	Rhythmic changes between 0 and 70 breaths/min.
Transthoracic impedance	Short spells of regular excursions are seen but in between there are periods of apnoea and deep inspirations.
Heart rate	Baseline heart rate was about 115 bpm with an amplitude of long-term variability mainly about 10 bpm.
tcPO_2	Fluctuating between 68 and 72 mm Hg (9.1 to 9.6 kPa).

Comments See Fig. 4.4.1.e.

Fig. 4.4.1.b

Birthweight: 3170 g

Apgar score: 8/8

Age (in hours) at recording: 3

Delivery: vaginal

Cord blood acid – base and blood gases							
	pH	PCO_2 mm Hg	kPa	PO_2 mm Hg	kPa	Base deficit mmol/l
Umbilical artery	7.19	41	5.5	23	3.1	11.1
Umbilical vein	7.28	40	5.3	11	1.5	6.5

Activity state	Active sleep.
Respiratory rate	Mainly between 40 and 70 breaths/min but was at one time down to 10 breaths/min.
Transthoracic impedance	Regular with occasional larger excursions.
Heart rate	Baseline heart rate was about 120 bpm with an amplitude of long-term variability $\leq$ 15 bpm.
tcPO_2	Fell from 88 to 75 mm Hg (11.7 to 10.0 kPa).

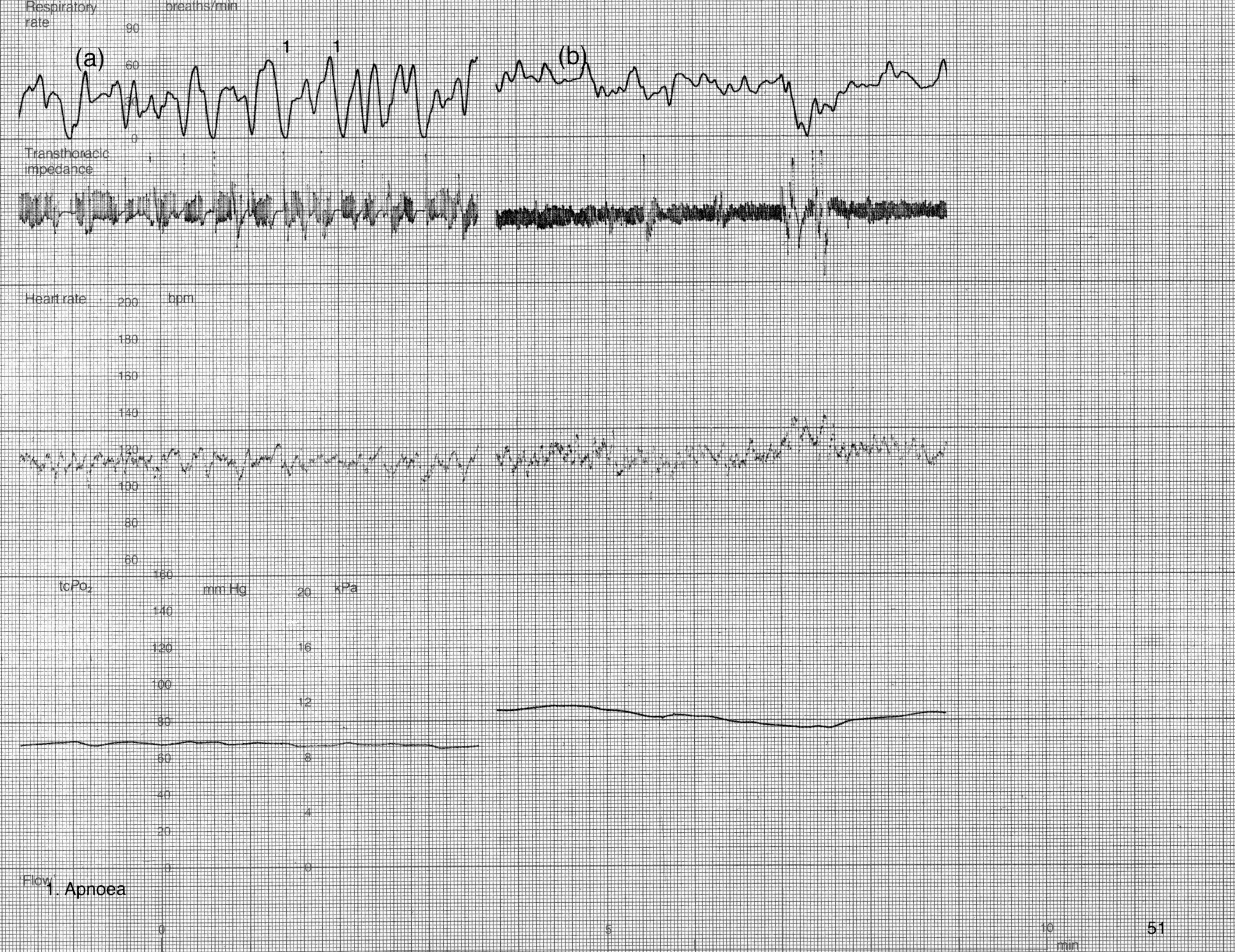

Respiratory rate
breaths/min
120
90
60
0
(a)
1
1
(b)
Transthoracic impedance
Heart rate
200
bpm
180
160
140
120
100
80
60
tcPo2
160
mm Hg
20
kPa
140
120
16
100
12
80
60
8
40
4
20
0
0
Flow
1. Apnoea
0
5
10
min

Fig. 4.4.1.c

Birthweight: 3480 g

Apgar score: 8/10/10

Age (in hours) at recording: 8

Delivery: vaginal

Activity state	Active sleep.
Respiratory rate	Rhythmic changes between 24 and 42 breaths/min.
Transthoracic impedance	Regular excursions with occasional deep inspirations.
Heart rate	Baseline heart rate was about 120 bpm with an amplitude of long-term variability $\leqslant$ 15 bpm.
tcPO_2	The level varied between 62 and 67 mm Hg (8.3 and 8.9 kPa).

Comments See Fig. 4.4.1.e.

Fig. 4.4.1.d

Birthweight: 3340 g

Apgar score: 8/10/10

Age (in hours) at recording: 2

Delivery: vaginal

Activity state	Active sleep.
Respiratory rate	Mostly about 30 breaths/min but part of the time varying between 12 and 48 breaths/min.
Transthoracic impedance	Mostly regular but with spells of irregular breathing.
Heart rate	Baseline heart rate was about 120 bpm with an amplitude of long-term variability $\leqslant$ 5 bpm except during the periods of irregular respiration when the variability was marked.
tcPO_2	Between 72 and 77 mm Hg (9.6 and 10.3 kPa).

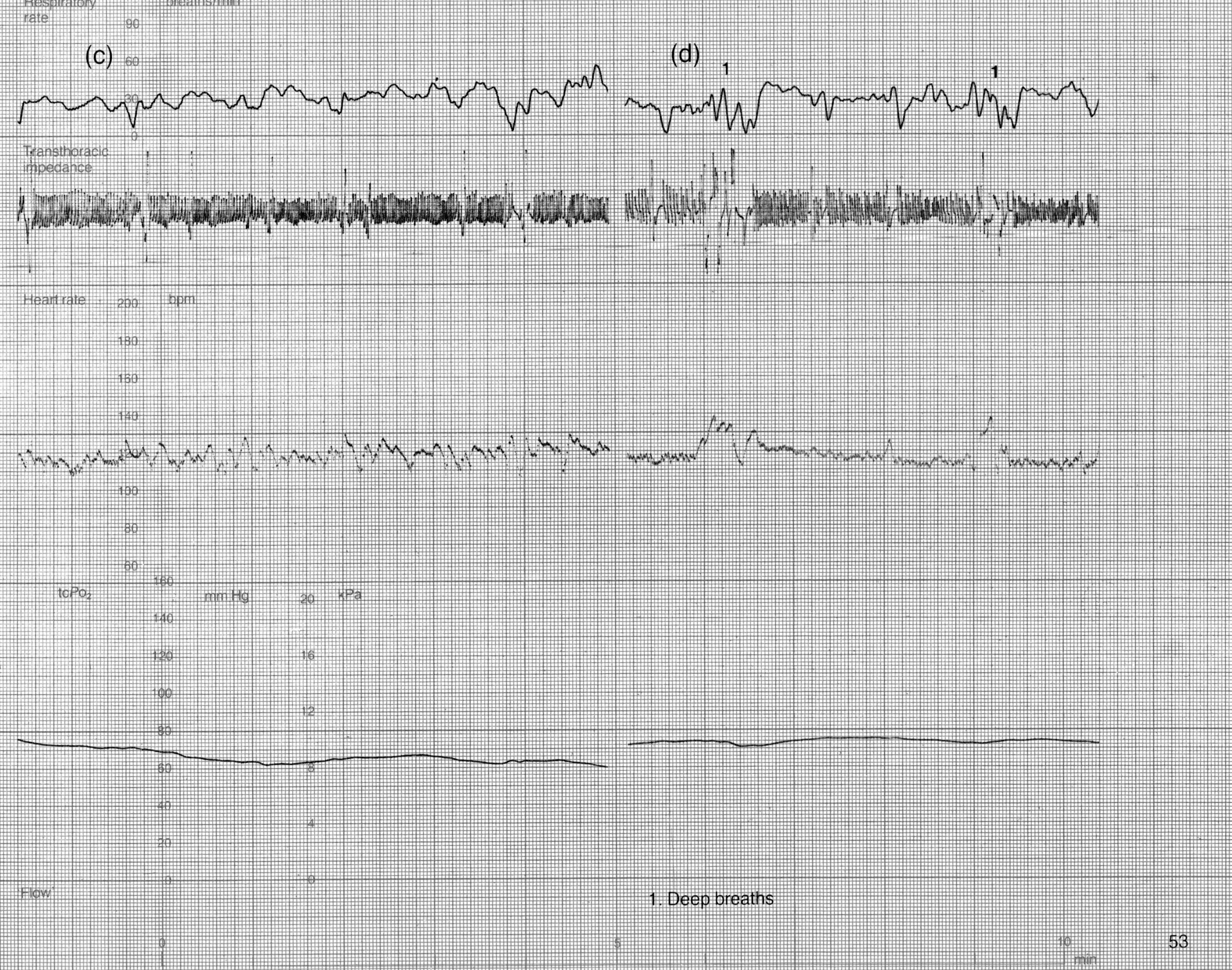
Respiratory rate
breaths/min
120
90
60
30
0
(c)
(d)
1
1
Transthoracic impedance
Heart rate
bpm
200
180
160
140
100
80
60
tcPo_2
mm Hg
kPa
160
140
120
100
80
60
40
20
0
20
16
12
8
4
0
Flow
1. Deep breaths
0
5
10
min

Fig. 4.4.1.e

Birthweight: 3380 g

Apgar score: 9/10

Age (in hours) at recording: >120

Delivery: vaginal

Activity state	Active sleep.
Respiratory rate	Between 0 and 55 breaths/min.
Transthoracic impedance	A very varied picture with different respiratory patterns within a few minutes. The excursions were sometimes regular and sometimes had a tendency to periodicity.
Heart rate	Baseline heart rate was about 110 bpm with an amplitude of long-term variability of $\leqslant$ 30 bpm but in the short quiet phase it was reduced to $\leqslant$ 5 bpm. During the deeper breaths there were accelerations to 150 bpm.
tcP_{O_2}	Between 80 and 86 mm Hg (10.7 and 11.3 kPa).
'Flow'	Increases parallel to the heart rate accelerations.

Comments (a–e) Active sleep is characterized by regular breathing interrupted by spells of very irregular breaths with different amplitude of the breathing excursions and different rates. The long-term heart rate variability is usually more pronounced than during quiet sleep. As Figs. **a–e** show the oxygen-cardio-respirograms may differ considerably from case to case. tcP_{O_2} usually fluctuates more than during quiet sleep although not much as also discussed in Chapters 10.5 –10.8. Moreover, in active sleep tcP_{O_2} has a tendency to fall.

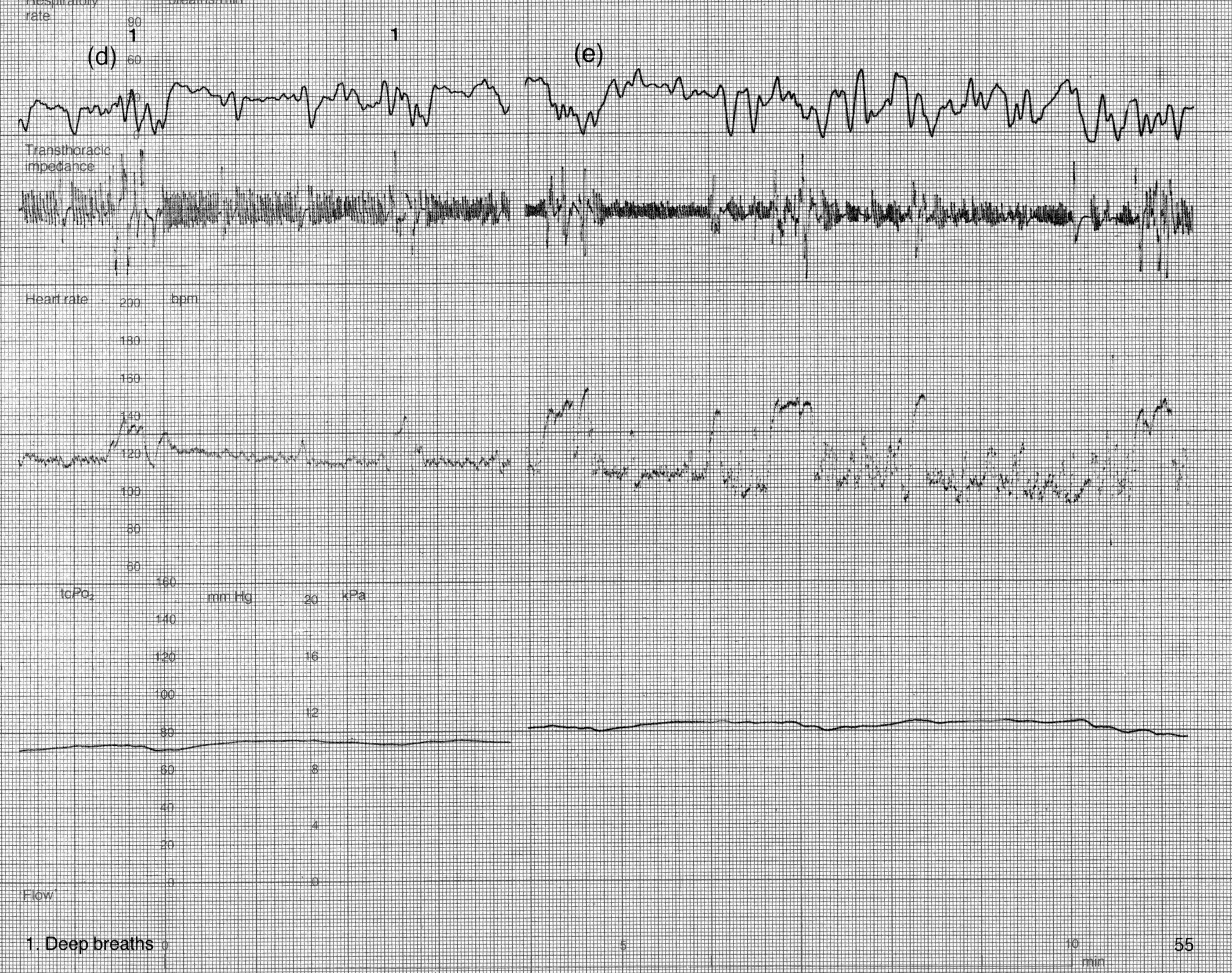

Respiratory rate
breaths/min
90
60
1
1
(d)
(e)
Transthoracic impedance
Heart rate
bpm
200
180
160
140
120
100
80
60
tcPo2
mm Hg
kPa
160
140
120
100
80
60
40
20
0
20
16
12
8
4
0
Flow
1. Deep breaths
0
5
10
min

Fig. 4.4.2

Birthweight: 3630 g
Apgar score: 8/9/10
Age (in hours) at recording: 36
Delivery: vaginal

Activity state	Active sleep.
Respiratory rate	Rhythmic changes of different amplitude from 0 to 85 breaths/min.
Transthoracic impedance	A varied picture – sometimes regular excursions, sometimes a tendency to periodicity, sometimes irregular excursions.
Heart rate	Baseline heart rate cannot be established because of the frequent accelerations and because of the large amplitude of the long-term variability. In the first and in the last part of the picture heart rate is slower and the amplitude of the long-term variability is $\leqslant$ 30 bpm.
tcP_{O_2}	The level of tcP_{O_2} varied between 80 and 90 mm Hg (10.7 and 12.0 kPa).
'Flow'	Changes synchronous to the deeper breaths.

Comments In this example the variations in respiratory rate and in the amplitude of the long-term variability of the heart rate are both particularly marked. Even in the more quiet phase the amplitude of the long-term variability is $\leqslant$ 30 bpm. This example illustrates how much the picture can vary even in sleep.

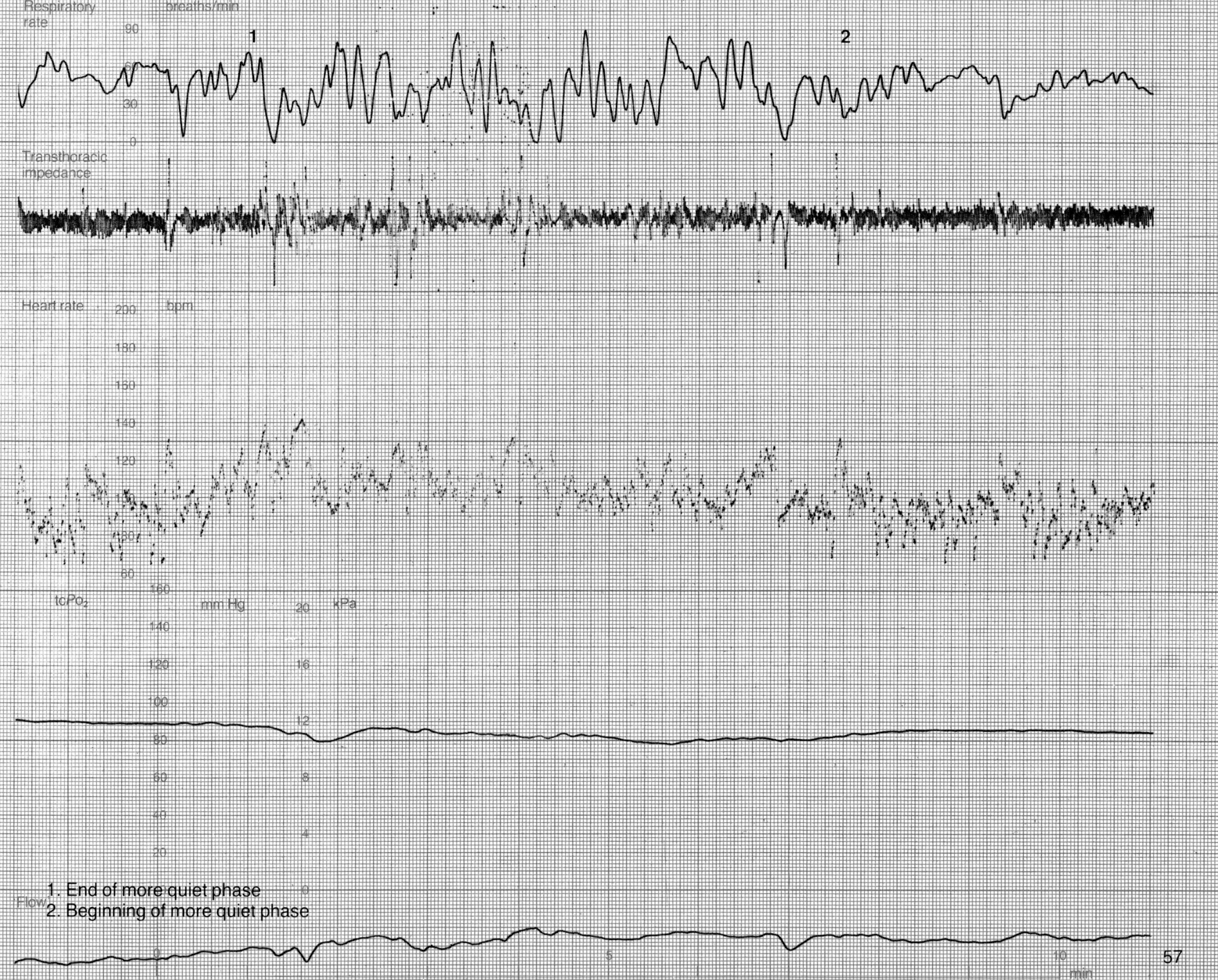
Respiratory rate
breaths/min
120
90
60
30
0
1
2
Transthoracic impedance
Heart rate
bpm
200
180
160
140
120
100
80
60
tcPo2
mm Hg
kPa
160
140
120
100
80
60
40
20
20
16
12
8
4
0
1. End of more quiet phase
2. Beginning of more quiet phase
Flow
0
5
10
min

Fig. 4.5.1.a

Birthweight: 2920 g

Apgar score: 9/10

Age (in hours) at recording:	2

Delivery: vaginal

Activity state	Awake, unquiet and crying.
Respiratory rate	Cyclic changes between 0 and 90 breaths/min.
Transthoracic impedance	Irregular excursions which were larger during crying.
Heart rate	Baseline heart rate about 120 bpm with an amplitude of long-term variability $\leq$ 20 bpm. During the crying, increase to 150 bpm interrupted by frequent short, deep decelerations.
tc$P\text{O}_2$	About 100 mm Hg (13.3 kPa) before crying. Fell to 70 mm Hg (9.3 kPa) after and then increased again to 88 mm Hg (11.7 kPa).
'Flow'	Concomitant with the crying and the increased heart rate there was an increase in 'flow'.

Comments See Fig. 4.5.1.c.

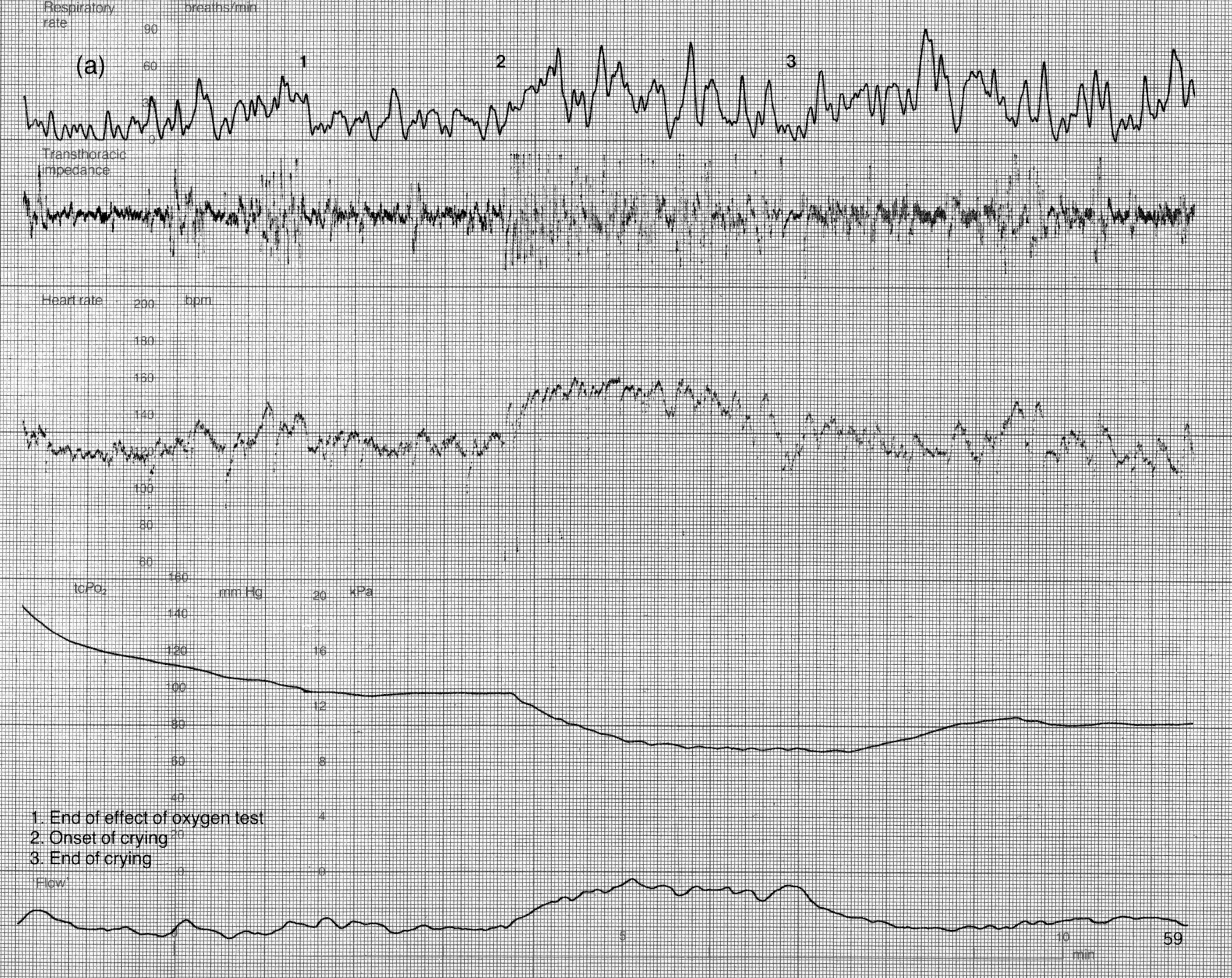

Respiratory rate
breaths/min
(a)
1
2
3
Transthoracic impedance
Heart rate
bpm
tcPo2
mm Hg
kPa
1. End of effect of oxygen test
2. Onset of crying
3. End of crying
'Flow'
min

Fig. 4.5.1.b

Birthweight: 3500 g

Apgar score: 9/10

Age (in hours) at recording: 3

Delivery: vaginal

Cord blood acid – base and blood gases							
	pH	$P\mathrm{CO}_2$	mm Hg	kPa	$P\mathrm{O}_2$ mm Hg	kPa	Base deficit mmol/l
Umbilical artery	7.24		41	5.5	28	3.7	8.2

Activity state	Quiet sleep succeeded by a period of crying.
Respiratory rate	About 50 breaths/min when asleep and variable during crying.
Transthoracic impedance	Regular excursions during the quiet phase and large irregular ones during the crying.
Heart rate	Increase in baseline heart rate from 120 to 200 bpm during the crying. The amplitude of the long-term variability was 5–15 bpm during quiet sleep.
tc$P\mathrm{O}_2$	Fell from 94 to 66 mm Hg (12.5 to 8.8 kPa) during the most active crying in spite of the administration of oxygen. Without the oxygen test it might have fallen more.

Fig. 4.5.1.c

Birthweight: 3630 g

Apgar score: 8/9/10

Age (in hours) at recording: 60

Delivery: vaginal

Activity state	Crying and active sleep.
Respiratory rate	During sleep respiratory rate was 50 – 60 breaths/min, but less during crying. Both states showed variation in respiratory rate.
Transthoracic impedance	Almost regular excursions during active sleep and increased excursions during crying.
Heart rate	Increase from 110 to 170 bpm during the most intense crying. The amplitude of the long-term variability was about 10 bpm at a heart rate of 160 bpm and $\leqslant$ 25 bpm during the quiet period when the rate was about 110 bpm.
tc$P\mathrm{O}_2$	From a level of 83 mm Hg (11.1 kPa) tc$P\mathrm{O}_2$ fell to 52 mm Hg (6.9 kPa) during crying only to increase to 86 mm Hg (11.5 kPa) when the infant went to sleep again.

Comments (a–c) The three illustrations show the most common oxygen-cardiorespirogram pattern seen during the first week of life during crying, i.e. the fall in tc$P\mathrm{O}_2$, the increased heart rate and *pari passu* reduced variability. 'Flow' also increases parallel to the increased activity and there is often a distinct covariation between heart rate changes and 'flow' changes.

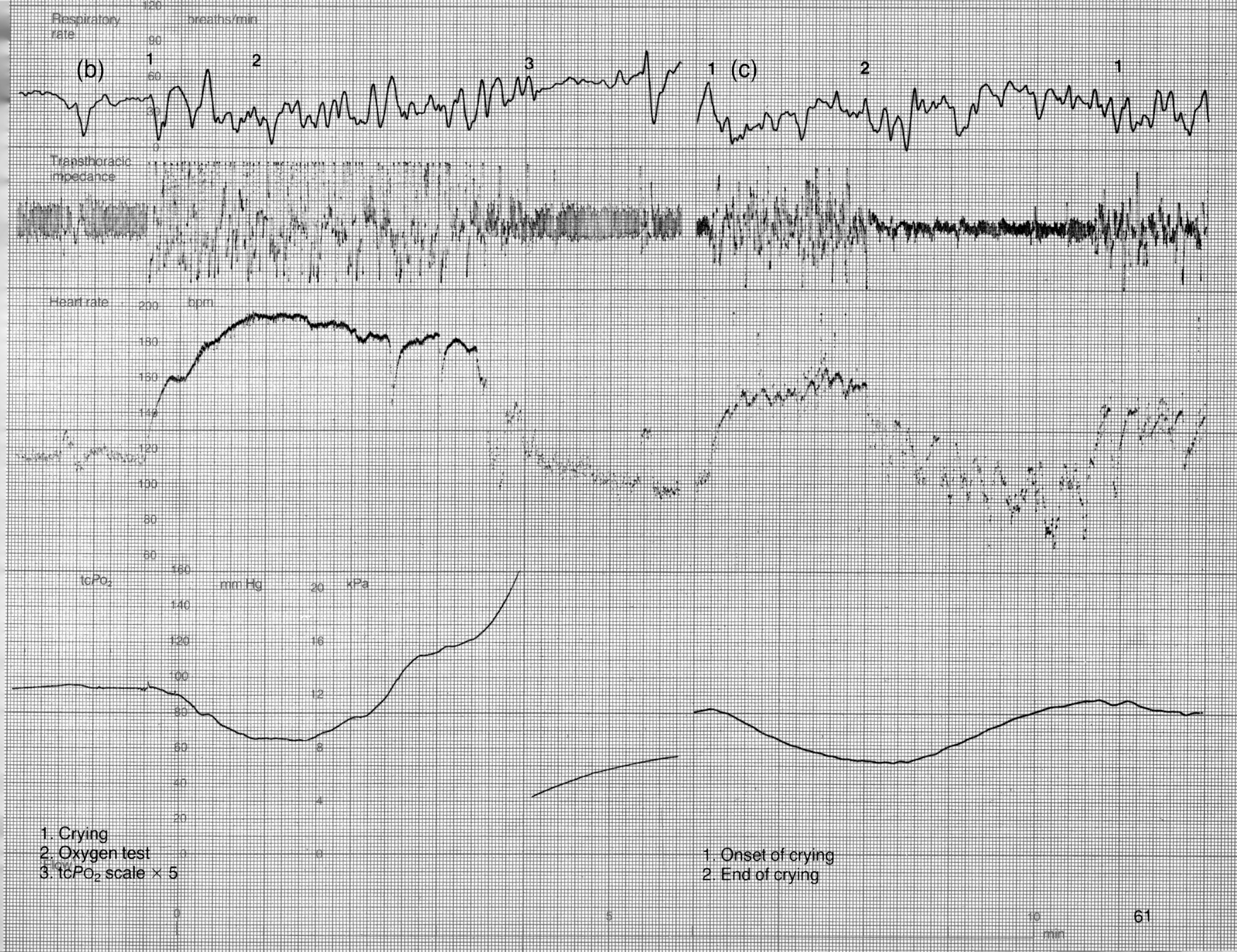

Respiratory rate
breaths/min
120
90
60
30
0
(b)
1
2
3
(c)
1
2
1
Transthoracic impedance
Heart rate
bpm
200
180
160
140
120
100
80
60
tcPo2
mm Hg
kPa
160
140
120
100
80
60
40
20
0
20
16
12
8
4
0
1. Crying
2. Oxygen test
3. tcPo2 scale × 5
1. Onset of crying
2. End of crying
0
5
10
min

Fig. 4.5.2.a

Birthweight: 3100 g

Apgar score: 9/10/10

Age (in hours) at recording: 2

Delivery: vaginal

Cord blood acid – base and blood gases							
	pH	$P\text{CO}_2$ mm Hg	kPa	$P\text{O}_2$ mm Hg	kPa	Base deficit mmol/l
Umbilical artery	7.38	36	4.8	13	1.7	3.4
Umbilical vein	7.41	33	4.4	13	1.7	3.6

Activity state	Crying with brief intervals.
Respiratory rate	Cyclic changes between 0 and 100 breaths/min.
Transthoracic impedance	Large irregular excursions interrupted by short spells of more regular excursions.
Heart rate	When quiet, baseline heart rate was about 135 bpm with an amplitude of long-term variability $\leqslant$ 10 bpm. During crying heart rate increased to 160 – 170 bpm. Heart rate fell temporarily during the short quiet intervals between crying. This gives an impression of a large amplitude of long-term variability.
tc$P\text{O}_2$	From an initial level of 95 mm Hg (12.7 kPa) the crying resulted in a fall to 78 mm Hg (10.4 kPa). The variations in activity were also reflected in the tc$P\text{O}_2$ curve. Simultaneous arterial and transcutaneous $P\text{O}_2$, 78 and 83 mm Hg (10.4 and 11.1 kPa) respectively.

Comments See Fig. 4.5.2.b.

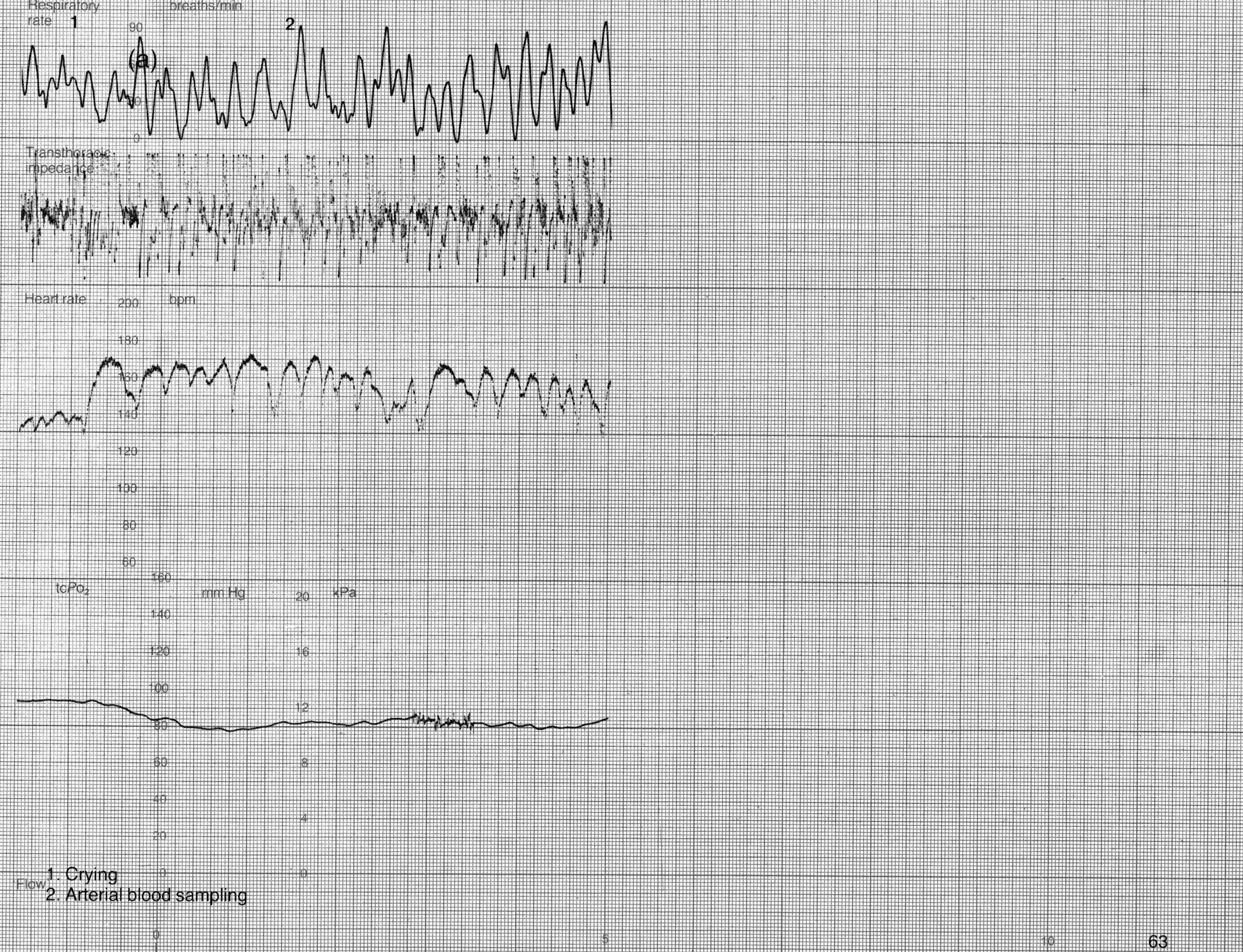

Respiratory rate
breaths/min
120
90
0
1
2
(a)
Transthoracic impedance
Heart rate
bpm
200
180
160
140
120
100
80
60
tcPo_2
mm Hg
kPa
160
140
120
100
80
60
40
20
0
20
16
12
8
4
0
Flow
1. Crying
2. Arterial blood sampling
0
5
10
min

Fig. 4.5.2.b

Birthweight: 2900 g

Apgar score: 7/9/10

Age (in hours) at recording: 3

Delivery: vaginal

Cord blood acid – base and blood gases							
	pH	$P\mathrm{CO_2}$ mm Hg	kPa	$P\mathrm{O_2}$ mm Hg	kPa	Base deficit mmol/l
Umbilical artery	7.25	52	6.9	14	1.9	4.2
Umbilical vein	7.28	43	5.7	19	2.5	6.1

Activity state	Awake, quiet at the beginning of the recording, then gradual increase in crying interrupted – as in **a** – by short quiet pauses.
Respiratory rate	Initially 40 to 50 breaths/min. During crying cyclic changes between 0 and 110 breaths/min.
Transthoracic impedance	Initially a regular pattern. The onset of the crying was manifested by larger and more irregular breathing excursions.
Heart rate	Baseline heart rate was about 115 bpm when the infant was quiet, increasing to 175 bpm during crying. In the quiet period long-term variability was distinct with an amplitude of $\leq$ 10 bpm. During crying the cyclic rate changes were largely due to the transition from crying to rest and the long-term variability cannot be read off at this period.
tc$P\mathrm{O_2}$	From a level of about 70 mm Hg (9.3 kPa) there was at first an increase but then a persistent fall in tc$P\mathrm{O_2}$ down to 56 mm Hg (7.5 kPa). The undulations in tc$P\mathrm{O_2}$ best seen late in this recording were also due to the change from crying to non-crying periods.

Comments (a and b) Basically similar patterns in both **a** and **b** to those shown in Figs 4.5.1.a – c but here the tc$P\mathrm{O_2}$ decrease was less marked during crying.

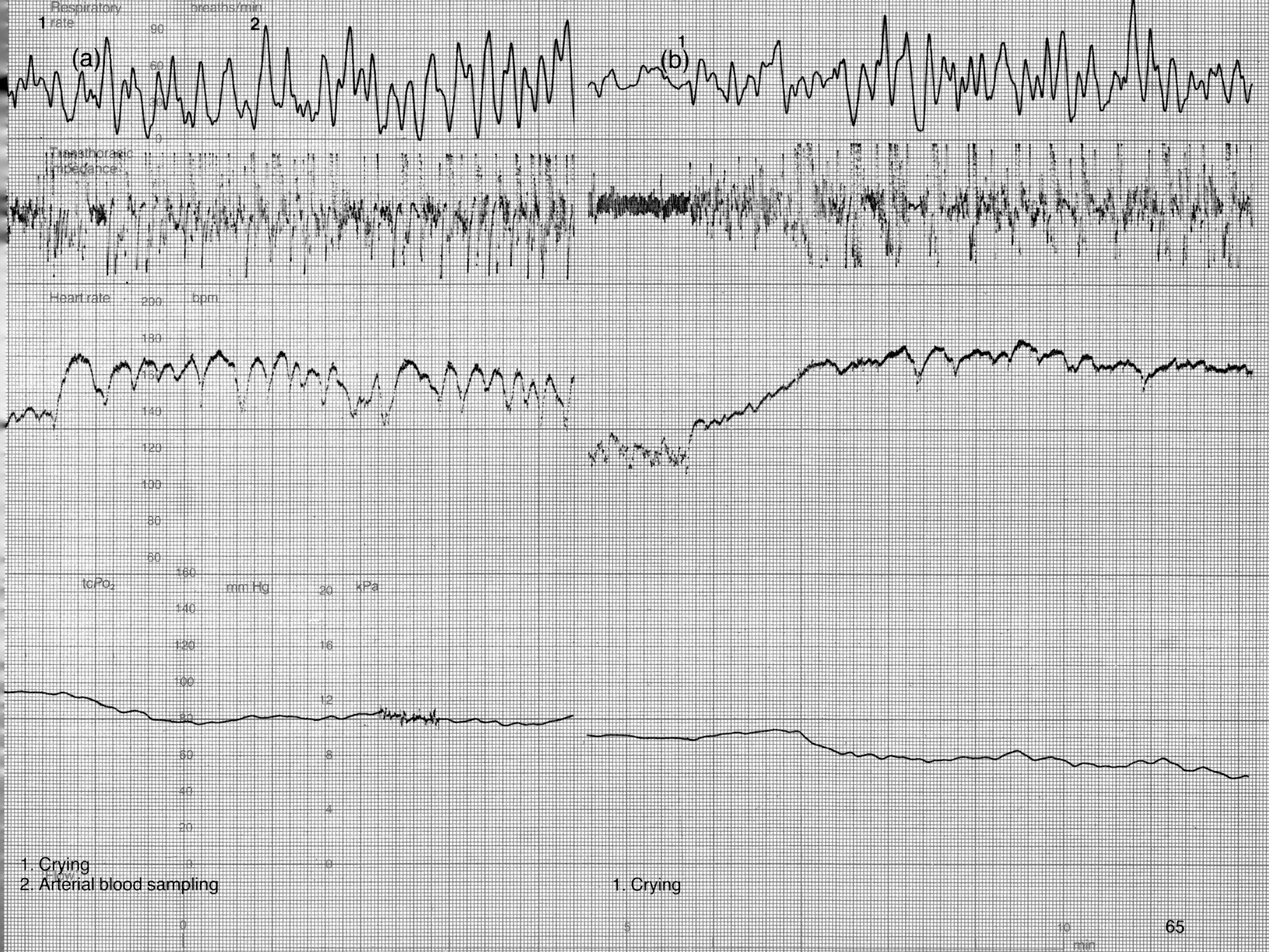
Respiratory rate
breaths/min
(a)
(b)
Transthoracic impedance
Heart rate
bpm
tcPo2
mm Hg
kPa
1. Crying
2. Arterial blood sampling
1. Crying
min

Fig. 4.5.3.a

Birthweight: 3900 g

Apgar score: 9/10/10

Age (in hours) at recording: 4

Delivery: vaginal

Cord blood acid – base and blood gases							
	pH	$P\mathrm{CO_2}$	mm Hg	kPa	$P\mathrm{O_2}$	mm Hg	kPa	Base deficit mmol/l
Umbilical artery	7.37		39	5.2		13	1.7	2.4
Umbilical vein	7.43		30	4.0		22	2.9	4.1

Activity state	Quiet sleep interrupted by crying.
Respiratory rate	About 40 breaths/min when quiet and 20 to 70 breaths/min during crying.
Transthoracic impedance	Regular with occasional deep breaths during the quiet period and irregular during the crying phase.
Heart rate	Baseline heart rate was 110–120 bpm with an amplitude of long-term variability during the quiet period of $\leqslant$ 10 bpm. Parallel to the crying activity heart rate increased to 160 bpm.
$\mathrm{tc}P\mathrm{O_2}$	Increased from 70 to 79 mm Hg (9.3 to 10.5 kPa) during crying.
'Flow'	Increase concomitant with that of heart rate during crying.

Fig. 4.5.3.b

Birthweight: 2820 g

Apgar score: 8/10/10

Age (in hours) at recording: 2

Delivery: vaginal

Activity state	Awake, quiet and periods of crying.
Respiratory rate	Cyclic variations between 25 and 110 breaths/min in the quiet period and between 0 and 95 breaths/min during crying.
Transthoracic impedance	Somewhat regular excursions in the quiet period, larger and irregular excursions during crying.
Heart rate	Baseline heart rate was about 130 bpm and the amplitude of the long-term variability was $\leqslant$ 15 bpm in the quiet phase. During crying heart rate increased to 175 bpm and long-term variability was $\leqslant$ 5 bpm.
$\mathrm{tc}P\mathrm{O_2}$	There was no change in $\mathrm{tc}P\mathrm{O_2}$ from the level of 85 mm Hg (11.3 kPa) regardless of the activity of the infant.

Comments (a and b) These two examples represent the exceptions to the rule that $\mathrm{tc}P\mathrm{O_2}$ falls during crying in the first week of life. See also Chapter 10.1.3 regarding the distribution of $\mathrm{tc}P\mathrm{O_2}$ fall during crying.

The reduced heart rate in between two crying periods in **b** should not be mistaken for a true deceleration of the type described in Chapter 2. Here as in Fig. 4.5.2.b it is a return to the baseline heart rate when quiet.

Respiratory rate
breaths/min
120
90
60
30
0
(a)
(b)
1
1
Transthoracic impedance
Heart rate
bpm
200
180
160
140
100
80
60
tcPo_2
mm Hg
kPa
160
140
120
100
80
60
40
20
0
20
16
12
8
4
0
Flow
0
5
10
min

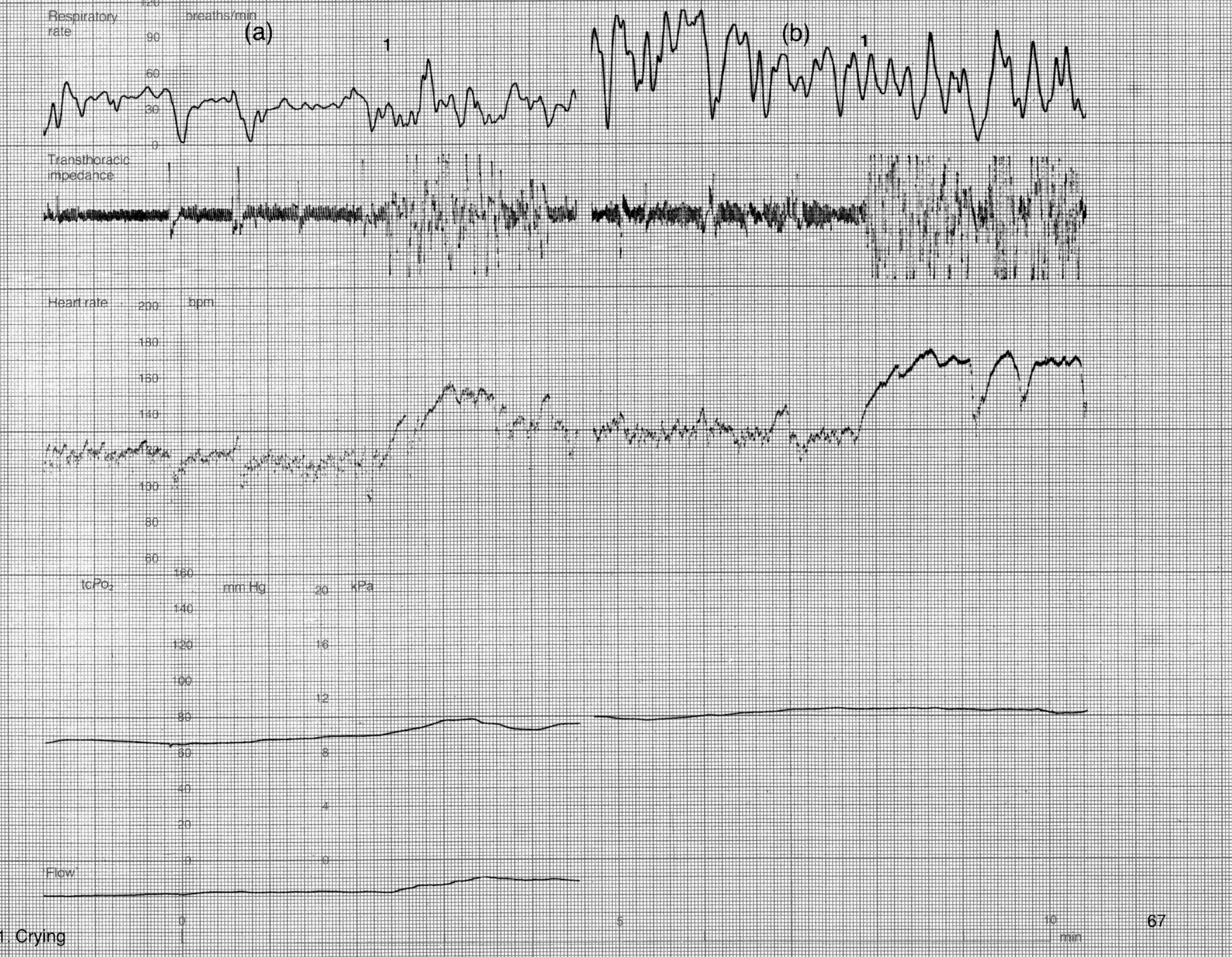

1. Crying

Fig. 4.6.1

Birthweight: 3280 g

Apgar score: 9/10/10

Age (in hours) at recording: 5

Delivery: vaginal

Cord blood acid – base and blood gases							
	pH	$P\text{CO}_2$	mm Hg	kPa	$P\text{O}_2$ mm Hg	kPa	Base deficit mmol/l
Umbilical artery	7.19		60	8.0	14	1.9	4.9

Activity state	Crying, suckling and then crying again.
Respiratory rate	Cyclic variations between 20 and 110 breaths/min. The periodicity is the same in heart rate.
Transthoracic impedance	Mostly regular excursions with often short apnoeas lasting 3 – 5 s. Again irregular excursions during the crying periods.
Heart rate	Baseline heart rate was about 115 bpm and the amplitude of the long-term variability ≤ 15 bpm. The undulations were synchronous to the suckling. During crying heart rate increased to 150 bpm.
$\text{tc}P\text{O}_2$	During crying $\text{tc}P\text{O}_2$ fell from 98 to 75 mm Hg (13.1 to 10.0 kPa).

Comments The waveform pattern seen best in the heart rate curve is typical for suckling and should not be mistaken for decelerations as described in Chapter 2.

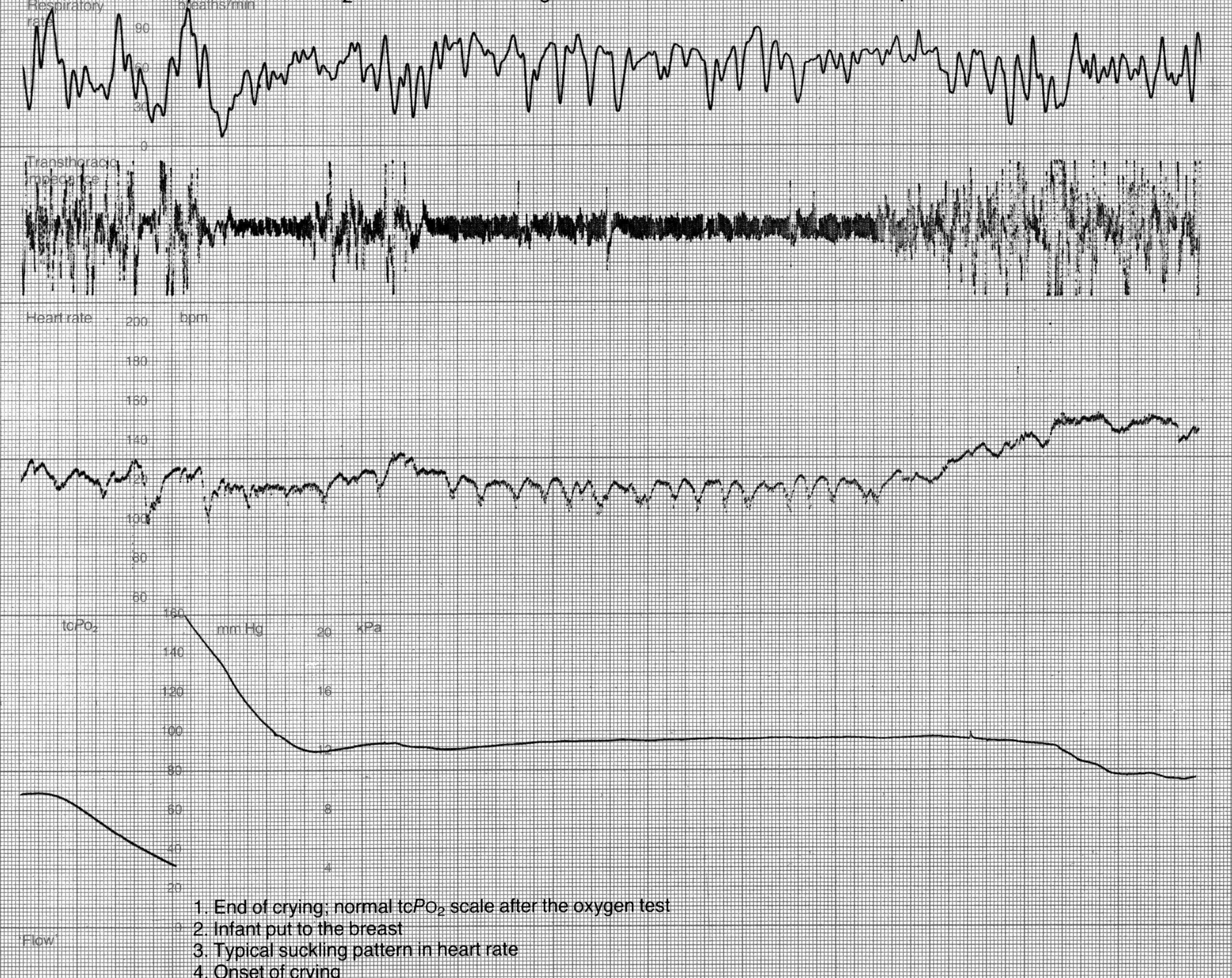

1. End of crying; normal tcP_{O_2} scale after the oxygen test
2. Infant put to the breast
3. Typical suckling pattern in heart rate
4. Onset of crying

Fig. 4.6.2.a

Birthweight: 3040 g

Apgar score: 10

Age (in hours) at recording: 4

Delivery: vaginal

Activity state	Suckling.
Respiratory rate	About 60 breaths/min with small cyclic variations.
Transthoracic impedance	Regular excursions with occasional deeper breaths.
Heart rate	Baseline heart rate was about 130 bpm with smooth waves with an amplitude $\leq$ 10 bpm.
tcP_{O_2}	The level increased gradually to 90 mm Hg (12.0 kPa).

Comments See Fig. 4.6.2.c.

Fig. 4.6.2.b

Birthweight: 3260 g

Apgar score: 9/10/10

Age (in hours) at recording: 2

Delivery: Caesarean section

Activity state	Initially awake, unquiet then suckling.
Respiratory rate	Cyclic changes with between 10 and 70 breaths/min with an irregular waveform.
Transthoracic impedance	Large irregular excursions during the unquiet phase and more regular excursions during the suckling period.
Heart rate	Baseline heart rate was about 125 bpm with large distinct waves synchronous to the suckling.
tcP_{O_2}	From a level of 61 mm Hg (8.1 kPa) tcP_{O_2} gradually increased to 95 mm Hg (12.7 kPa).
'Flow'	Waveform changes synchronous to that of the heart rate and the suckling.

(a)
(b)
Respiratory rate
breaths/min
90
60
30
0
1
Transthoracic impedance
Heart rate
bpm
200
180
160
140
120
100
80
60
tcPo2
mm Hg
kPa
160
140
120
100
80
60
40
20
0
20
16
12
8
4
0
Flow
0
5
10
min
1. Suckling

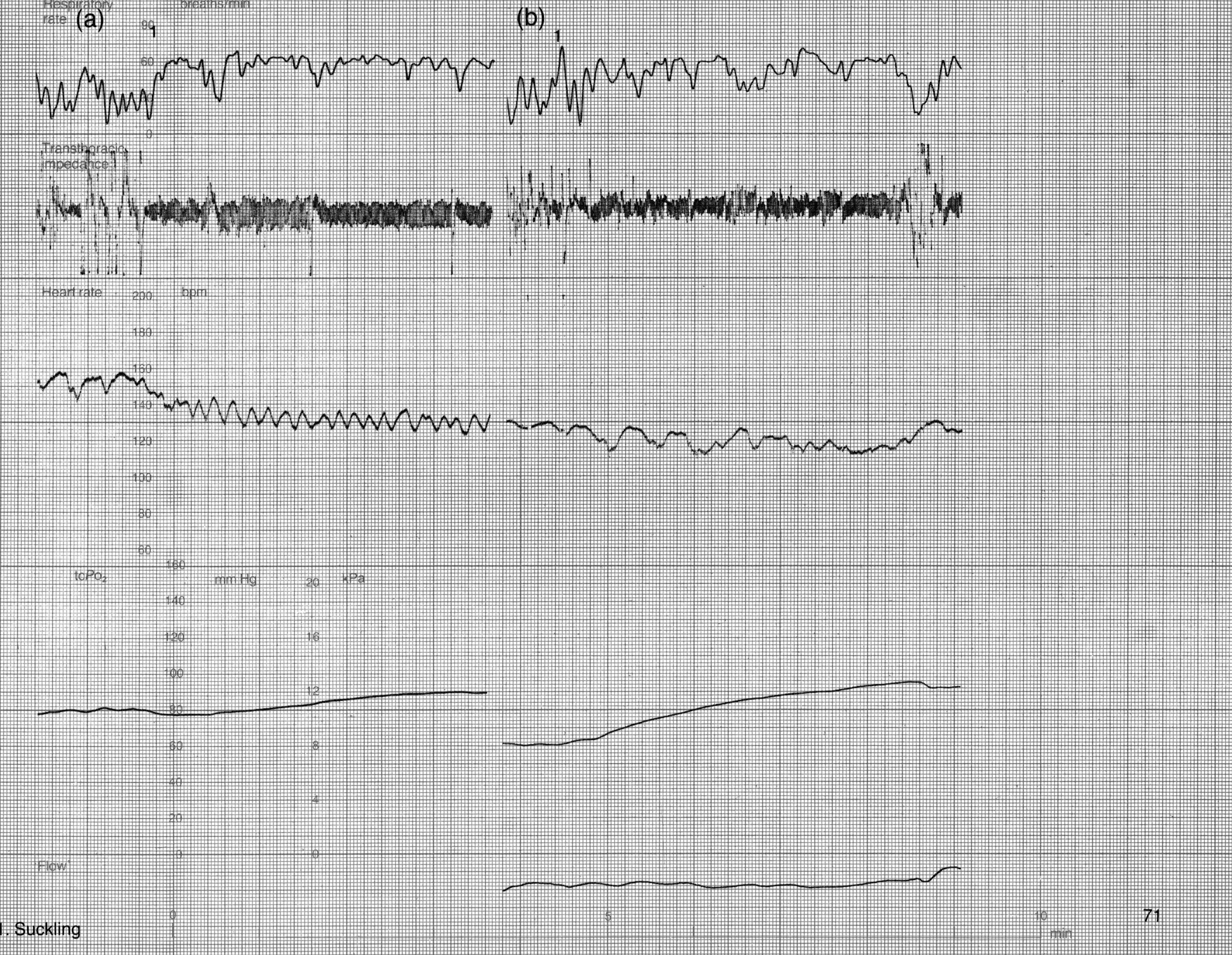

Fig. 4.6.2.c

Birthweight: 3850 g

Apgar score: 9/10/10

Age (in hours) at recording: 2

Delivery: vaginal

Cord blood acid – base and blood gases							
	pH	PCO_2 mm Hg	kPa	PO_2 mm Hg	kPa	Base deficit mmol/l
Umbilical artery	7.29	41	5.5	28	3.7	5.9
Umbilical vein	7.31	37	5.0	35	4.7	6.9

Activity state	Suckling.
Respiratory rate	Irregular cyclic changes between 30 and 75 breaths/min.
Transthoracic impedance	A tendency to periodicity in the amplitude of the excursions parallel to the heart rate changes.
Heart rate	Baseline heart rate about 130 bpm with regular waves having an amplitude of $\leq$ 20 bpm and synchronous to the suckling.
tcPO_2	Remained stable between 110 and 108 mm Hg (14.7 and 14.4 kPa).

Comments (a – c) Suckling is always recognized in the oxygen-cardiorespirogram by the smooth waveform of the heart rate as seen in these three examples. However, as illustrated here, both the amplitude and the frequency of these waves may differ. The same waves may also be present in 'flow', in respiratory rate and in the excursions of the transthoracic impedance. Even the tcPO_2 curve may show these changes but then a larger scale must be used.

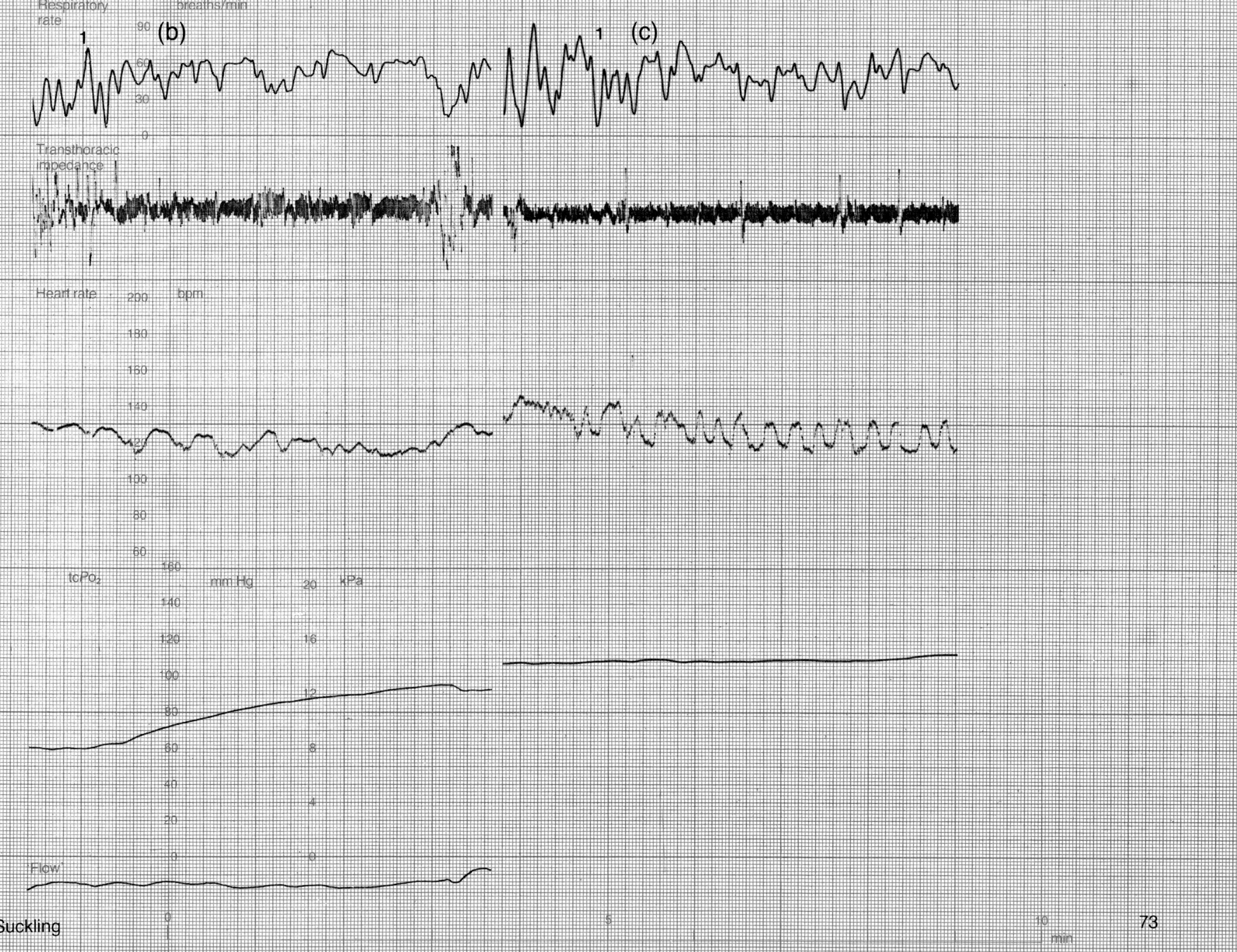
Respiratory rate
breaths/min
120
90
60
30
0
1
(b)
1
(c)
Transthoracic impedance
Heart rate
bpm
200
180
160
140
120
100
80
60
tcPo₂
mm Hg
kPa
160
140
120
100
80
60
40
20
0
20
16
12
8
4
0
Flow
Suckling
0
5
10
min

Fig. 4.6.3

Birthweight: 3860 g

Apgar score: 10

Age (in hours) at recording: 1

Delivery: Caesarean section

Cord blood acid – base and blood gases							
	pH	PCO_2	mm Hg	kPa	PO_2 mm Hg	kPa	Base deficit mmol/l
Umbilical artery	7.27		55	7.3			1.0
Umbilical vein	7.32		44	5.9			2.8

Activity state	Initially awake, unquiet then awake, quiet (feeding).
Respiratory rate	About 30 breaths/min in the unquiet phase and 40 breaths/min during feeding (Monitor II).
Transthoracic impedance	Irregular excursions in the unquiet phase and almost regular ones in the quiet phase.
Heart rate	In the awake, unquiet period heart rate varies with activity from 130 to 170 bpm. During feeding heart rate was about 150 bpm with undulations.
$tcPO_2$	The peak value during the oxygen test was 390 mm Hg (52.0 kPa) from which a shunt of 20 per cent is calculated. During feeding $tcPO_2$ gradually fell from 78 to 68 mm Hg (10.4 to 9.1 kPa).

Comments During feeding the infant became quiet. The undulating heart rate is similar to that seen during suckling.

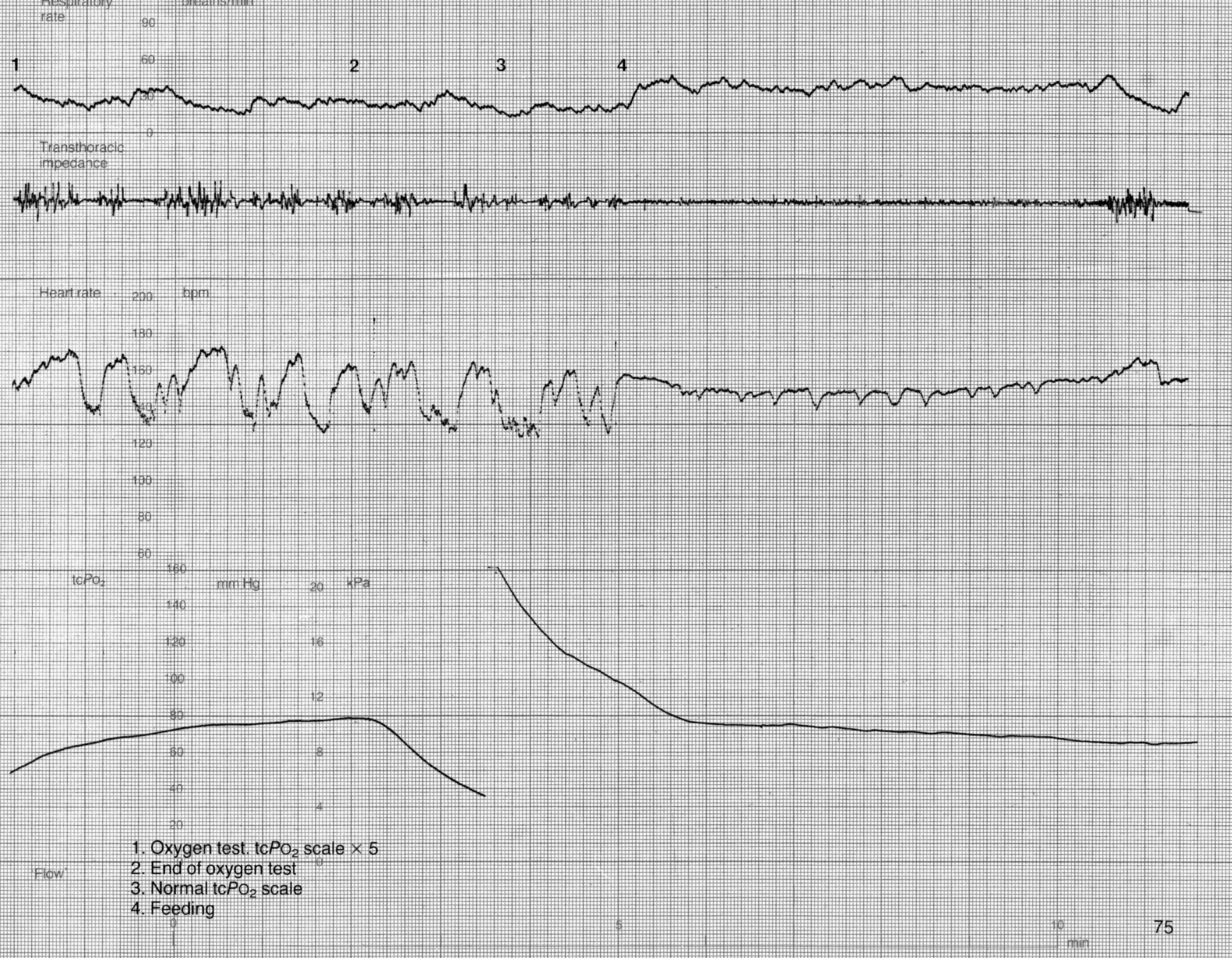
Respiratory rate
breaths/min
90
60
30
0
1
2
3
4
Transthoracic impedance
Heart rate
bpm
200
180
160
140
120
100
80
60
tcPo2
mm Hg
kPa
160
140
120
100
80
60
40
20
20
16
12
8
4
0
Flow
1. Oxygen test. tcPo2 scale × 5
2. End of oxygen test
3. Normal tcPo2 scale
4. Feeding
0
5
10
min

Fig. 4.6.4

Birthweight: 2890 g
Apgar score: 4/8/8
Age (in hours) at recording: 120
Delivery: vaginal

Activity state	Crying, awake, quiet (feeding).
Respiratory rate	Between 60 and 80 breaths/min during crying and then between 30 and 60 breaths/min.
Transthoracic impedance	Large irregular excursions during crying. Smaller, almost regular ones during the first feeding period and in the awake, quiet phase.
Heart rate	During crying baseline heart rate was up to 170 bpm with an amplitude of long-term variability $\leq$ 20 bpm. At the onset of feeding heart rate fell at first to about 100 bpm and then stayed around 130 bpm. The amplitude of long-term variability then was 20 to 35 bpm. After feeding heart rate returned to 120 bpm.
tc$P\text{O}_2$	During crying tc$P\text{O}_2$ increased to 70 mm Hg (9.3 kPa) and initially fell to 56 mm Hg (7.5 kPa) during feeding, but gradually increased to 76 mm Hg (10.1 kPa).

Comments This oxygen-cardiorespirogram shows the following features which are characteristic for feeding. 1, A higher heart rate level. 2, Initial fall in tc$P\text{O}_2$ and then a gradual return.

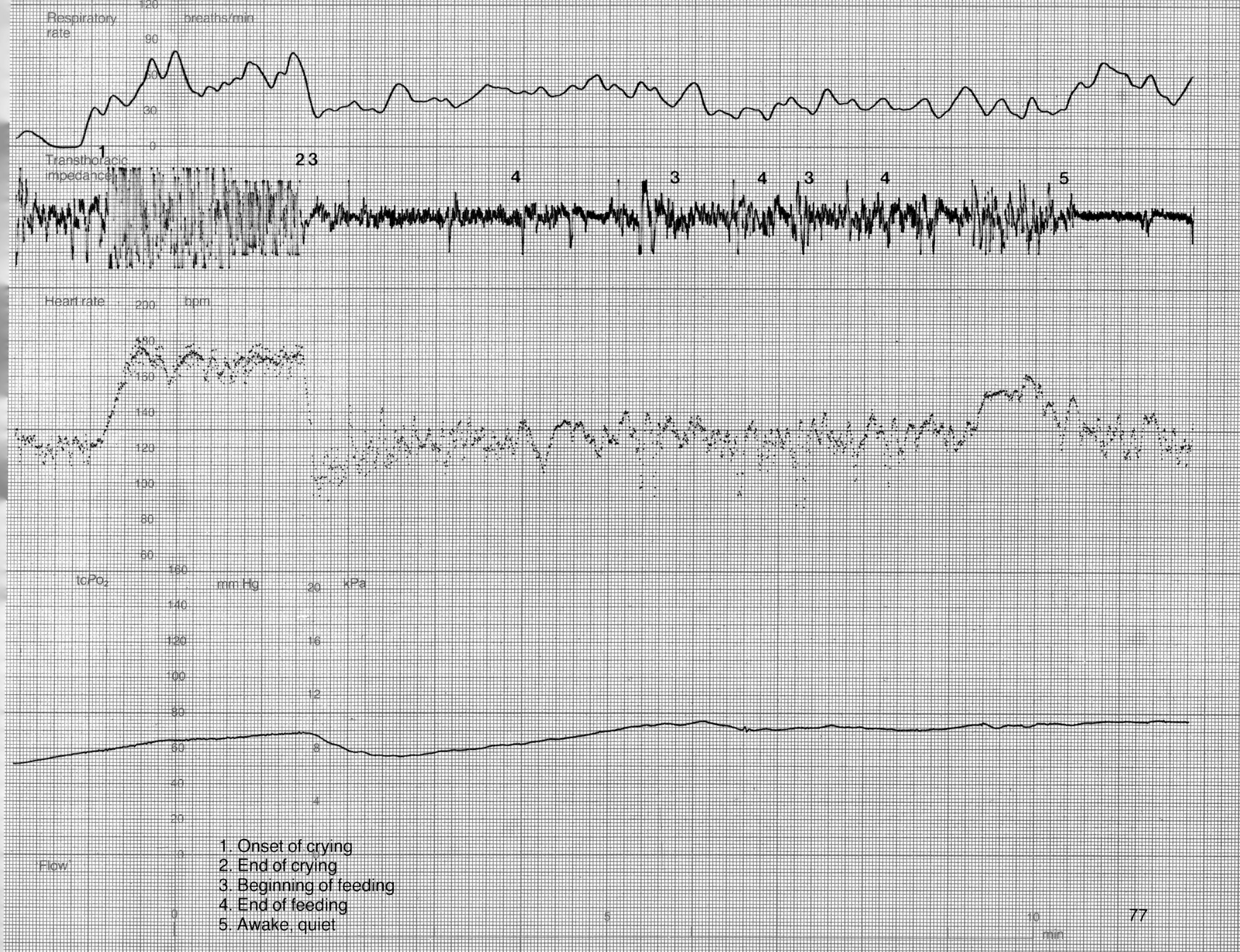

Respiratory rate
breaths/min
120
90
60
30
0
Transthoracic impedance
1
2 3
4
3
4
3
4
5
Heart rate
200
bpm
180
160
140
120
100
80
60
$tcPo_2$
160
mm Hg
20
kPa
140
120
16
100
12
80
60
8
40
4
20
0
Flow
0
5
10
min
1. Onset of crying
2. End of crying
3. Beginning of feeding
4. End of feeding
5. Awake, quiet

Fig. 4.6.5

Birthweight: 2240 g

Apgar score: 5/8/8

Age (in hours) at recording: >120

Delivery: vaginal

Cord blood acid – base and blood gases							
	pH	$P\text{CO}_2$	mm Hg	kPa	$P\text{O}_2$	mm Hg	kPa	Base deficit mmol/l
Umbilical artery	7.29		51	6.8		12	1.6	1.2
Umbilical vein	7.44		33	4.4		37	4.9	2.2

Activity state	Awake, unquiet (feeding) and awake, quiet.
Respiratory rate	Variable between 15 and 75 breaths/min.
Transthoracic impedance	Small, somewhat irregular excursions interrupted by short apnoeas at the onset of feeding; larger, irregular excursions afterwards.
Heart rate	Baseline heart rate between 150 and 155 bpm during feeding falling to 145 bpm afterwards. The amplitude of the long-term variability $\leq$ 15 bpm.
tc$P\text{O}_2$	At the onset of the first feeding period tc$P\text{O}_2$ fell from 70 to 60 mm Hg (9.3 to 8.0 kPa) and at the onset of the second period from 75 to 60 mm Hg (10.0 to 8.0 kPa). After this there was a gradual return to the initial tc$P\text{O}_2$ level in both instances.

Comments This oxygen-cardiorespirogram illustrates as Fig. 4.6.4 the initial tc$P\text{O}_2$ fall during feeding.

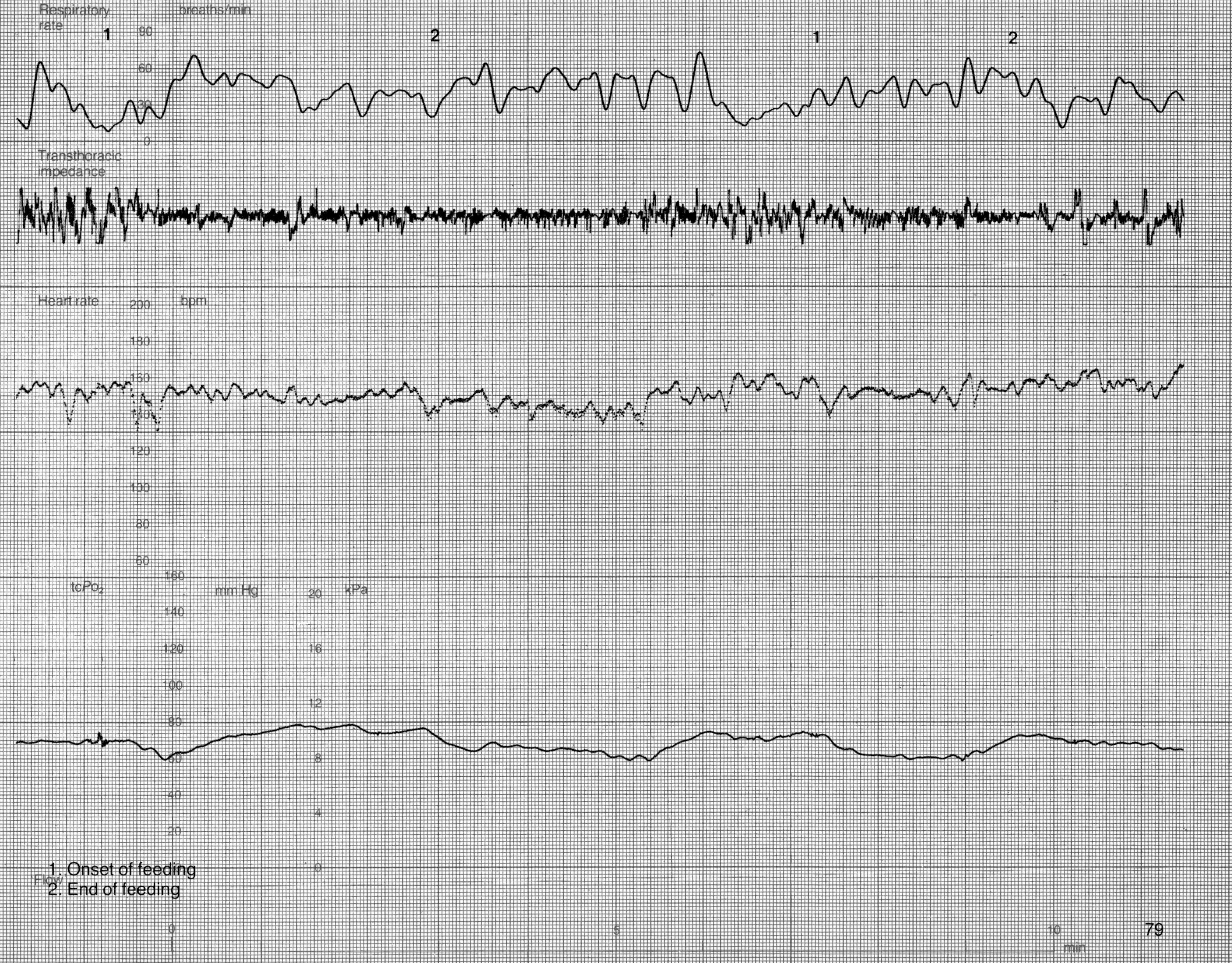
Respiratory rate
breaths/min
120
90
60
30
0
1
2
1
2
Transthoracic impedance
Heart rate
bpm
200
180
160
140
120
100
80
60
tcP_{O_2}
mm Hg
kPa
160
140
120
100
80
60
40
20
20
16
12
8
4
0
Flow
0
5
10
min
1. Onset of feeding
2. End of feeding

Fig. 4.7.1

Birthweight: 3780 g

Apgar score: 6/8/10

Age (in hours) at recording: 15

Delivery: vaginal

Cord blood acid – base and blood gases						
	pH	$P\text{CO}_2$ mm Hg	kPa	$P\text{O}_2$ mm Hg	kPa	Base deficit mmol/l
Umbilical artery	7.25	58	7.7	12	1.6	1.9

Activity state	Quiet sleep.
Respiratory rate	From a level of 40 breaths/min respiratory rate increased gradually to 50 breaths/min during oxygen breathing.
Transthoracic impedance	Regular excursions of the same amplitude when the infant breathes air and when the infant breathes oxygen.
Heart rate	Baseline heart rate about 110 bpm and with an amplitude of long-term variability $\leq$ 10 bpm. Baseline heart rate decreased to 105 bpm during the first part of the oxygen breathing.
$\text{tc}P\text{O}_2$	From a level of 75 mm Hg (10.0 kPa) $\text{tc}P\text{O}_2$ increased consistently to about 300 mm Hg (40.0 kPa). From this a shunt of 25 per cent is calculated. The $\text{tc}P\text{O}_2$ increase was fast.

Comments The changes seen in the oxygen-cardiorespirogram when oxygen is administered vary somewhat according to the activity state. The most distinct changes are seen during quiet sleep as this figure illustrates. There is a rapid increase in $\text{tc}P\text{O}_2$, respiratory rate increases and heart rate decreases. See also Chapter 10.5.5.

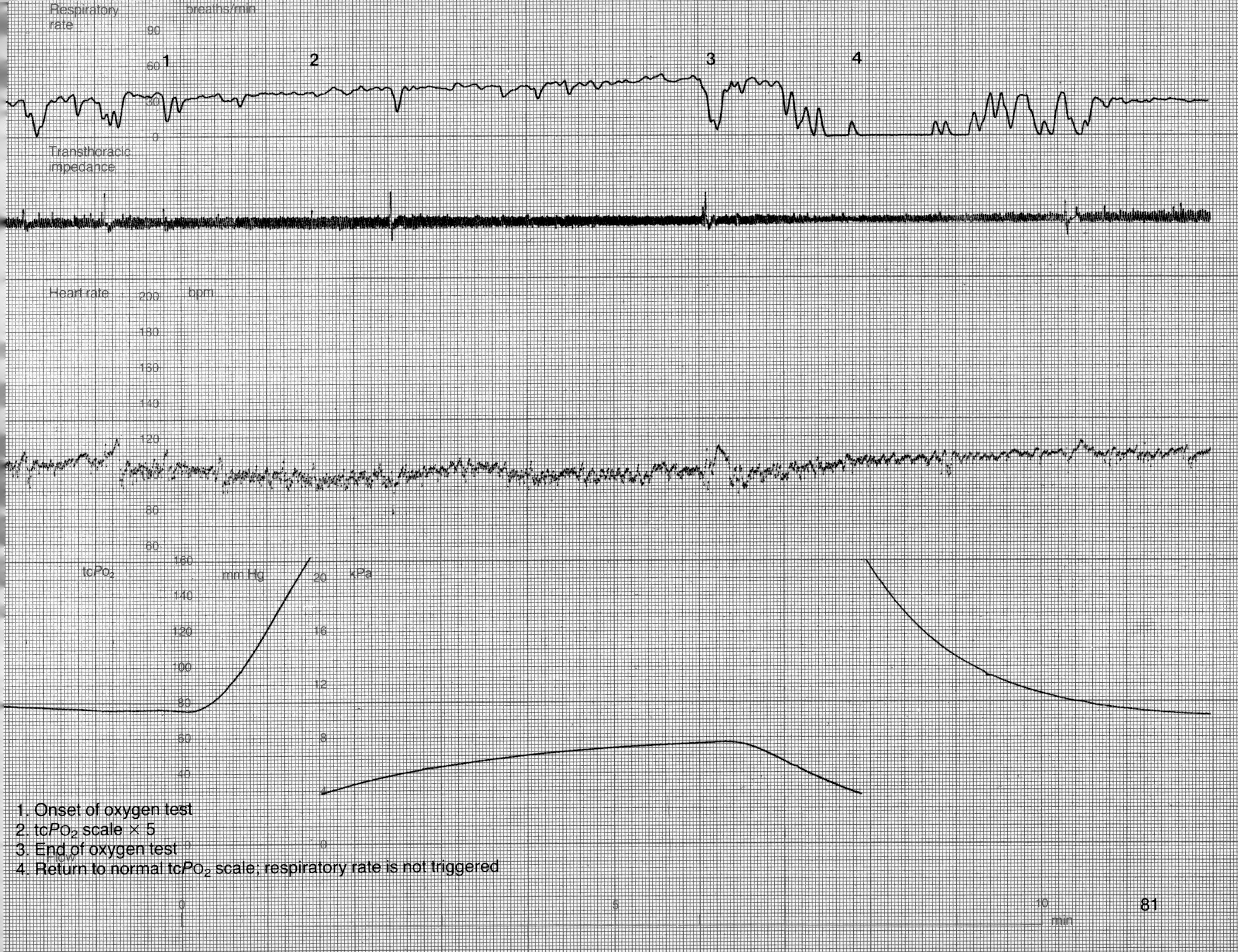
Respiratory rate
breaths/min
90
60
30
0
1
2
3
4
Transthoracic impedance
Heart rate
bpm
200
180
160
140
120
100
80
60
tcPo2
mm Hg
kPa
160
140
120
100
80
60
40
20
16
12
8
4
0
Flow
1. Onset of oxygen test
2. tcPo2 scale × 5
3. End of oxygen test
4. Return to normal tcPo2 scale; respiratory rate is not triggered
0
5
10
min

Fig. 4.7.2.a

Birthweight: 3260 g

Apgar score: 9/10

Age (in hours) at recording:	28

Delivery: vaginal

Cord blood acid – base and blood gases							
	pH	PCO_2 mm Hg	kPa	PO_2 mm Hg	kPa	Base deficit mmol/l
Umbilical artery	7.20	46	6.1	23	3.1	9.4
Umbilical vein	7.27	40	5.3	29	3.9	7.9

Activity state	Quiet sleep.
Respiratory rate	60 to 110 breaths/min with some cyclic changes.
Transthoracic impedance	Regular excursions except for occasional deeper breaths. There was a tendency to smaller amplitude of the excursions during oxygen breathing.
Heart rate	Baseline heart rate was reduced from 160 to 150 bpm during oxygen breathing. The amplitude of the long-term variability was $\leq$ 10 bpm.
tcPO_2	From a level of about 65 mm Hg (8.7 kPa) tcPO_2 increased to 315 mm Hg (42.0 kPa) during oxygen breathing. From this a shunt of 24 per cent is calculated. 180 mm Hg (24.0 kPa) was reached in less than 2 min.

Comments See Fig. 4.7.2.b.

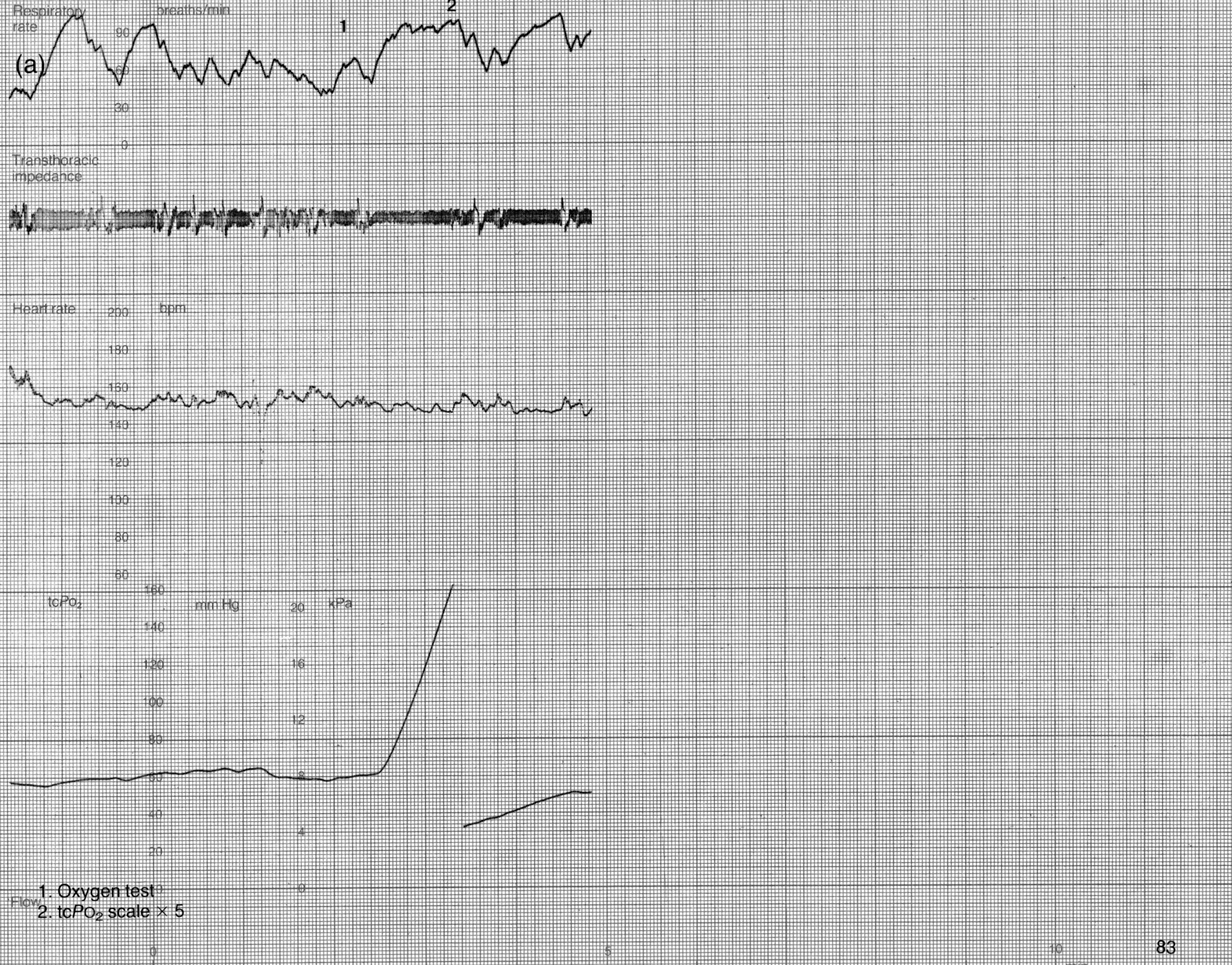
Respiratory rate
breaths/min
(a)
1
2
90
60
30
0
Transthoracic impedance
Heart rate
bpm
200
180
160
140
120
100
80
60
tcPo_2
mm Hg
kPa
160
140
120
100
80
60
40
20
0
20
16
12
8
4
0
Flow
1. Oxygen test
2. tcPo_2 scale × 5
0
5
10
min

Fig. 4.7.2.b

Birthweight: 3750 g

Apgar score: 9/9/10

Age (in hours) at recording: 17

Delivery: Caesarean section

Cord blood acid – base and blood gases							
	pH	$P\text{CO}_2$	mm Hg	kPa	$P\text{O}_2$	mm Hg	kPa	Base deficit mmol/l
Umbilical artery	7.25		58	7.7		21	2.8	2.1
Umbilical vein	7.28		48	6.4		29	3.9	4.0

Activity state	Quiet sleep.
Respiratory rate	From a level of 40 breaths/min there was a gradual increase to 70 breaths/min during oxygen breathing.
Transthoracic impedance	Regular excursions with gradually diminishing amplitude during oxygen breathing.
Heart rate	Baseline heart rate about 105 bpm with accelerations during the occasional deep breaths. The amplitude of the long-term variability was $\lesssim$10 bpm. During oxygen breathing baseline heart rate became about 5 bpm lower than before.
tc$P\text{O}_2$	From a level of 75 mm Hg (10.0 kPa) tc$P\text{O}_2$ increased to 300 mm Hg (40.0 kPa) during the oxygen test. From this a shunt of 25 per cent is calculated.

Comments (a and b) As in Fig. 4.7.1 the infants were in quiet sleep during the oxygen test. The increase in tc$P\text{O}_2$ was fast and uninterrupted in both instances. Only in **b** was there a distinct increase in respiratory rate but in both there was a small decrease in heart rate.

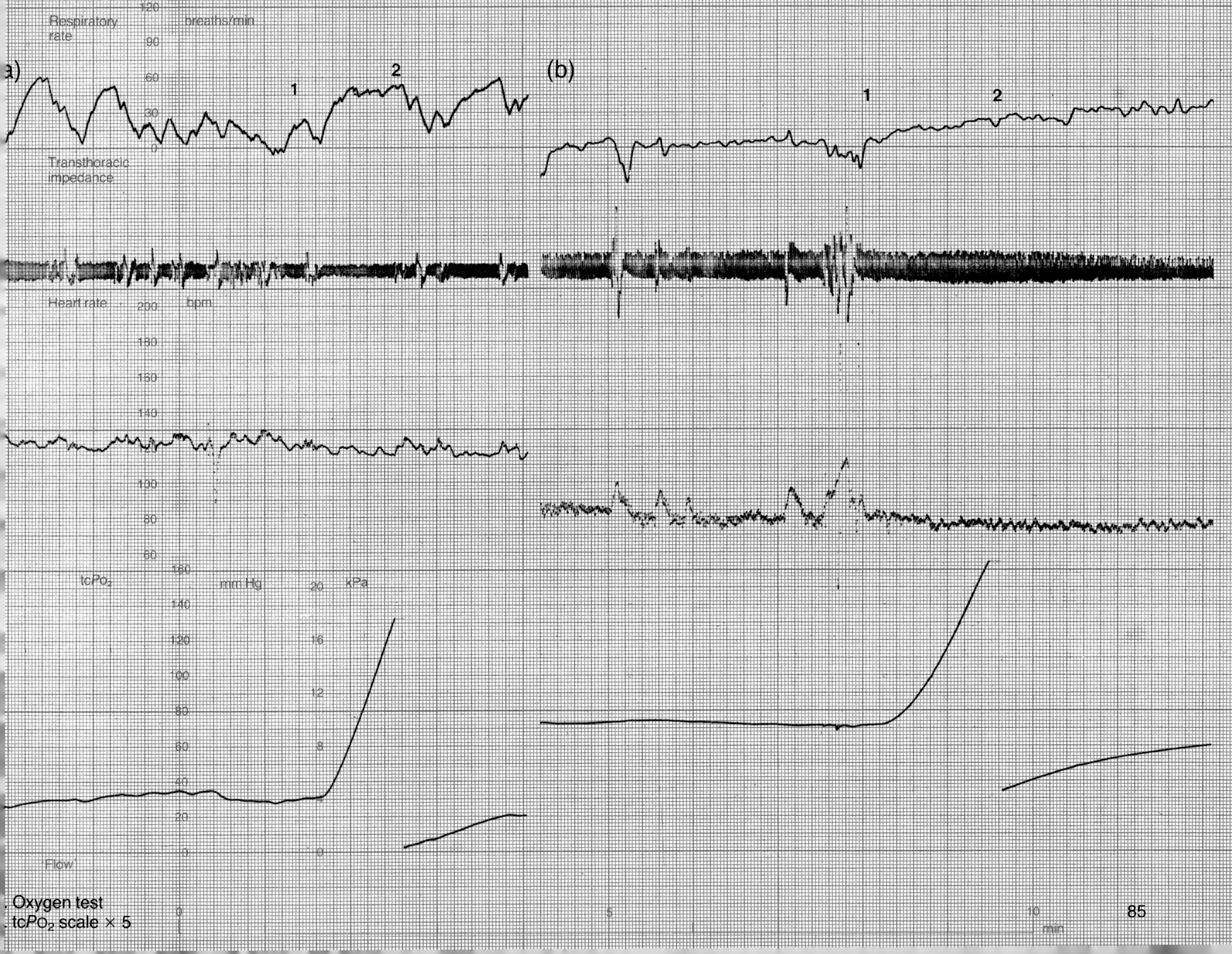

. Oxygen test
tcPo_2 scale × 5

Fig. 4.7.3.a

Birthweight: 2560 g

Apgar score: 8/10/10

Age (in hours) at recording: 2

Delivery: vaginal

Activity state	Crying.
Respiratory rate	Cyclic changes between 25 and 65 breaths/min and not affected by the oxygen administration.
Transthoracic impedance	Irregular, mostly large excursions of the same type whether oxygen was given or not.
Heart rate	Baseline heart rate was 150 bpm falling to 140 bpm during oxygen administration. The amplitude of long-term variability was ≤15 bpm.
tcPO_2	From a level of about 60 mm Hg (8.0 kPa) tcPO_2 after four minutes of oxygen administration, had not yet reached 180 mm Hg (24.0 kPa). The peak value was 190 mm Hg (25.3 kPa) from which a shunt of 30 per cent is obtained.

Comments (a and b) During crying oxygen breathing results in a slow and irregular increase in tcPO_2. Also the final level reached is lower than if the infants are quiet. No change is seen in the respiratory rate but heart rate is decreased during oxygen administration.

Fig. 4.7.3.b

Birthweight: 2480 g

Apgar score: 9/10/10

Age (in hours) at recording: 2

Delivery: vaginal

Cord blood acid – base and blood gases							
	pH	PCO_2 mm Hg	kPa	PO_2	mm Hg	kPa	Base deficit mmol/l
Umbilical artery	7.25	50	6.7		17	2.3	4.9
Umbilical vein	7.34	39	5.2				4.5

Activity state	Intermittent crying.
Respiratory rate	During crying periods respiratory rate was between 10 and 70 breaths/min. In the quiet phases it was about 60 breaths/min before and 90 breaths/min during oxygen administration.
Transthoracic impedance	Regular excursions during the quiet periods. Large irregular excursions during crying.
Heart rate	Baseline heart rate was about 115 bpm with an amplitude of long-term variability ≤15 bpm and an increase during crying to 150 bpm. In the quiet phase during the oxygen test at the end of the figure baseline heart rate was down to 100 bpm.
tcPO_2	The crying resulted in a fall in tcPO_2 to 62 mm Hg (8.3 kPa) and then a stepwise slow increase during oxygen administration. The peak value was 260 mm Hg (34.7 kPa) from which a shunt of 27 per cent is calculated.

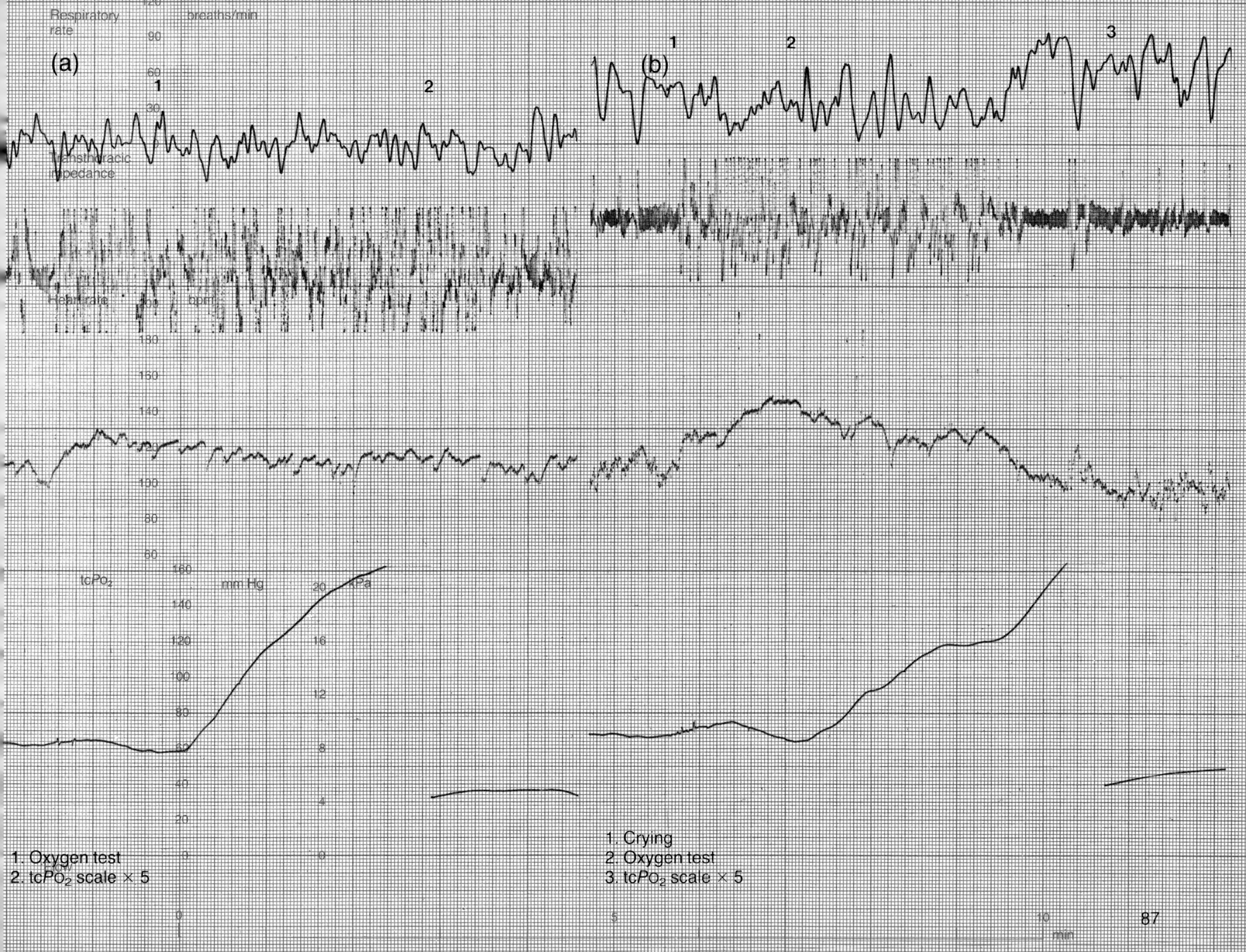

Respiratory rate
breaths/min
120
90
60
30
(a)
1
2
(b)
1
2
3
ransthoracic
mpedance
Heartrate
bpm
180
160
140
100
80
60
tcP_{O_2}
mm Hg
kPa
160
140
120
100
80
60
40
20
0
20
16
12
8
4
0
1. Oxygen test
2. tcP_{O_2} scale × 5
1. Crying
2. Oxygen test
3. tcP_{O_2} scale × 5
Flow
0
5
10
min

Fig. 4.7.4.1

Birthweight: 3860 g

Apgar score: 10/10/10

Age (in hours) at recording: 1

Delivery: vaginal

Cord blood acid – base and blood gases

	pH	$P\text{CO}_2$ mm Hg	kPa	$P\text{O}_2$ mm Hg	kPa	Base deficit mmol/l
Umbilical artery	7.28	45	6.0	21	2.8	4.1
Umbilical vein	7.42	35	4.7	31	4.1	1.3

Activity state	Awake, unquiet, crying and awake, quiet.
Respiratory rate	Rapid changes between 5 and 100 breaths/min. The most rapid respiratory rate is seen during crying.
Transthoracic impedance	Sometimes a tendency to regular excursions during the awake, non-crying periods. Larger always irregular excursions during crying.
Heart rate	Baseline heart rate about 130 bpm in the awake non-crying periods with an amplitude of long-term variability ≤ 20 bpm. During crying accelerations to 160 – 170 bpm.
tc$P\text{O}_2$ (chest)	About 80 mm Hg (10.7 kPa). During the oxygen test it increased to 390 mm Hg (52.0 kPa). From this a shunt of 20 per cent is calculated.
tc$P\text{O}_2$ (abdomen)	About 80 mm Hg (10.7 kPa). During the oxygen test it increased to 365 mm Hg (48.7 kPa). From this a shunt of 21 per cent is calculated.

Comments An oxygen-cardiorespirogram from a full-term infant with normal Apgar score obtained in the first hour of life. A second tc$P\text{O}_2$ electrode was positioned below the ductus. In air and during the oxygen test almost identical tc$P\text{O}_2$ curves were obtained.

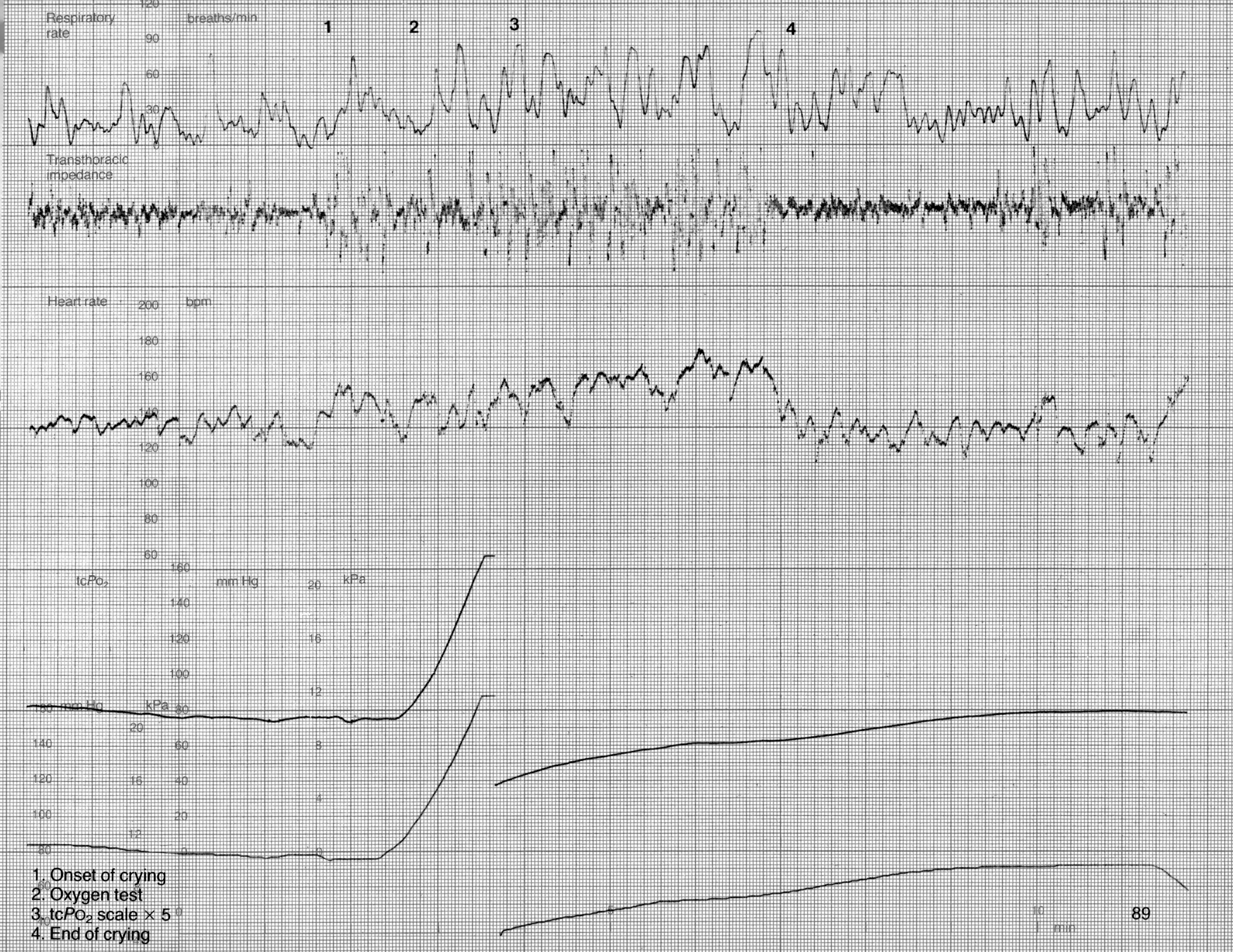
Respiratory rate
breaths/min
120
90
60
30
0
1
2
3
4
Transthoracic impedance
Heart rate
bpm
200
180
160
140
120
100
80
60
tcPo_2
mm Hg
kPa
160
140
120
100
80
60
40
20
0
20
16
12
8
4
0
10
min
1. Onset of crying
2. Oxygen test
3. tcPo_2 scale × 5
4. End of crying

Fig. 4.7.4.2

Birthweight: 3540 g

Apgar score: 8/10/10

Age (in hours) at recording: 1

Delivery: vaginal

Cord blood acid – base and blood gases							
	pH	$P\text{CO}_2$	mm Hg	kPa	$P\text{O}_2$ mm Hg	kPa	Base deficit mmol/l
Umbilical artery	7.21		47	6.3			8.3
Umbilical vein	7.27		37	4.9	24	3.2	8.2

Activity state	Awake, unquiet, crying and awake, quiet.
Respiratory rate	Cannot be estimated because of repeated trigger errors.
Transthoracic impedance	Irregular all the time.
Heart rate	Baseline heart rate about 150 bpm in the awake, unquiet period and about 140 bpm in the awake, quiet period. The amplitude of the long-term variability was ≤10 and ≤15 bpm respectively. Accelerations during crying.
tc$P\text{O}_2$ (chest)	Between 85 and 71 mm Hg (11.3 and 9.5 kPa). Increase to 420 mm Hg (56.0 kPa) during the oxygen test. From this a shunt of 18 per cent is calculated.
tc$P\text{O}_2$ (abdomen)	Between 70 and 64 mm Hg (9.3 and 8.5 kPa) increasing to 290 mm Hg (38.7 kPa) during the oxygen test. From this a shunt of 25 per cent is calculated.

Comments An oxygen-cardiorespirogram from a full-term infant with normal Apgar score obtained during the first hour of life. A second tc$P\text{O}_2$ electrode was positioned below the ductus. Both in air and during the oxygen test the electrode below the ductus showed lower values indicating a right – left shunt in the ductus.

Respiratory rate
breaths/min
120
90
60
30
0
Transthoracic impedance
1
2
3
1
Heart rate
bpm
200
180
160
140
120
100
80
60
tcPo_2
mm Hg
kPa
160
140
120
100
80
60
40
20
0
20
16
12
8
4
0
4
4
5
10
min
1 Onset of crying
2 Oxygen test
3 End of crying
4 tcPo_2 scale × 5

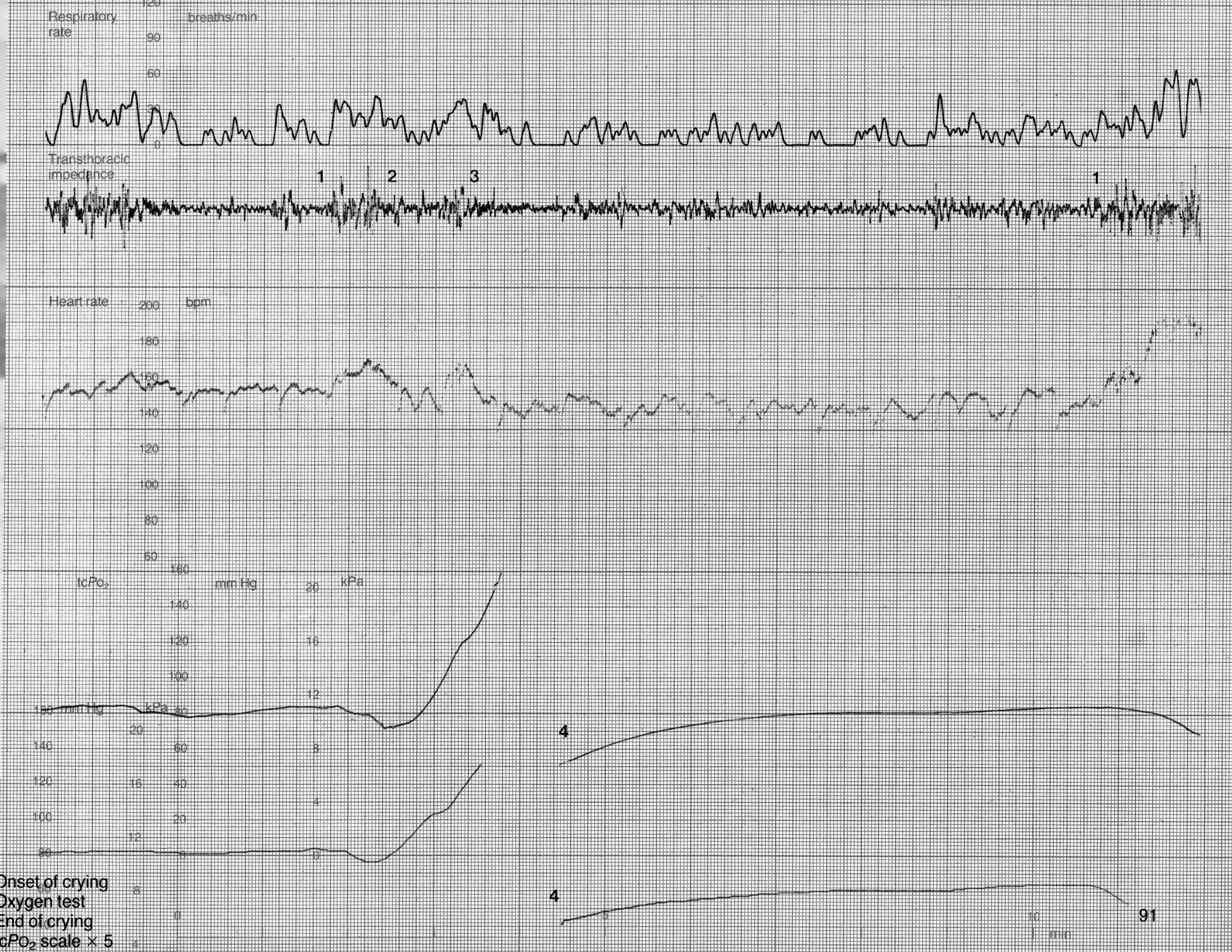

91

Fig. 4.8.1

Birthweight: 3120 g

Apgar score: 9/10/10

Age (in hours) at recording: 2

Delivery: vaginal

Cord blood acid – base and blood gases							
	pH	$P\text{CO}_2$	mm Hg	kPa	$P\text{O}_2$ mm Hg	kPa	Base deficit mmol/l
Umbilical artery	7.18		57	7.6	9	1.2	6.7
Umbilical vein	7.29		36	4.8	34	4.5	8.8

Activity state	Awake, unquiet.
Respiratory rate	Very variable from 0 to 80 breaths/min.
Transthoracic impedance	Mainly large irregular excursions often interrupted by periods of apnoea lasting some 20 – 30 s or small regular excursions. Parts of the record show periodicity.
Heart rate	The baseline heart rate drifts so much that no representative value may be given. At a heart rate of 180 bpm the amplitude of long-term variability was ≤10 bpm. Distinct undulations with an amplitude ≤ 20 bpm during the periodic breathing.
tc$P\text{O}_2$	Between 72 and 80 mm Hg (9.6 and 10.7 kPa).
'Flow'	Undulations in the 'flow' curve synchronous to that of heart rate and an increase parallel to the more marked tachycardia.

Comments In this oxygen-cardiorespirogram there is a repeated tendency to large excursions followed by apnoea and/or small regular excursions. The clinical course was uneventful.

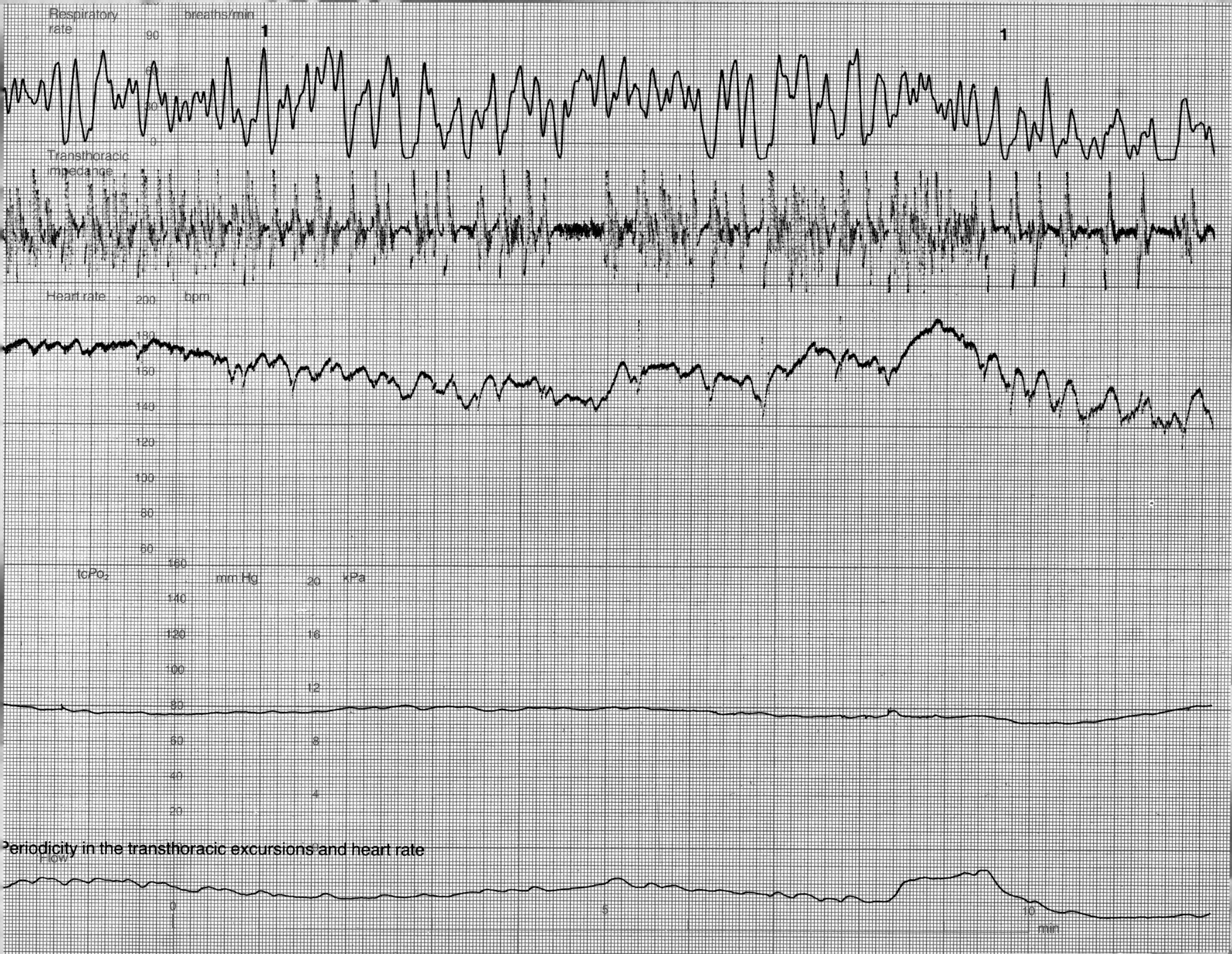

Periodicity in the transthoracic excursions and heart rate

Fig. 4.8.2

Birthweight: 2700 g

Apgar score: 9/10/10

Age (in hours) at recording: 120

Delivery: vaginal

Activity state	Awake, unquiet.
Respiratory rate	Periodic breathing. Cyclic changes round a mean level of about 30 breaths/min (Monitor II).
Transthoracic impedance	Short spells of breathing movements, at different levels, interrupted by apnoea lasting some 20 seconds. Periodicity.
Heart rate	Baseline heart rate about 110 bpm with marked long-term variability with an amplitude sometimes $>$25 bpm.
tcP_{O_2}	About 75 mm Hg (10.0 kPa) with marked waves with the same periodicity as the breathing excursions and the heart rate.
'Flow'	Cyclic changes parallel to those of the respiration and heart rate.

Comments The periodicity is marked with breathing phases interrupted by apnoea. The same frequency of periodicity is seen in respiratory rate, long-term variability of heart rate, tcP_{O_2} and in 'flow'.

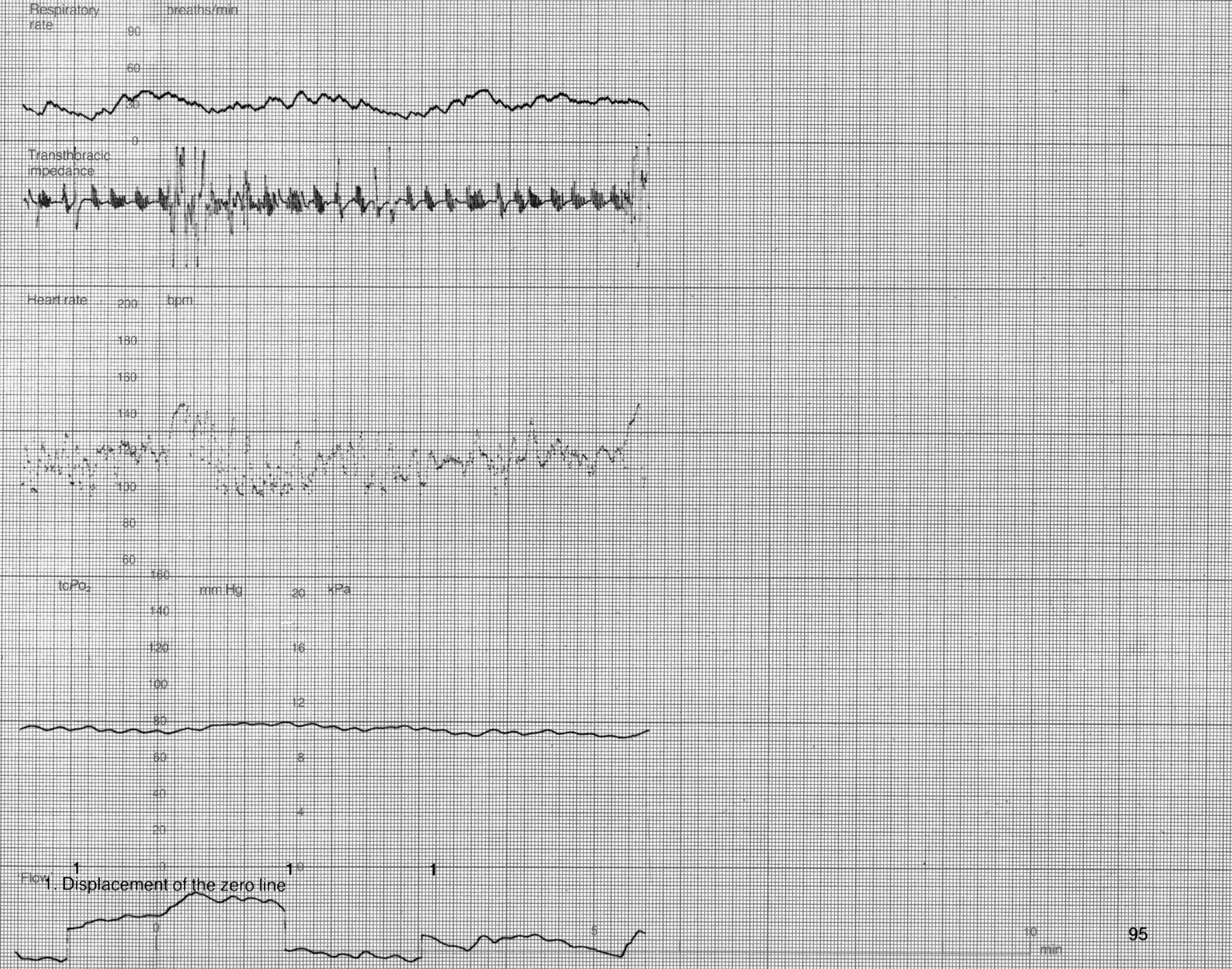

Respiratory rate
breaths/min
90
60
30
0
Transthoracic impedance
Heart rate
bpm
200
180
160
140
120
100
80
60
tcPo2
mm Hg
kPa
160
140
120
100
80
60
40
20
0
20
16
12
8
4
0
Flow
1
1
1
1. Displacement of the zero line
0
5
10
min

Fig. 4.8.3

Birthweight: 1990 g

Apgar score: 7/10/10

Age (in hours) at recording:	1

Delivery: Caesarean section

Cord blood acid – base and blood gases							
	pH	$P\text{CO}_2$	mm Hg	kPa	$P\text{O}_2$	mm Hg	kPa	Base deficit mmol/l
Umbilical artery	7.26		51	6.8		21	2.8	4.2
Umbilical vein	7.28		45	6.0				5.3

Activity state	Awake, unquiet and frequent periods of crying.
Respiratory rate	Often 60 – 80 breaths/min but in between periods of apnoea.
Transthoracic impedance	Large irregular excursions during the crying spells, in between apnoea or rather regular excursions.
Heart rate	During crying heart rate was about 185 bpm but was down to 165 bpm when the infant was more quiet. The amplitude of long-term variability in that period was $\leqslant$ 5 bpm. Clusters of spikes.
$\text{tc}P\text{O}_2$	Between 52 and 78 mm Hg (6.9 and 11.2 kPa) falling after each apnoea, but increasing again after a spell of crying.

Comments This oxygen-cardiorespirogram contains a certain periodicity because of the crying-apnoea intervals.

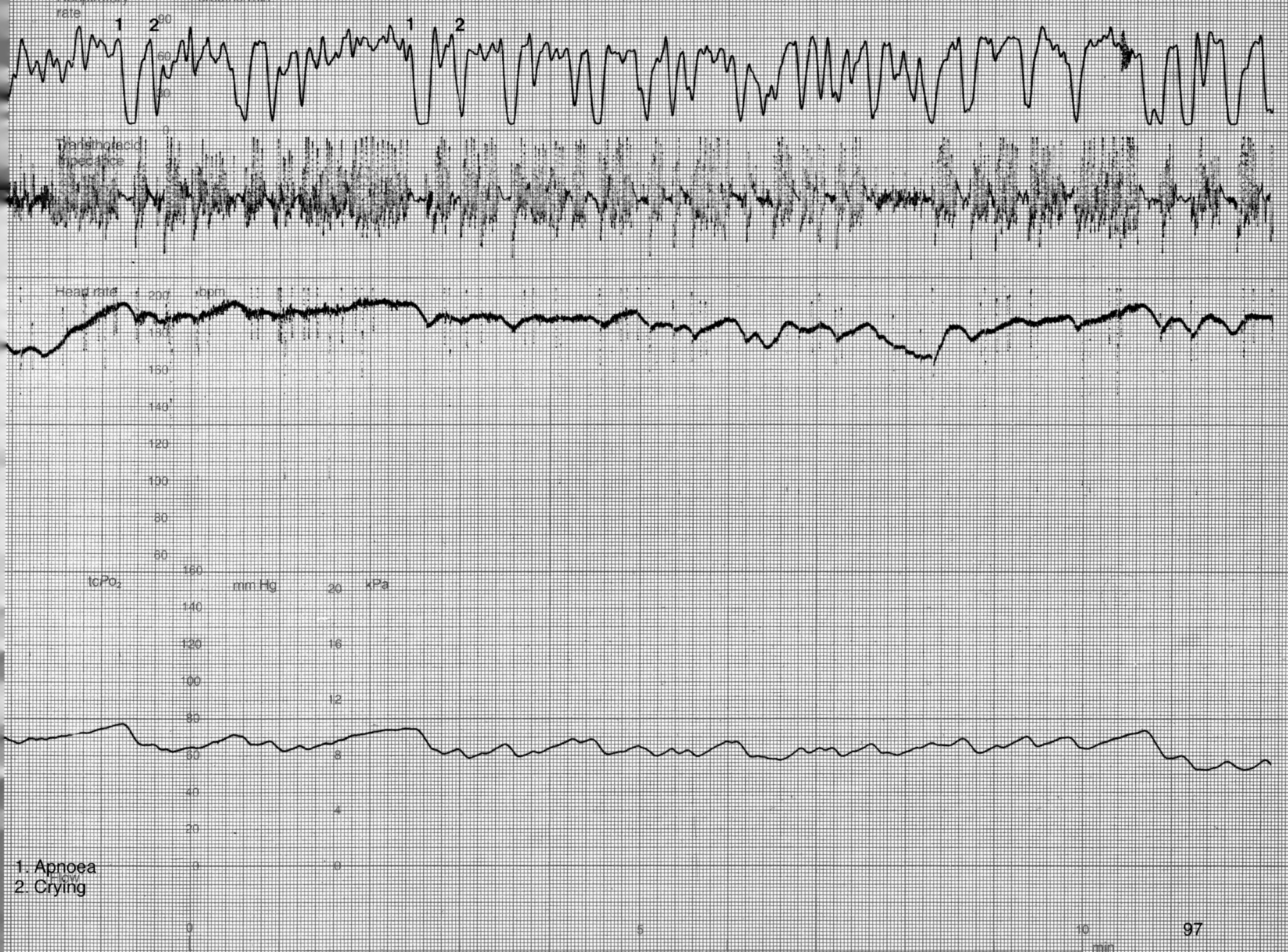
Respiratory rate
breaths/min
1
2
80
60
40
20
0
Transthoracic impedance
Heart rate
bpm
200
180
160
140
120
100
80
60
tcPo2
160
mm Hg
20
kPa
140
120
16
100
12
80
60
8
40
4
20
0
0
1. Apnoea
2. Crying
0
5
10
min

Fig. 4.9.1

Birthweight: 3900 g

Apgar score: 5/9/10

Age (in hours) at recording: 19

Delivery: vaginal

Activity state	Quiet sleep and short cry.
Respiratory rate	Small cyclic changes at three different levels, 110, 95 and 65 breaths/min interrupted by short spells of bradypnoea.
Transthoracic impedance	Regular excursions with an amplitude which was smaller when the respiratory rate was faster and vice versa. Intermittent bursts of larger breathing excursions synchronous to heart rate accelerations.
Heart rate	Baseline heart rate was about 120 bpm with accelerations at the time of the deep breaths. The amplitude of the long-term variability was $\leqslant$10 bpm.
tcP_{O_2}	There is a small fall in tcP_{O_2} from 87 to 80 mm Hg (11.6 to 10.7 kPa) and a further drop to 74 mm Hg (9.9 kPa) during crying.
'Flow'	Distinct increase in 'flow' synchronous to the larger breathing excursions and heart rate accelerations.

Comments Quiet sleep is usually interrupted by short phases with changes in respiratory rate, breathing pattern and heart rate. Often, as here, 'flow' also increases. In this example tcP_{O_2} was unaffected. The covariation of the different parameters is usually best seen in quiet sleep because the changes then are sudden and clearcut.

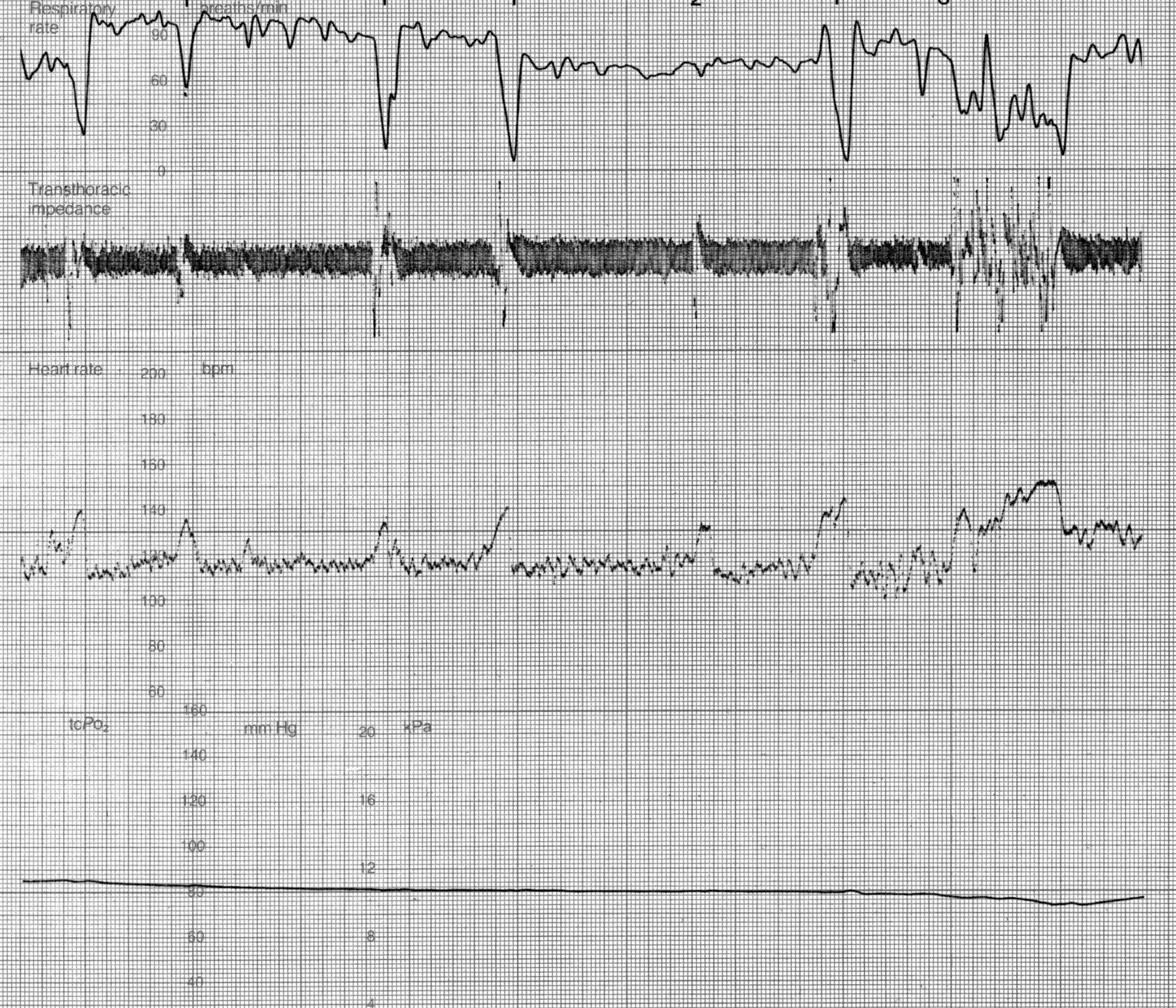

1. Simultaneous changes in four variables
2. The deep breath was less marked than in 1. and no changes were seen in respiratory rate
3. Crying

Fig. 4.9.2

Birthweight: 2920 g

Apgar score: 4/8/10

Age (in hours) at recording: 11

Delivery: Caesarean section

Cord blood acid – base and blood gases							
	pH	$P\text{CO}_2$	mm Hg	kPa	$P\text{O}_2$	mm Hg	kPa	Base deficit mmol/l
Umbilical artery	7.09		78	10.4		6	0.8	6.3
Umbilical vein	7.13		68	9.1		13	1.7	6.2

Activity state	Quiet sleep.
Respiratory rate	Mostly about 30 breaths/min, but short periods at slower rate.
Transthoracic impedance	Basically regular excursions but short periods of deeper, irregular breaths.
Heart rate	Baseline heart rate was about 110 bpm with small accelerations concomitant with the large breathing excursions. Occasionally decelerations occurred at these periods. Amplitude of long-term variability was $\leq$ 5 bpm.
tc$P\text{O}_2$	During the quiet periods tc$P\text{O}_2$ slowly fell to 64 mm Hg (8.5 kPa) and increased after the deep intermittent breaths. The peak value was 76 mm Hg (10.3 kPa).
'Flow'	'Flow' was reduced during the periods of irregular breathing.

Comments The infant was in quiet sleep as in Fig. 4.9.1 and the deep sighs are reflected in all the parameters displayed.

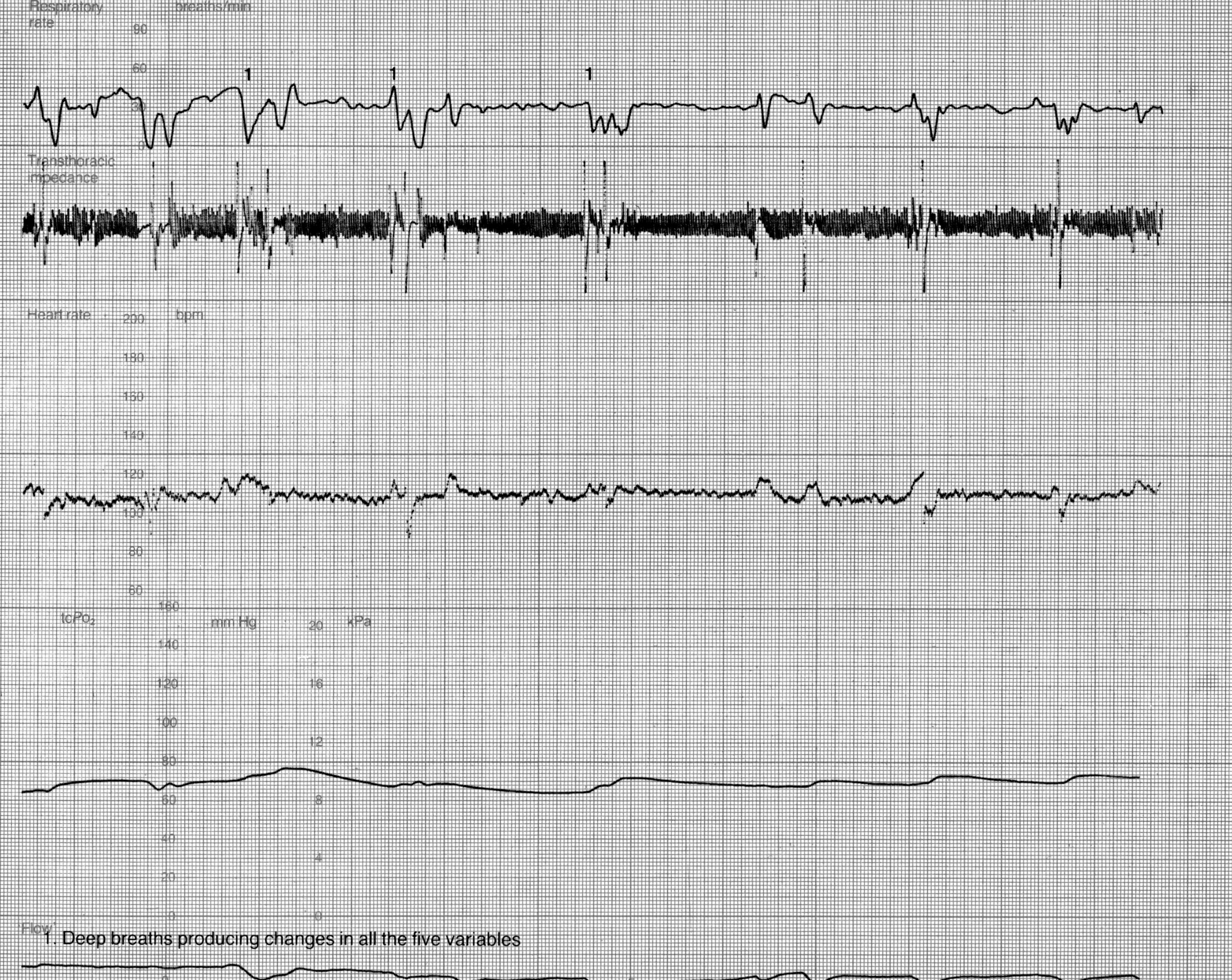

1. Deep breaths producing changes in all the five variables

Fig. 4.9.3

Birthweight: 3640 g

Apgar score: 9/10/10

Age (in hours) at recording:	10

Delivery: vaginal

Activity state	Active sleep.
Respiratory rate	In the quiet phases about 40 breaths/min and in the active phases rates between 5 and 60 breaths/min.
Transthoracic impedance	Regular excursions in the quiet phases, otherwise irregular ones.
Heart rate	Baseline heart rate was about 90 bpm with an amplitude of long-term variability $\leqslant$ 15 bpm. During the bursts of deep breaths there were accelerations with occasional short decelerations.
tcP_{O_2}	Close to 80 mm Hg (10.7 kPa).
'Flow'	Increase in 'flow' concomitant with the deep breaths and the heart rate acceleration.

Comments As in Figs 4.9.1 and 4.9.2 this illustrates covariability of respiratory rate, transthoracic impedence, heart rate and 'flow' all initiated by deep breaths.

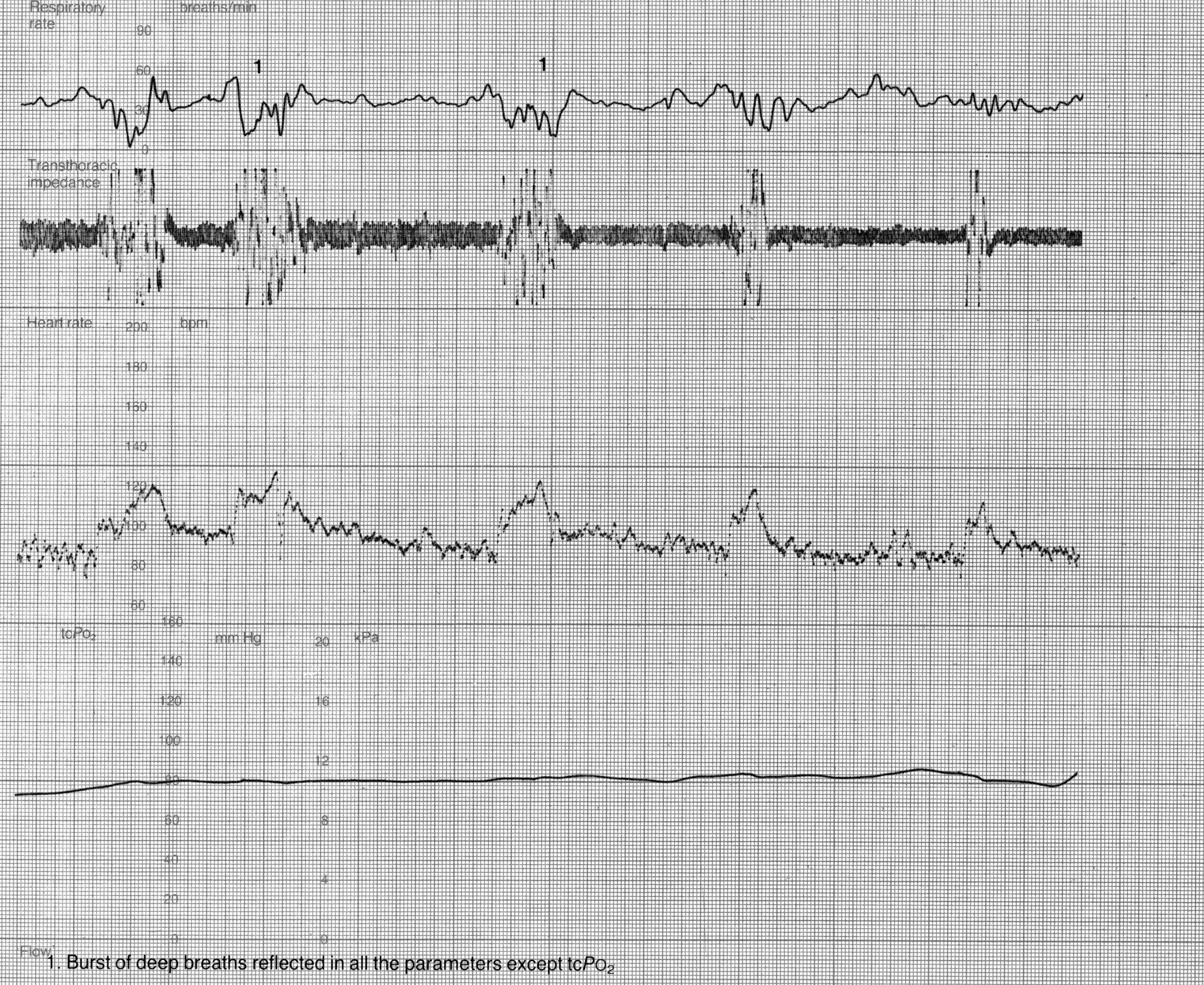

1. Burst of deep breaths reflected in all the parameters except $tcPo_2$

Fig. 4.9.4

Birthweight: 4080 g

Apgar score: 9/10

Age (in hours) at recording: 2

Delivery: vaginal

Cord blood acid – base and blood gases							
	pH	$P\text{CO}_2$	mm Hg	kPa	$P\text{O}_2$	mm Hg	kPa	Base deficit mmol/l
Umbilical vein	7.38		34	4.5		33	4.4	4.5

Activity state	Crying, initially continuously, later interrupted by quiet phases.
Respiratory rate	Cyclic changes during crying between 50 and 70 breaths/min.
Transthoracic impedance	Irregular excursions during crying, in between more regular ones.
Heart rate	Baseline heart rate cannot be seen except in the quiet phase when it is about 130 bpm. There were marked accelerations during crying. The amplitude of long-term variability in the quiet phase was $\leqslant$10 bpm.
$\text{tc}P\text{O}_2$	Between 83 and 92 mm Hg (11.1 and 12.3 kPa) and hardly any decrease during the crying.
'Flow'	Increase in 'flow' parallel to the heart rate accelerations.

Comments The activity of the crying is seen in the respiratory rate, the transthoracic impedance, the heart rate and in 'flow'.

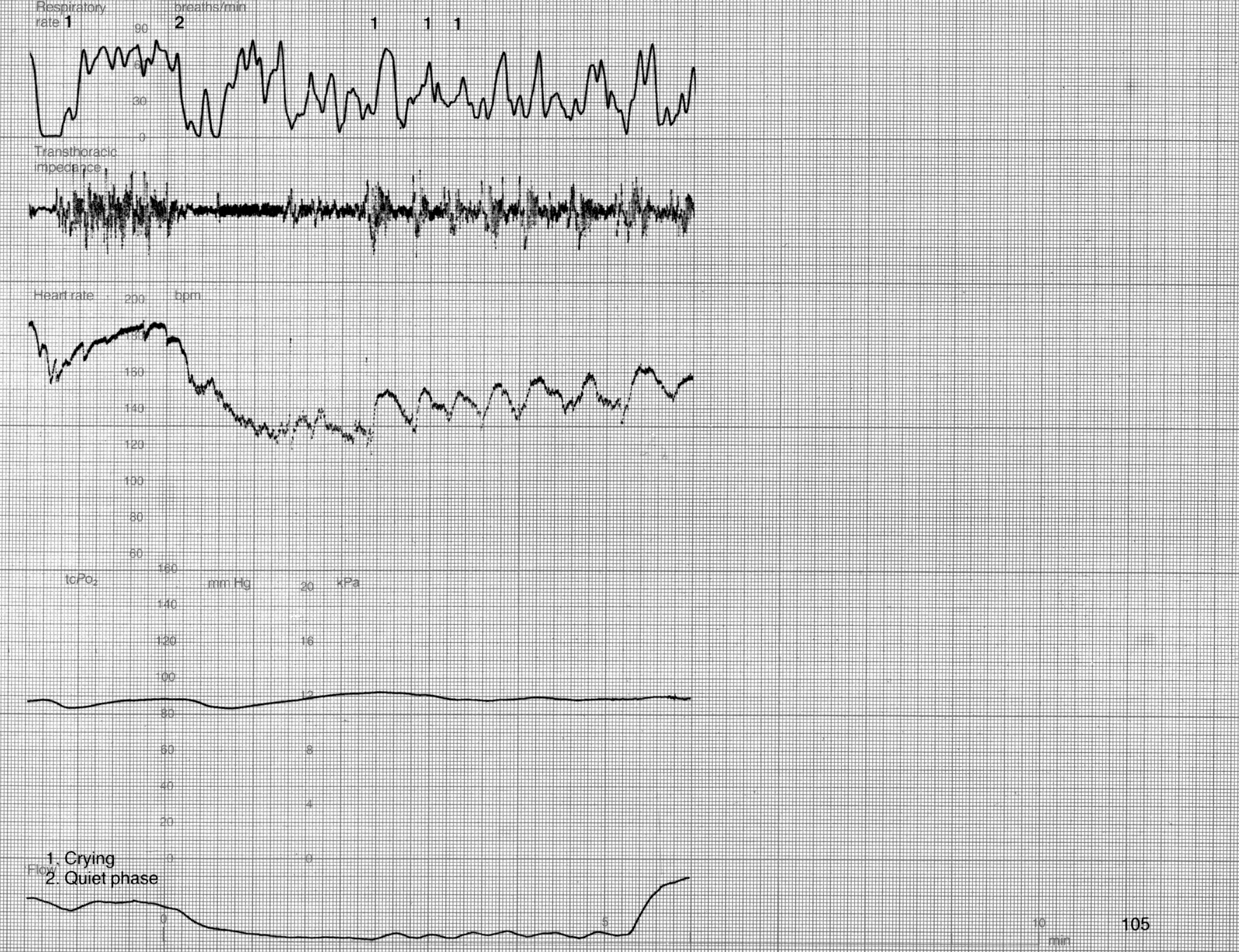

Respiratory rate
breaths/min
120
90
60
30
0
1
2
1
1
1
Transthoracic impedance
Heart rate
bpm
200
180
160
140
120
100
80
60
tcPo2
mm Hg
kPa
160
140
120
100
80
60
40
20
0
20
16
12
8
4
0
Flow
1. Crying
2. Quiet phase
0
5
10
min

5 The first hour of life

Fig. 5.1.1

Birthweight: 3020 g

Apgar score: 8/9/10

Age at recording: 10 min

Delivery: vaginal

Cord blood acid – base and blood gases							
	pH	PCO_2 mm Hg	kPa	PO_2 mm Hg	kPa	Base deficit mmol/l
Umbilical artery	7.28	54	7.2	15	2.0	0.4
Umbilical vein	7.39	34	4.5	31	4.1	3.6

Activity state	Awake, unquiet.
Respiratory rate	Variable mainly between 30 and 70 breaths/min.
Transthoracic impedance	Irregular excursions.
Heart rate	Baseline heart rate was about 150 bpm with an amplitude of long-term variability $\leq$10 bpm. Occasionally very short decelerations.
tcPO_2	Between 85 and 93 mm Hg (11.3 and 12.4 kPa).

Comments The oxygen-cardiorespirogram of this unquiet infant has a high tcPO_2 level already at 10 min. There were some fluctuations in tcPO_2 which could not be correlated visually with the respiration.

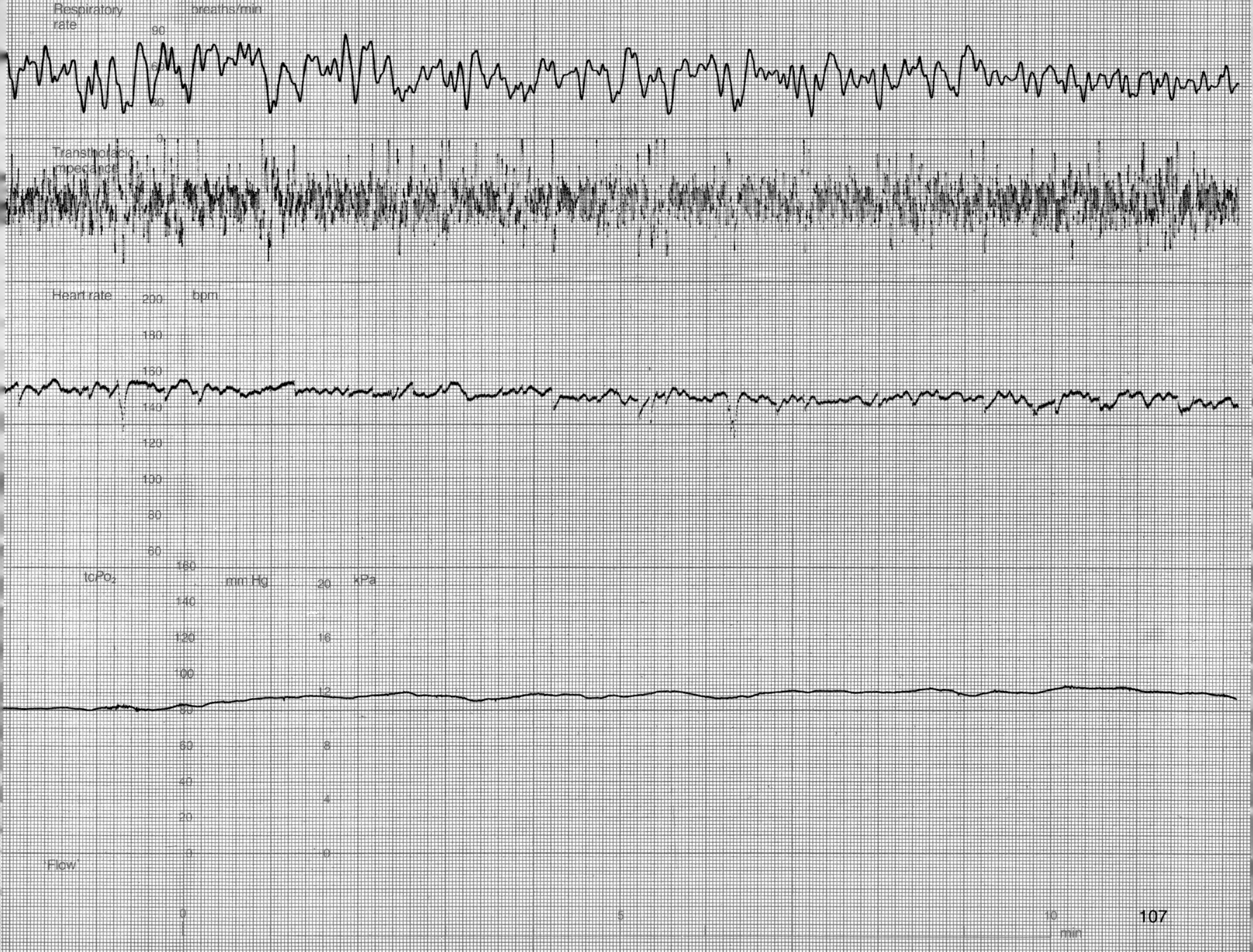

Respiratory rate
breaths/min
120
90
60
30
0
Transthoracic impedance
Heart rate
200
bpm
180
160
140
120
100
80
60
tcPo2
160
mm Hg
20
kPa
140
120
16
100
12
80
60
8
40
20
4
0
0
Flow
0
5
10
min

Fig. 5.1.2

Birthweight: 3900 g

Apgar score: 9/10

Age at recording: 30 min

Delivery: vaginal

Cord blood acid – base and blood gases							
	pH	$P\text{CO}_2$	mm Hg	kPa	$P\text{O}_2$	mm Hg	kPa	Base deficit mmol/l
Umbilical artery	7.27		44	5.9		25	3.3	4.9
Umbilical vein	7.32		32	4.3		34	4.5	6.7

Activity state	At first awake, unquiet and then crying.
Respiratory rate	Cyclic change between 0 and 60 breaths/min.
Transthoracic impedance	Before crying some phases were more regular and some more irregular with large excursions. During crying the excursions were large and irregular.
Heart rate	It is difficult to ascertain baseline heart rate even in the first part of the figure, i.e. before the crying. Probably it was about 125 bpm with an amplitude of long-term variability $\leqslant$10 bpm and interrupted by short decelerations. There were frequent accelerations up to 155 bpm. During crying heart rate was about 160 bpm.
tc$P\text{O}_2$	In the awake, unquiet phase tc$P\text{O}_2$ varied between 56 and 76 mm Hg (7.5 and 10.1 kPa) with waves coinciding with the heart rate accelerations. During crying tc$P\text{O}_2$ fell to 48 mm Hg (6.4 kPa).

Comments There is nothing to distinguish this oxygen-cardiorespirogram from those obtained some hours later in life showing the same activity state.

Respiratory rate
breaths/min
90
60
0
1
Transthoracic impedance
Heart rate
200
bpm
180
160
140
120
100
80
60
tcPo_2
160
mm Hg
20
kPa
140
120
16
100
12
80
60
8
40
4
20
0
0
Flow
0
5
10
min
1. Crying

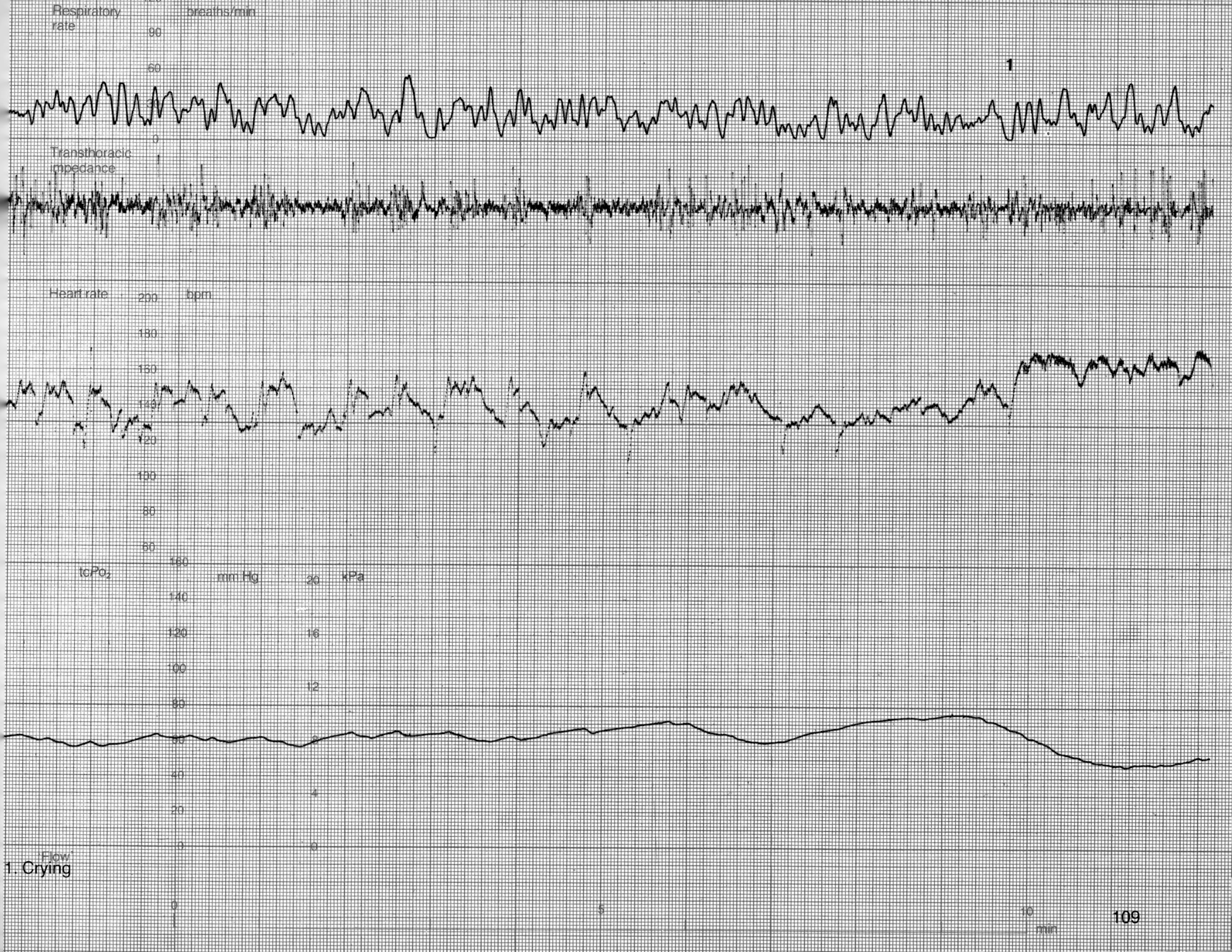

Fig. 5.1.3

Birthweight: 2550 g

Apgar score: 9/10

Age at recording: 15 min

Delivery: vaginal

Cord blood acid – base and blood gases

	pH	PCO_2 mm Hg	PCO_2 kPa	PO_2 mm Hg	PO_2 kPa	Base deficit mmol/l
Umbilical artery	7.30	45	6.0	15	2.0	3.0
Umbilical vein	7.34	36	4.8	26	3.5	5.3

Activity state	At first awake, unquiet, then crying.
Respiratory rate	Cyclic changes between 15 and 90 breaths/min.
Transthoracic impedance	In the awake, unquiet period there was a certain pattern with undulating baseline and sometimes larger excursions. During crying there were larger irregular excursions.
Heart rate	Baseline heart rate was about 130 bpm with an amplitude of long-term variability $\leq$10 bpm and frequent deep but short decelerations. During crying heart rate was about 145 bpm.
tcPO_2	Undulated and gradually increased from 73 to 83 mm Hg (9.7 to 11.1 kPa) before crying and then fell to 70 mm Hg (9.3 kPa).

Comments As in the other oxygen-cardiorespirograms obtained soon after birth there is nothing to distinguish this one from those obtained some hours later showing the same activity state.

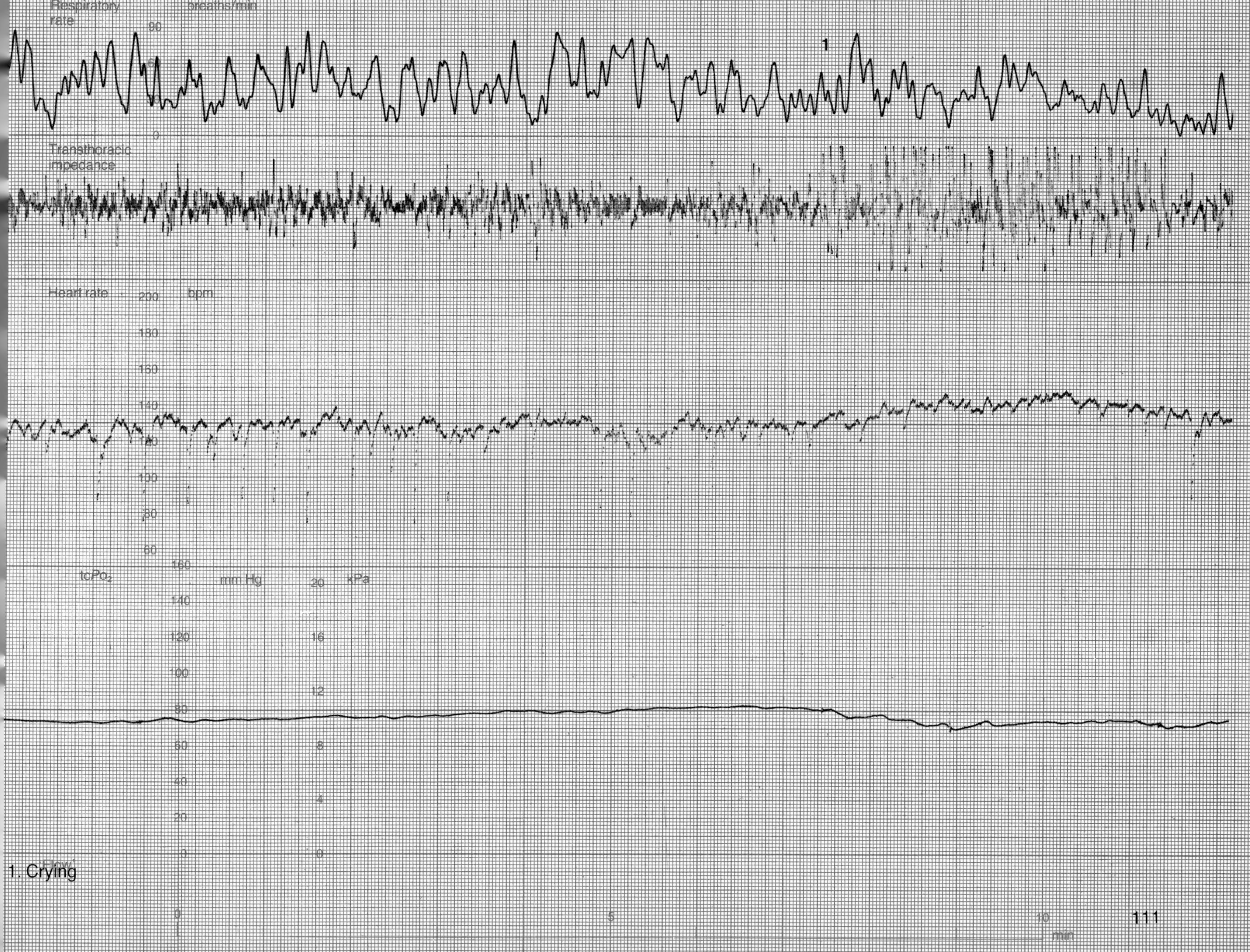

Respiratory rate
breaths/min
90
60
0
1
Transthoracic impedance
Heart rate
bpm
200
180
160
140
120
100
80
60
tcPo2
mm Hg
kPa
160
140
120
100
80
60
40
20
0
20
16
12
8
4
0
Flow
1. Crying
0
5
10
min

Fig. 5.1.4

Birthweight: 3040 g

Apgar score: 9/10

Age at recording:	30 min

Delivery: vaginal

Cord blood acid – base and blood gases								
	pH	$P\mathrm{CO}_2$	mm Hg	kPa	$P\mathrm{O}_2$	mm Hg	kPa	Base deficit mmol/l
Umbilical artery	7.26		47	6.3		12	1.6	4.6
Umbilical vein	7.36		31	4.1		27	3.6	6.7

Activity state	Awake, unquiet, then crying and again awake, unquiet.
Respiratory rate	About 35 – 40 breaths/min (Monitor II).
Transthoracic impedance	The excursions were irregular all the time. Here and there a tendency to periodicity.
Heart rate	Baseline heart rate was about 140 bpm with an amplitude of long-term variability ≤10 bpm and occasionally short decelerations during the awake, unquiet periods. During crying heart rate increased to about 160 bpm with short decelerations.
tc$P\mathrm{O}_2$	Small fluctuations between 102 and 108 mm Hg (13.6 and 14.4 kPa) in the unquiet period. During crying tc$P\mathrm{O}_2$ fell slowly to 98 mm Hg (13.1 kPa).

Comments As in the previous oxygen-cardiorespirograms obtained in the first hour of life there is nothing characteristic to distinguish this one from those recorded later in the same activity state.

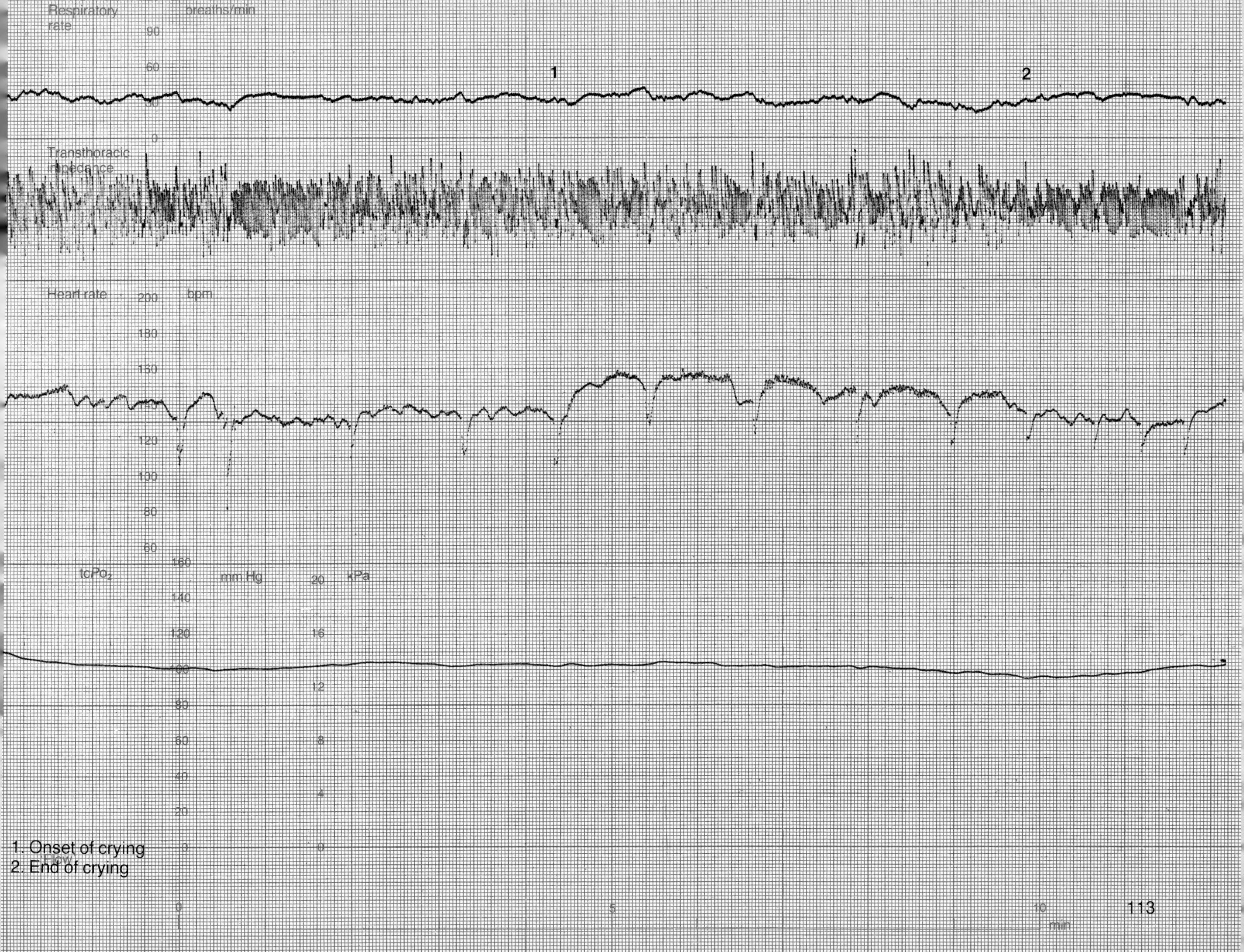

Respiratory rate
breaths/min
90
60
30
0
1
2
Transthoracic impedance
Heart rate
bpm
200
180
160
140
120
100
80
60
tcPo2
mm Hg
kPa
160
140
120
100
80
60
40
20
0
20
16
12
8
4
0
1. Onset of crying
2. End of crying
0
5
10
min

Fig. 5.1.5

Birthweight: 3240 g

Apgar score: 7/10/10

Age (in hours) at recording: 1

Delivery: vaginal (breech)

Cord blood acid – base and blood gases							
	pH	$P\text{CO}_2$ mm Hg	kPa	$P\text{O}_2$ mm Hg	kPa	Base deficit mmol/l
Umbilical artery	7.23	49	6.5	10	1.3	5.4
Umbilical vein	7.25	36	4.8	29	3.9	10.2

Activity state	At first awake, unquiet, then crying and finally again awake, unquiet.
Respiratory rate	Cyclic changes from 15 to 90 breaths/min.
Transthoracic impedance	Fairly regular excursions in the awake, unquiet phases, but larger and irregular excursions during crying.
Heart rate	Baseline heart rate was about 140 bpm with an amplitude of long-term variability $\leq$15 bpm. During crying there was an increase to 165 bpm and the long-term variability was $\leq$10 bpm.
tc$P\text{O}_2$	Close to 100 mm Hg (13.3 kPa) until crying began when it fell to 76 mm Hg (10.1 kPa). Subsequently tc$P\text{O}_2$ increased to 114 mm Hg (15.2 kPa).

Comments This is an oxygen-cardiorespirogram from a newborn infant born after a breech delivery. There is nothing to distinguish this from oxygen-cardiorespirograms from vertex deliveries.

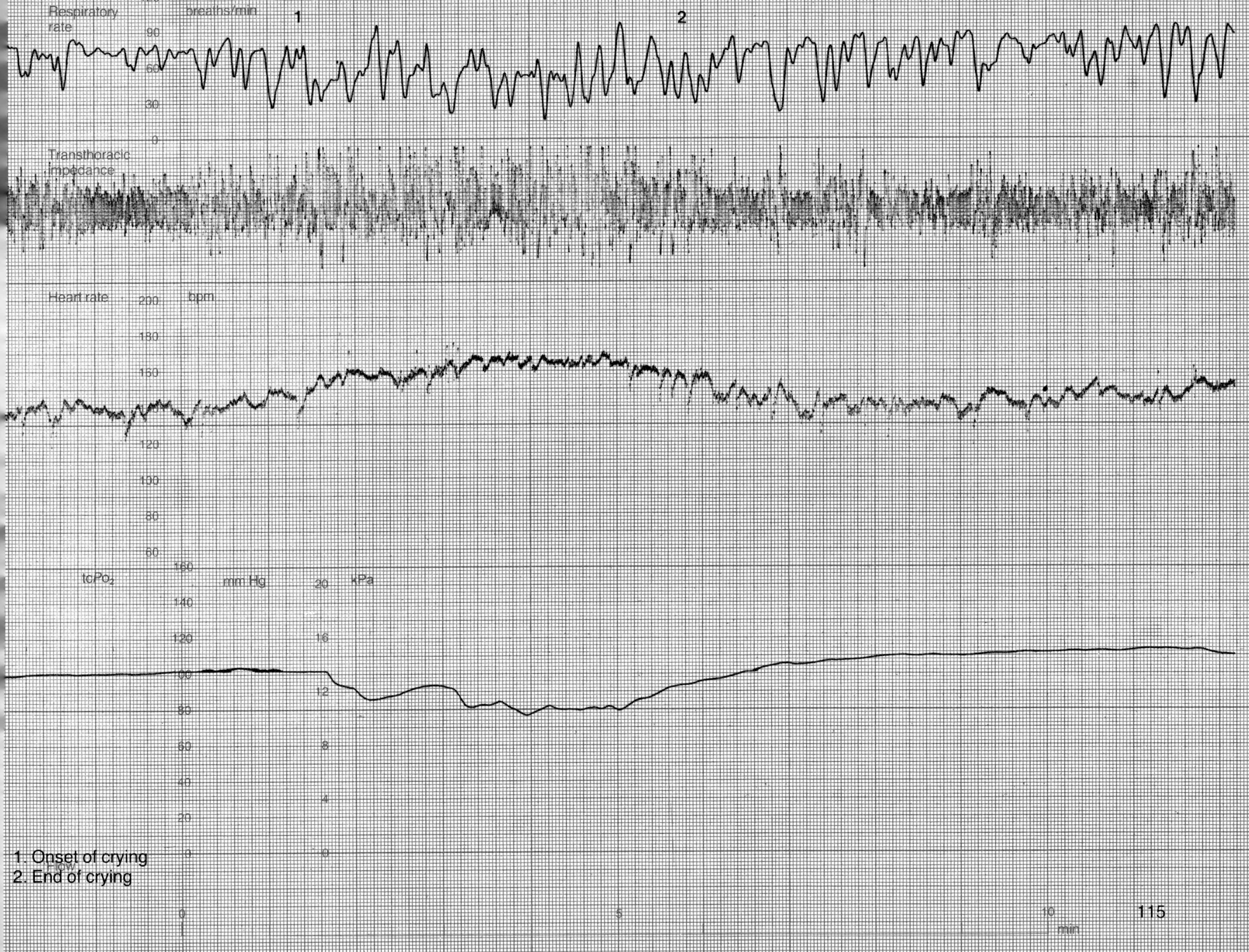
Respiratory rate
breaths/min
1
2
90
60
30
0
Transthoracic impedance
Heart rate
200
bpm
180
160
120
100
80
60
tcPo_2
160
mm Hg
20
kPa
140
120
16
100
12
80
60
8
40
4
20
0
0
1. Onset of crying
2. End of crying
0
5
10
min

Fig. 5.2.1.a

Birthweight: 2610 g

Apgar score: 9/10

Age at recording: 30 min

Delivery: vaginal

Cord blood acid – base and blood gases							
	pH	$P\text{CO}_2$ mm Hg	kPa	$P\text{O}_2$ mm Hg	kPa	Base deficit mmol/l
Umbilical artery	7.24	41	5.5	19	2.5	8.9
Umbilical vein	7.25	40	5.3	26	3.5	9.0

Activity state	Awake, unquiet.
Respiratory rate	Cyclic changes between 0 and 110 breaths/min.
Transthoracic impedance	Periodic breathing with alternating small rapid breaths and deep infrequent ones.
Heart rate	Baseline heart rate was about 165 bpm with an amplitude of long-term variability $\leq$10 bpm.
tc$P\text{O}_2$	Close to 70 mm Hg (9.3 kPa) with minute fluctuations synchronous to the periodicity of the respiration.

Fig. 5.2.1.b

Age (in hours) at recording: 24

Activity state	Awake, unquiet.
Respiratory rate	Cyclic changes between 7 and 95 breaths/min.
Transthoracic impedance	Irregular. There are phases with larger and phases with smaller excursions.
Heart rate	Baseline heart rate about 130 bpm and amplitude of long-term variability $\leq$ 20 bpm.
tc$P\text{O}_2$	A gradual increase from 59 to 71 mm Hg (7.9 to 9.5 kPa).

Comments See Fig. 5.2.1.d.

For neonatal data see Fig. 5.2.1.a.

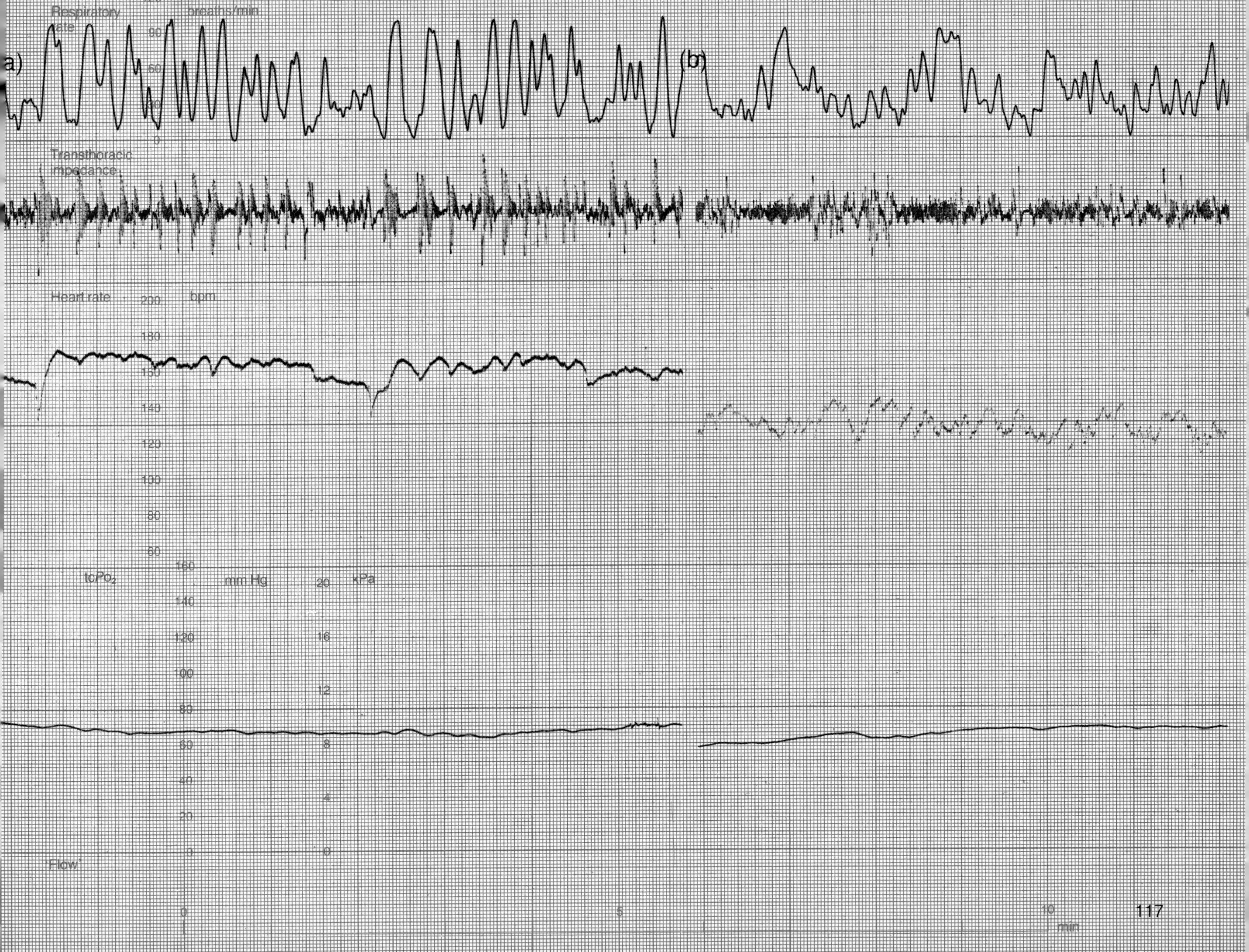
(a)
(b)
Respiratory rate
breaths/min
120
90
60
30
0
Transthoracic impedance
Heart rate
bpm
200
180
160
140
120
100
80
60
tcPo_2
mm Hg
kPa
160
140
120
100
80
60
40
20
0
20
16
12
8
4
0
Flow
0
5
10
min

Fig. 5.2.1.c

Age (in hours) at recording:	75

Activity state	Awake, unquiet.
Respiratory rate	Cyclic changes between 0 and 90 breaths/min.
Transthoracic impedance	Irregular excursions.
Heart rate	Baseline heart rate about 120 bpm with an amplitude of long-term variability $\leq$ 25 bpm.
tcP_{O_2}	Undulating between 70 and 81 mm Hg (9.3 and 10.8 kPa).

Fig. 5.2.1.d

Age (in hours) at recording:	98

Activity state	Awake, unquiet.
Respiratory rate	Cyclic changes between 12 and 90 breaths/min.
Transthoracic impedance	Irregular excursions.
Heart rate	Baseline heart rate about 120 bpm with an amplitude of long-term variability $\geq$ 25 bpm.
tcP_{O_2}	Undulating between 61 and 74 mm Hg (8.1 and 9.9 kPa).

Comments (a–d) The only clear-cut evolution of the oxygen-cardiorespirogram seen in this series is the reduction of the heart rate from the initial tachycardia and the gradual increases in the amplitude of the long-term variability. See also Chapter 10.5.3.

For neonatal data see Fig. 5.2.1.a.

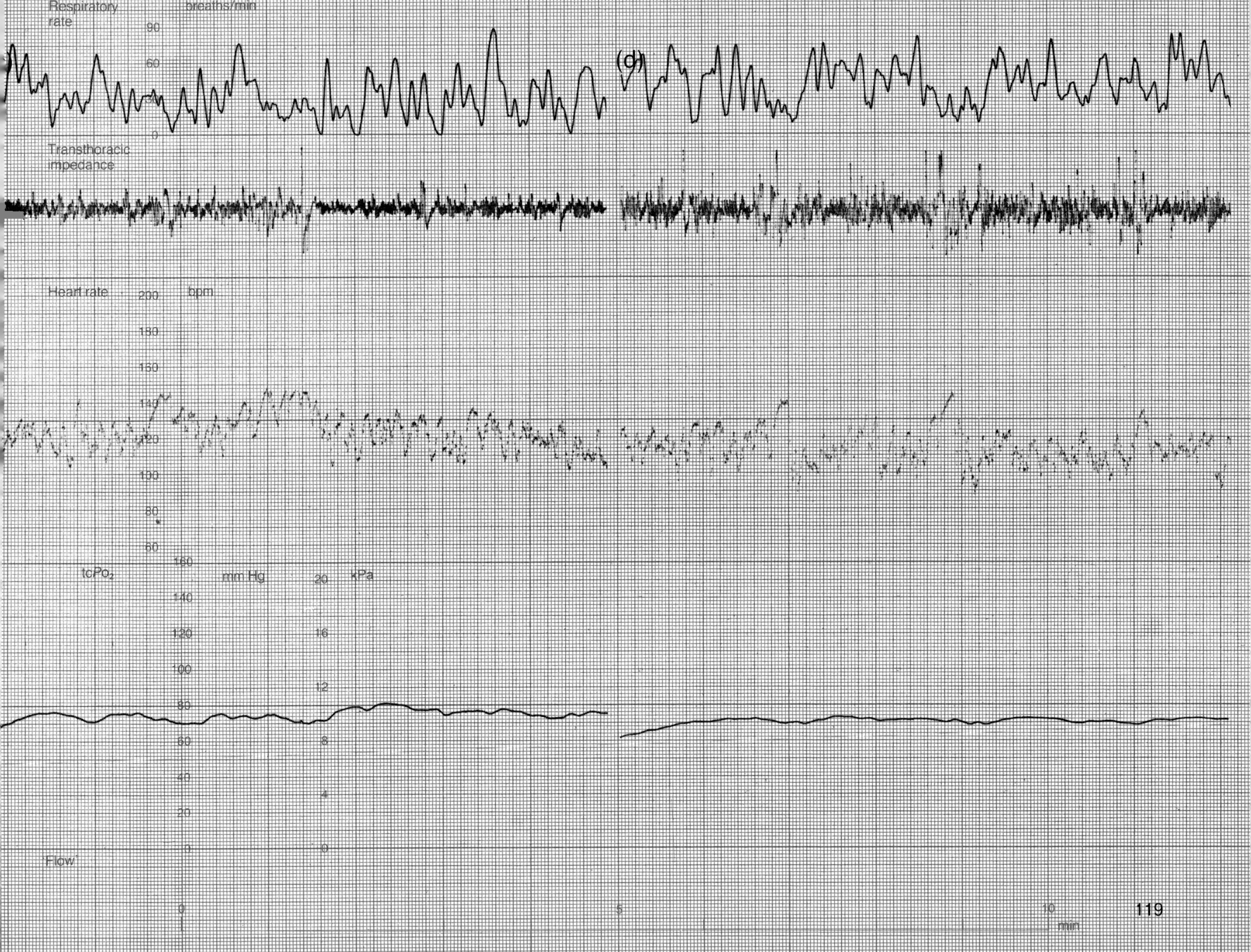
Respiratory rate
breaths/min
90
60
0
(d)
Transthoracic impedance
Heart rate
bpm
200
180
160
140
120
100
80
60
$tcPo_2$
mm Hg
160
140
120
100
80
60
40
20
0
kPa
20
16
12
8
4
0
'Flow'
0
5
10
min

Fig. 5.2.2.a

Birthweight: 3390 g

Apgar score: 9/10

Age (in hours) at recording: 1

Delivery: vaginal

Cord blood acid – base and blood gases							
	pH	$P\text{CO}_2$	mm Hg	kPa	$P\text{O}_2$	mm Hg	kPa	Base deficit mmol/l
Umbilical artery	7.26		52	6.9		10	1.3	3.8
Umbilical vein	7.29		44	5.9		19	2.5	5.3

Activity state	Awake, unquiet or crying.
Respiratory rate	Cyclic changes between 5 and >100 breaths/min.
Transthoracic impedance	Before crying the excursions were almost regular with occasional large ones. During crying there were large, irregular excursions with a tendency to periodicity.
Heart rate	Baseline heart rate was about 135 bpm with an amplitude of long-term variability mostly ≤ 10 bpm but occasionally ≤ 20 bpm. During crying heart rate increased to 155 bpm.
tc$P\text{O}_2$	Between 86 and 93 mm Hg (11.5 and 12.4 kPa) regardless of the activity state.

Comments See Fig. 5.2.2.c.

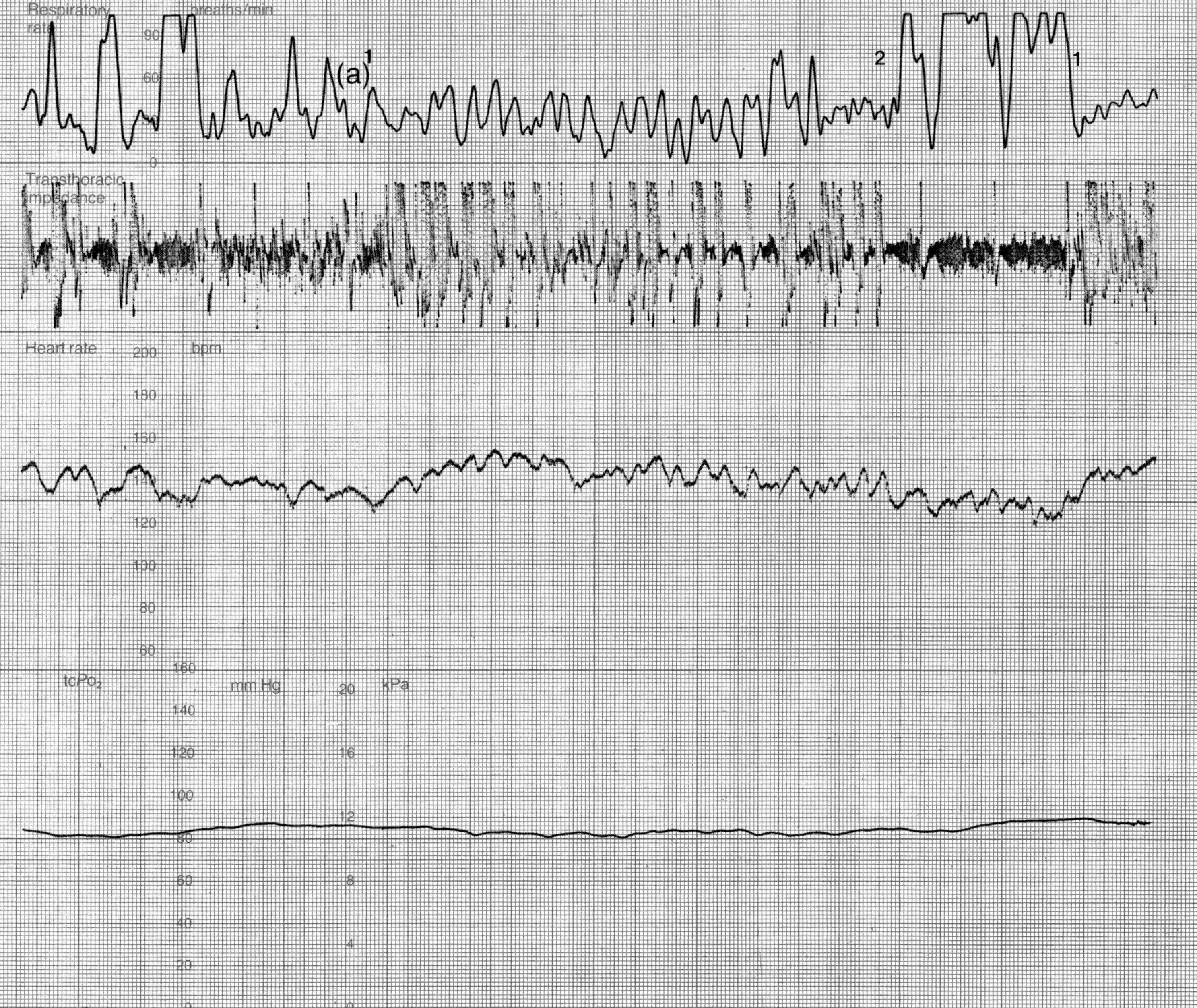

Respiratory rate
breaths/min
120
90
60
0
(a)
1
2
1
Transthoracic impedance
Heart rate
bpm
200
180
160
140
120
100
80
60
tcP_{O_2}
mm Hg
kPa
160
140
120
100
80
60
40
20
20
16
12
8
4
0
Flow
1. Onset of crying
2. End of crying
0
5
10
min

Fig. 5.2.2.b

Age (in hours) at recording:	28

Activity state	Transition from awake, quiet to quiet sleep.
Respiratory rate	Undulating about 40 breaths/min from 30 to 68 breaths/min.
Transthoracic impedance	Mostly regular excursions.
Heart rate	Baseline heart rate was about 110 bpm with an amplitude of long-term variability $\leqslant$ 15 bpm.
tcP_{O_2}	A gradual increase from 64 to 76 mm Hg (8.5 to 10.1 kPa).

Fig. 5.2.2.c

Age (in hours) at recording:	100

Activity state	Quiet sleep.
Respiratory rate	Cyclic changes between 35 and 45 breaths/min.
Transthoracic impedance	Regular excursions and occasionally deep breaths.
Heart rate	Baseline heart rate was about 115 bpm with an amplitude of long-term variability about 10 bpm, but difficult to ascertain because of artifacts.
tcP_{O_2}	A gradual increase in tcP_{O_2} from 69 to 77 mm Hg (9.2 to 10.3 kPa).

Comments (a–c) As in Figs 5.2.1. a–d this series of oxygen-cardiorespirograms from the same infant showed initial tachycardia, and tcP_{O_2} was also higher during the first hour of life than in the subsequent measurements. See also Chapter 10.1.3.

For neonatal data see Fig. 5.2.2.a.

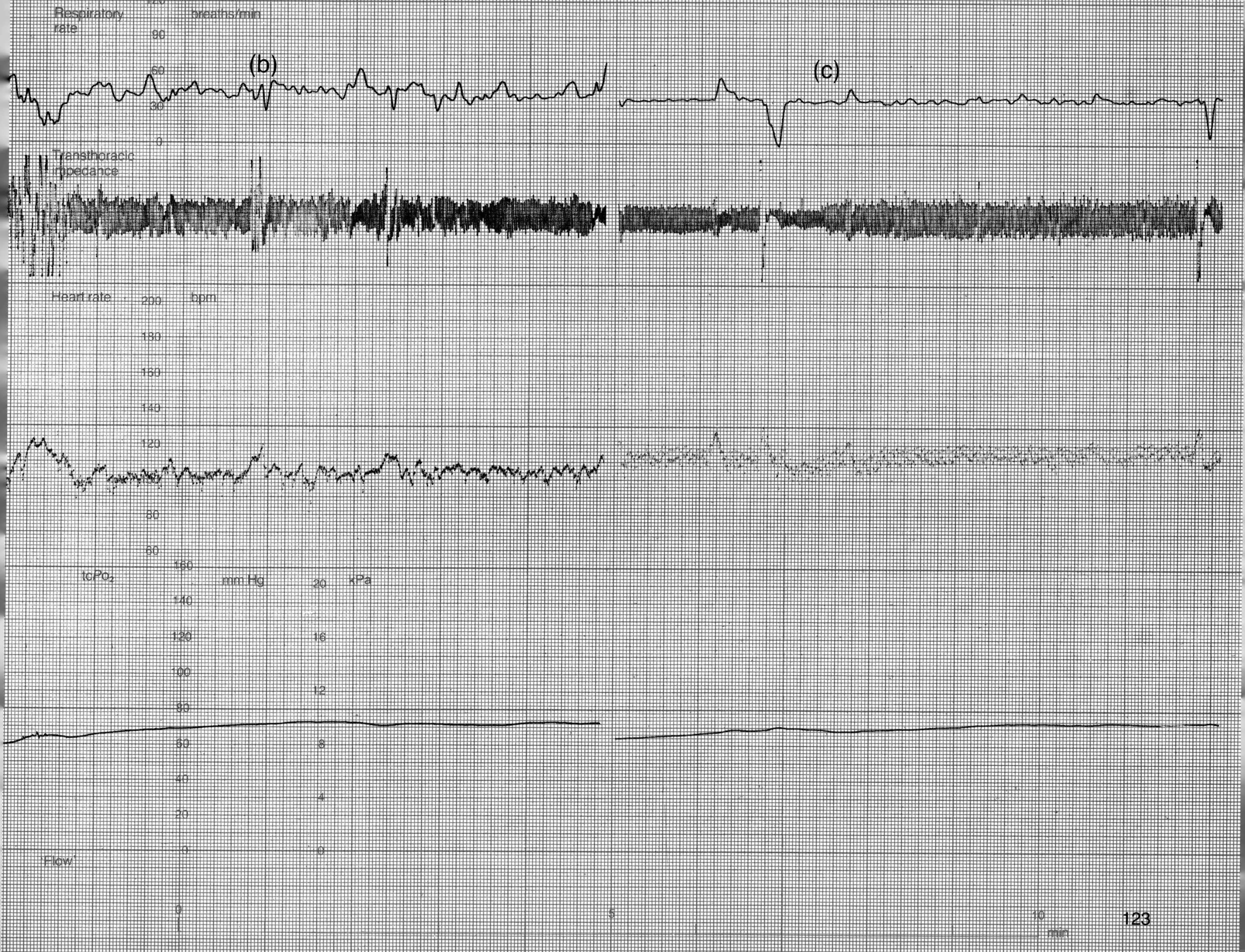
Respiratory rate
breaths/min
90
60
30
0
(b)
(c)
Transthoracic
mpedance
Heart rate
200
bpm
180
160
140
120
80
60
$tcPo_2$
160
mm Hg
20
kPa
140
120
16
100
12
80
60
8
40
4
20
0
0
'Flow'
0
5
10
min

Fig. 5.2.3.a

Birthweight: 2400 g

Apgar score: 8/10/10

Age (in hours) at recording: 1

Delivery: vaginal

Cord blood acid – base and blood gases									
	pH	PCO_2	mm Hg	kPa	PO_2	mm Hg	kPa	Base deficit mmol/l
Umbilical artery	7.38		30	4.0		22	2.9	7.0
Umbilical vein	7.40		25	3.3		26	3.5	8.4

Activity state	Awake, unquiet.
Respiratory rate	Cyclic changes partly around 20, partly around 50 breaths/min.
Transthoracic impedance	Irregular excursions, which were larger when the rate was slower.
Heart rate	Baseline heart rate was about 150 bpm and the amplitude of long-term variability ≤10 bpm.
tcPO_2	Small undulations in tcPO_2 between 86 and 83 mm Hg (11.5 and 11.1 kPa).

Fig. 5.2.3.b

Age (in hours) at recording: 19

Activity state	Awake, unquiet and awake, quiet.
Respiratory rate	About 30 breaths/min (Monitor II).
Transthoracic impedance	Regular excursions in the short quiet period, otherwise irregular ones.
Heart rate	Baseline heart rate was 130 bpm with an amplitude of long-term variability ≤ 10 bpm. During the unquiet phase heart rate was about 150 bpm.
tcPO_2	The level of tcPO_2 varied between 75 and 62 mm Hg (10.0 and 8.3 kPa).

For neonatal data see Fig. 5.2.3.a.

For comments see Fig. 5.2.3.c.

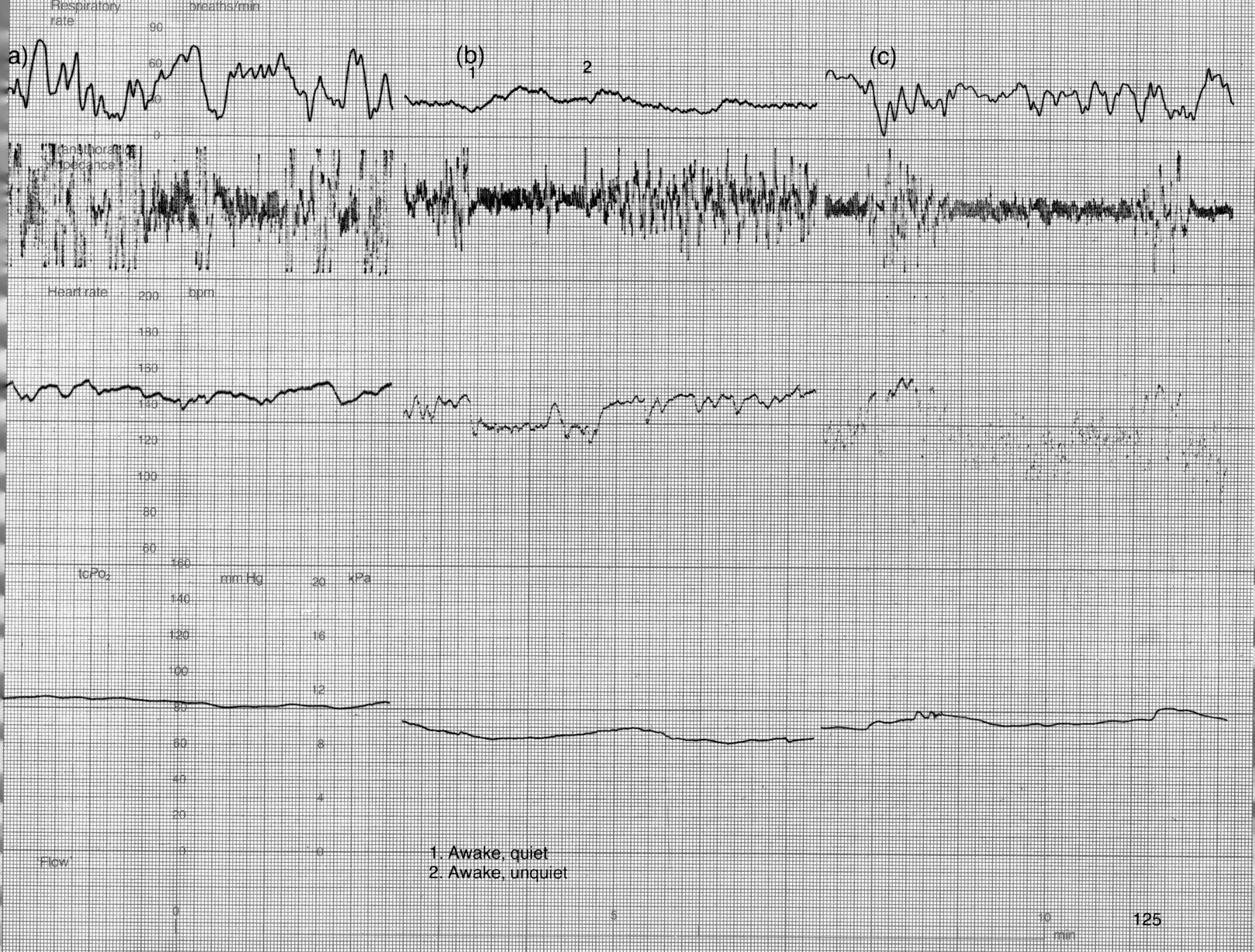
Respiratory rate
breaths/min
a)
(b)
(c)
1
2
Transthoracic impedance
Heart rate
bpm
tcPo2
mm Hg
kPa
Flow
1. Awake, quiet
2. Awake, unquiet
min

Fig. 5.2.3.c

Age (in hours) at recording:	90

Activity state	Active sleep.
Respiratory rate	Undulating between 25 and 45 breaths/min.
Transthoracic impedance	Mostly regular excursions, but bursts of larger irregular breaths.
Heart rate	Baseline heart rate about 115 bpm with an amplitude of long-term variability ⩾ 25 bpm. Coinciding with the deep breaths there were accelerations to 155 bpm.
tcPO_2	Between 70 and 82 mm Hg (9.3 and 10.9 kPa).

For neonatal data see Fig. 5.2.3.a.

Comments (a – c) As in Figs 5.2.2 a – c tcPO_2 was highest during the first hour of life. See also Chapter 10.1.3.

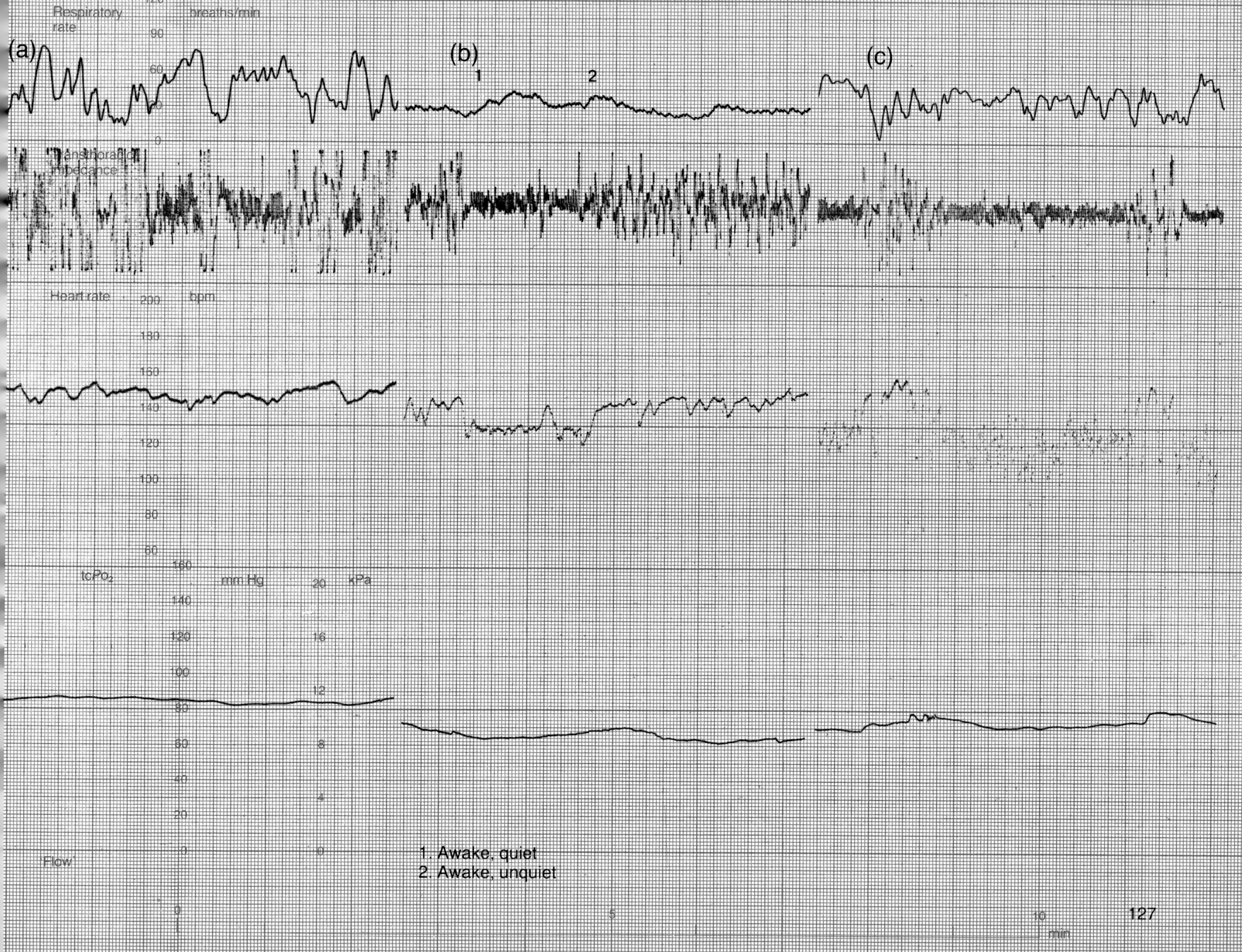

Respiratory rate
breaths/min
120
90
60
0
(a)
(b)
1
2
(c)
Transthoracic impedance
Heart rate
bpm
200
180
160
140
120
100
80
60
$tcPo_2$
mm Hg
kPa
160
140
120
100
80
60
40
20
0
20
16
12
8
4
0
Flow
1. Awake, quiet
2. Awake, unquiet
0
5
10
min

6 Anaesthesia and analgesia

Fig. 6.1.1.a

Birthweight: 3500 g

Apgar score: 8/10

Age (in hours) at recording: 1

Delivery: Caesarean section

Cord blood acid – base and blood gases							
	pH	P_{CO_2}	mm Hg	kPa	P_{O_2} mm Hg	kPa	Base deficit mmol/l
Umbilical artery	7.29		59	7.9	16	2.1	1.4
Umbilical vein	7.31		44	5.9	29	3.9	3.8

Activity state	Awake, unquiet and crying.
Respiratory rate	Undulating between 50 and 90 breaths/min before crying and about 25 breaths/min in the crying periods.
Transthoracic impedance	Some periods of regular excursions in between crying and larger irregular excursions during crying.
Heart rate	During the longest quiet period baseline heart rate was about 125 bpm with an amplitude of long-term variability about 10 bpm. During crying there were increases up to 170 bpm sometimes interrupted by decelerations.
tcP_{O_2}	Close to 65 mm Hg (8.7 kPa) and fell to 56 mm Hg (7.5 kPa) after the most intense crying.

Fig. 6.1.1.b

Age (in hours) at recording: 100

Activity state	Active sleep.
Respiratory rate	Cyclic changes between 15 and 70 breaths/min.
Transthoracic impedance	Partly irregular excursions, partly more regular ones with a tendency to periodicity.
Heart rate	Baseline heart rate was about 115 bpm and later about 105 bpm and the amplitude of long-term variability $\leqslant 20 - \leqslant 30$.
tcP_{O_2}	Between 77 and 82 mm Hg (10.3 and 10.9 kPa).

Comments (a and b) In contrast to Figs 5.2.2 and 5.2.3 this oxygen-cardio-respirogram showed a tcP_{O_2} value which was lowest in the first hour of life but then the neonate was crying all the time.

For neonatal data see Fig. 6.1.1.a.

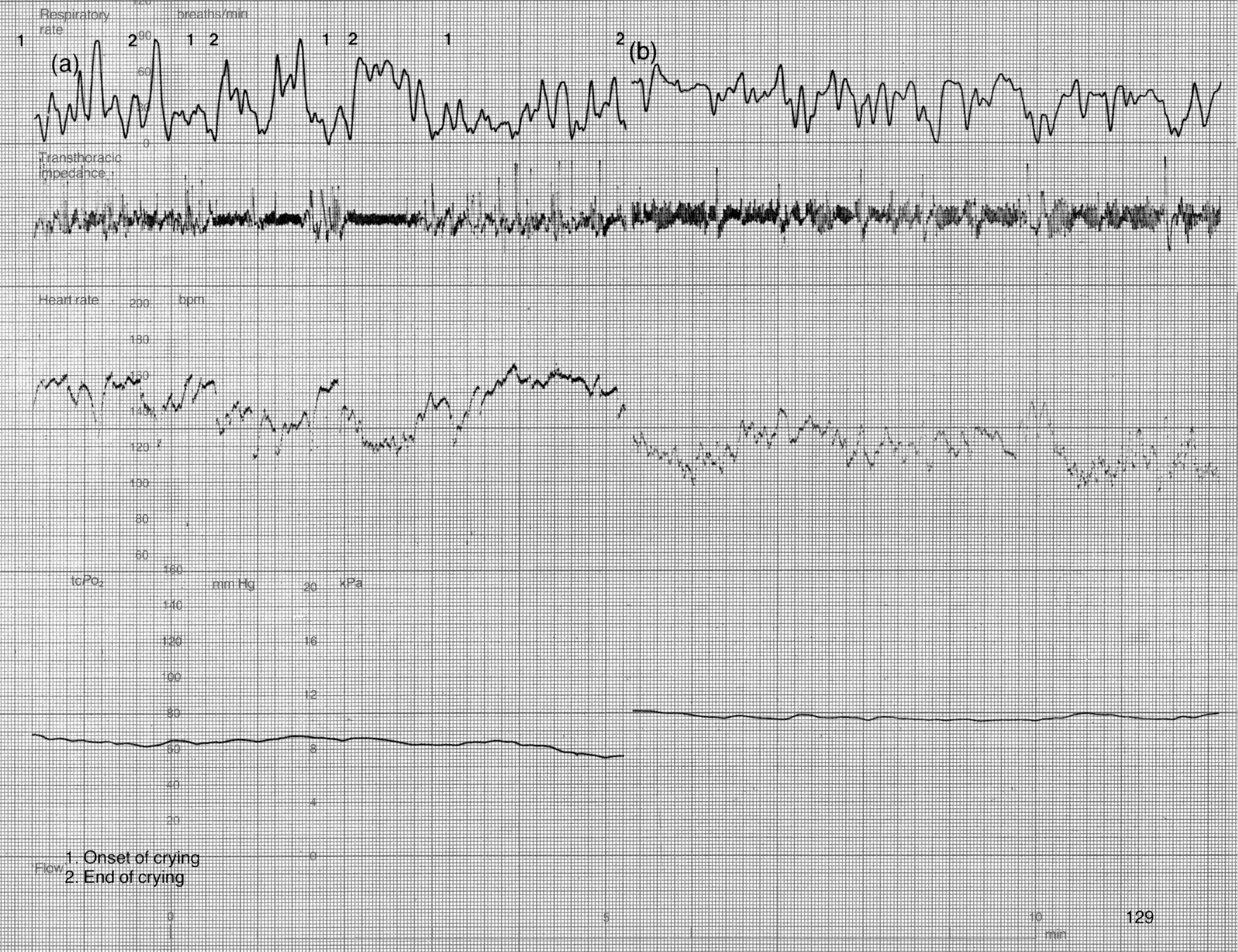

Respiratory rate
breaths/min
(a)
(b)
1
2
1
2
1
2
1
2
Transthoracic impedance
Heart rate
bpm
tcPo2
mm Hg
kPa
Flow
1. Onset of crying
2. End of crying
0
5
10
min

Fig. 6.1.2.a

Birthweight: 2790 g

Apgar score: 8/10/10

Age (in hours) at recording: 1

Delivery: Caesarean section

Cord blood acid – base and blood gases							
	pH	$P\text{CO}_2$	mm Hg	kPa	$P\text{O}_2$	mm Hg	kPa	Base deficit mmol/l
Umbilical artery	7.31		45	6.0		20	2.7	3.7
Umbilical vein	7.33		40	5.3		29	3.9	4.5

Activity state	Crying.
Respiratory rate	Cyclic changes between 10 and 75 breaths/min.
Transthoracic impedance	Irregular, often large excursions.
Heart rate	Baseline heart rate was about 170 bpm with an amplitude of long-term variability $\leqslant$ 10 bpm.
tc$P\text{O}_2$	Between 107 and 94 mm Hg (14.3 and 12.6 kPa).

Comments See Fig. 6.1.2.c.

Fig. 6.1.2.b

Age (in hours) at recording: 4

Activity state	Vomiting, then sleeping.
Respiratory rate	Cyclic changes between 10 and 50 breaths/min during vomiting. Mainly between 25 and 35 breaths/min during sleeping.
Transthoracic impedance	Large irregular excursions during vomiting and almost regular excursions during sleeping.
Heart rate	Baseline heart rate about 160 bpm in sleep with an amplitude of long-term variability $\leqslant$ 10 bpm. Changing heart rate during vomiting from 130 to 175 bpm.
tc$P\text{O}_2$	From about 90 mm Hg (12.0 kPa) tc$P\text{O}_2$ fell to 73 mm Hg (9.7 kPa) during vomiting and then gradually increased to 105 mm Hg (14.0 kPa) during sleep.

For neonatal data see Fig. 6.1.2.a.

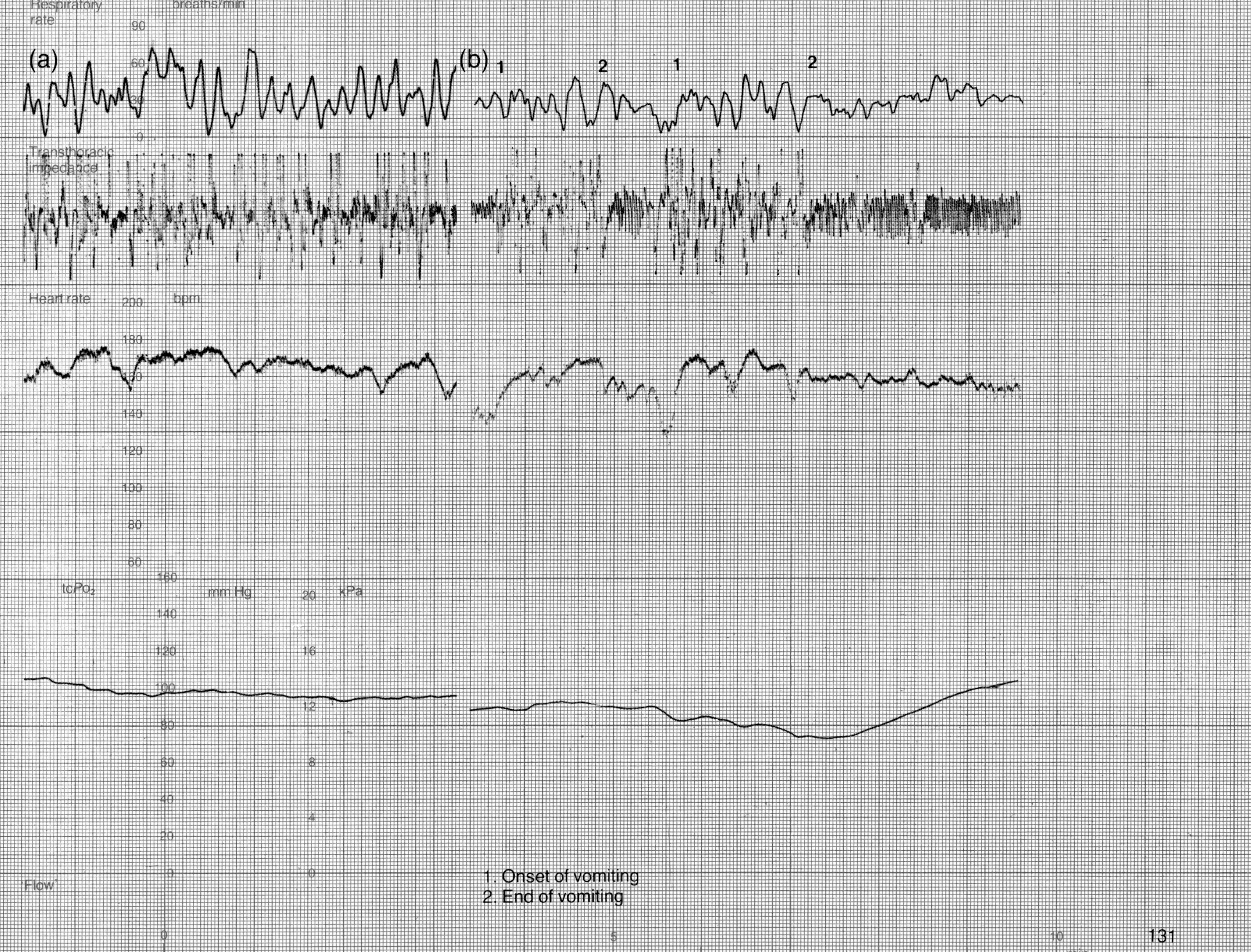
Respiratory rate
breaths/min
120
90
60
30
0
(a)
(b)
1
2
1
2
Transthoracic impedance
Heart rate
bpm
200
180
160
140
120
100
80
60
$tcPo_2$
mm Hg
kPa
160
140
120
100
80
60
40
20
0
20
16
12
8
4
0
'Flow'
1. Onset of vomiting
2. End of vomiting
0
5
10
min

Fig. 6.1.2.c

Age (in hours) at recording:	>120

Activity state	Awake, unquiet and crying.
Respiratory rate	About 30 breaths/min (Monitor II).
Transthoracic impedance	Partly rather regular excursions, partly periodic breathing with apnoea. There were two periods of large irregular excursions during crying.
Heart rate	Baseline heart rate was around 130 bpm with an amplitude of long-term variability $\leq$ 20 bpm. During crying there were accelerations to 165 bpm.
tcP_{O_2}	The periodic breathing resulted in a gradually falling tcP_{O_2} from 86 to 68 mm Hg (11.5 to 9.1 kPa).

For neonatal data see Fig. 6.1.2.a.

Comments (a – c) This example demonstrates how difficult it is to identify time trends in the oxygen-cardiorespirograms because it may not be possible to obtain recordings from comparable activity states. The increased long-term variability is largely a factor of the slower heart rate in **c** than in **a** and **b**.

The fall in tcP_{O_2} during vomiting is further illustrated in Fig. 8.4.1. The short phase of periodic breathing is typical as such. For other examples of periodic breathing see Chapter 4.8.

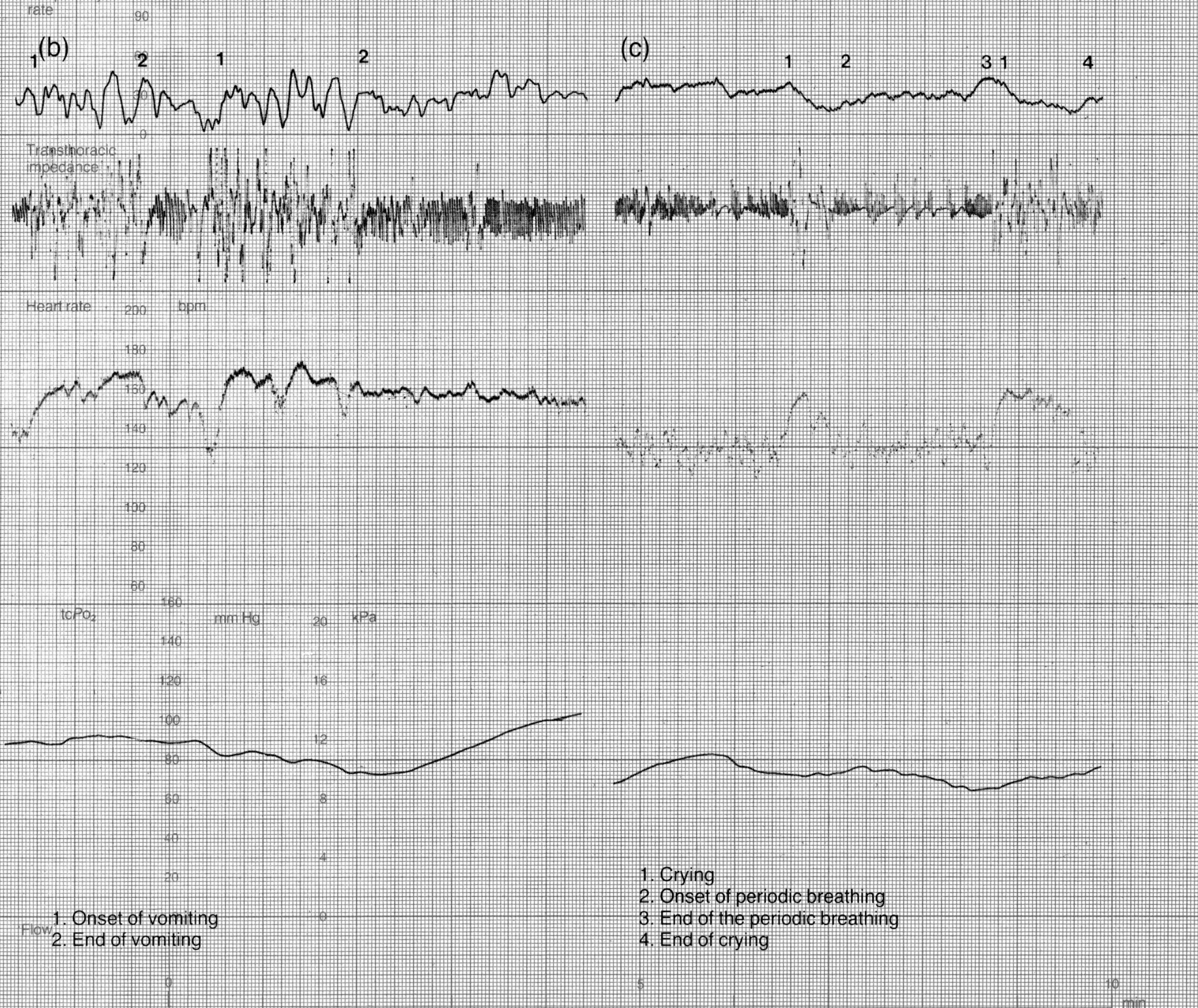

Respiratory rate
breaths/min
90
(b)
1
2
1
2
(c)
1
2
3 1
4
0
Transthoracic impedance
Heart rate
200
bpm
180
160
140
120
100
80
60
160
$tcPo_2$
mm Hg
20
kPa
140
120
16
100
12
80
60
8
40
4
20
0
Flow
1. Onset of vomiting
2. End of vomiting
1. Crying
2. Onset of periodic breathing
3. End of the periodic breathing
4. End of crying
0
5
10
min

Fig. 6.1.3.a

Birthweight: 3180 g

Apgar score: 7/10

Age (in hours) at recording: 1

Delivery: Caesarean section

Cord blood acid – base and blood gases							
	pH	$P\text{CO}_2$ mm Hg	kPa	$P\text{O}_2$ mm Hg	kPa	Base deficit mmol/l
Umbilical artery	7.22	49	6.5	29	3.9	7.1
Umbilical vein	7.28	33	4.4			10.5

Activity state	Active sleep.
Respiratory rate	Cyclic, somewhat irregular changes mainly between 60 and 75 breaths/min.
Transthoracic impedance	Fairly regular excursions and few periods of apnoea lasting about 10 seconds.
Heart rate	Baseline heart rate was around 140 bpm with an amplitude of long-term variability $\leq$ 5 bpm and small deceleration at the time of the apnoea.
tc$P\text{O}_2$	There was a gradual increase in tc$P\text{O}_2$ during the whole figure from 47 to 54 mm Hg (6.3 to 7.2 kPa).

Fig. 6.1.3.b

Age (in hours) at recording: 29

Activity state	Active sleep and crying.
Respiratory rate	About 60 breaths/min during active sleep and between 5 and 50 breaths/min during crying.
Transthoracic impedance	Fairly regular excursions during active sleep and larger irregular excursions during crying.
Heart rate	Baseline heart rate about 120 bpm with an amplitude of long-term variability $\leq$ 10 bpm and accelerations during crying.
tc$P\text{O}_2$	Undulated around 70 mm Hg (9.3 kPa) irrespective of the activity state.

For neonatal data see Fig. 6.1.3.a.

Comments (a and b) This is a case which may be termed prepathological in the adaptation because of the low tc$P\text{O}_2$ value of 50 mm Hg (6.7 kPa) at 1 hour after birth. However, neither the heart rate nor the breathing recordings indicated any abnormality and the clinical course was uneventful.

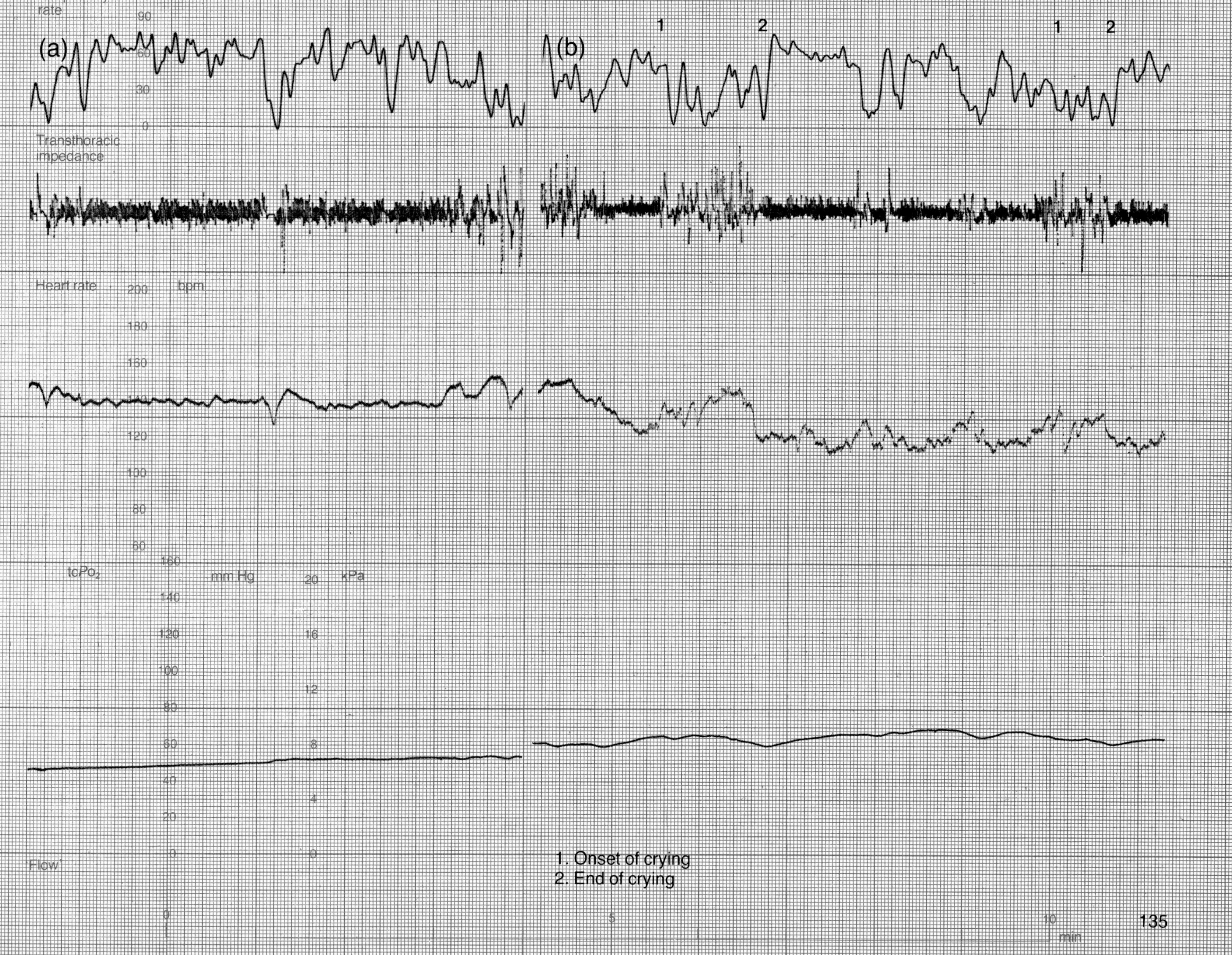

Respiratory rate
breaths/min
90
60
30
0
(a)
(b)
1
2
1
2
Transthoracic impedance
Heart rate
200
bpm
180
160
120
100
80
60
tcPo_2
160
mm Hg
20
kPa
140
120
16
100
12
80
60
8
40
4
20
0
0
Flow
1. Onset of crying
2. End of crying
0
5
10
min

Fig. 6.1.4.a

Birthweight: 3220 g

Apgar score: 4/9/10

Age (in hours) at recording: 1

Delivery: Caesarean section

Cord blood acid – base and blood gases							
	pH	PCO_2	mm Hg	kPa	PO_2	mm Hg	kPa	Base deficit mmol/l
Umbilical artery	6.94		72	9.6		12	1.6	16.0
Umbilical vein	6.97		64	8.5		19	2.5	16.1

Activity state	Awake, unquiet.
Respiratory rate	Cyclic changes about a mean of 40 breaths/min (Monitor II).
Transthoracic impedance	Irregular excursion.
Heart rate	Baseline heart rate about 135 bpm with an amplitude of long-term variability $\leqslant$ 15 bpm and frequent deep spikes.
tcPO_2	Between 106 and 104 mm Hg (14.1 and 13.9 kPa). Simultaneous arterial blood and transcutaneous PO_2 were 100 and 104 mm Hg respectively (13.3 and 13.9 kPa).
	Neonatal arterial acid–base and blood gases: pH, 7.37; PCO_2, 28 mm Hg (3.7 kPa); PO_2, 100 mm Hg (13.3 kPa); base deficit, 8.1 mmol/l.

Fig. 6.1.4.b

Age (in hours) at recording: 4

Activity state	Quiet sleep.
Respiratory rate	About 40 breaths/min (Monitor II).
Transthoracic impedance	Regular excursions except after deep inspirations when there was apnoea lasting about 10 seconds.
Heart rate	Baseline heart rate about 115 bpm with an amplitude of long-term variability $\leqslant$ 10 bpm.
tcPO_2	Between 64 and 68 mm Hg (8.5 and 9.1 kPa).

For neonatal data see Fig. 6.1.4.a.

Comments See Fig. 6.1.4.c.

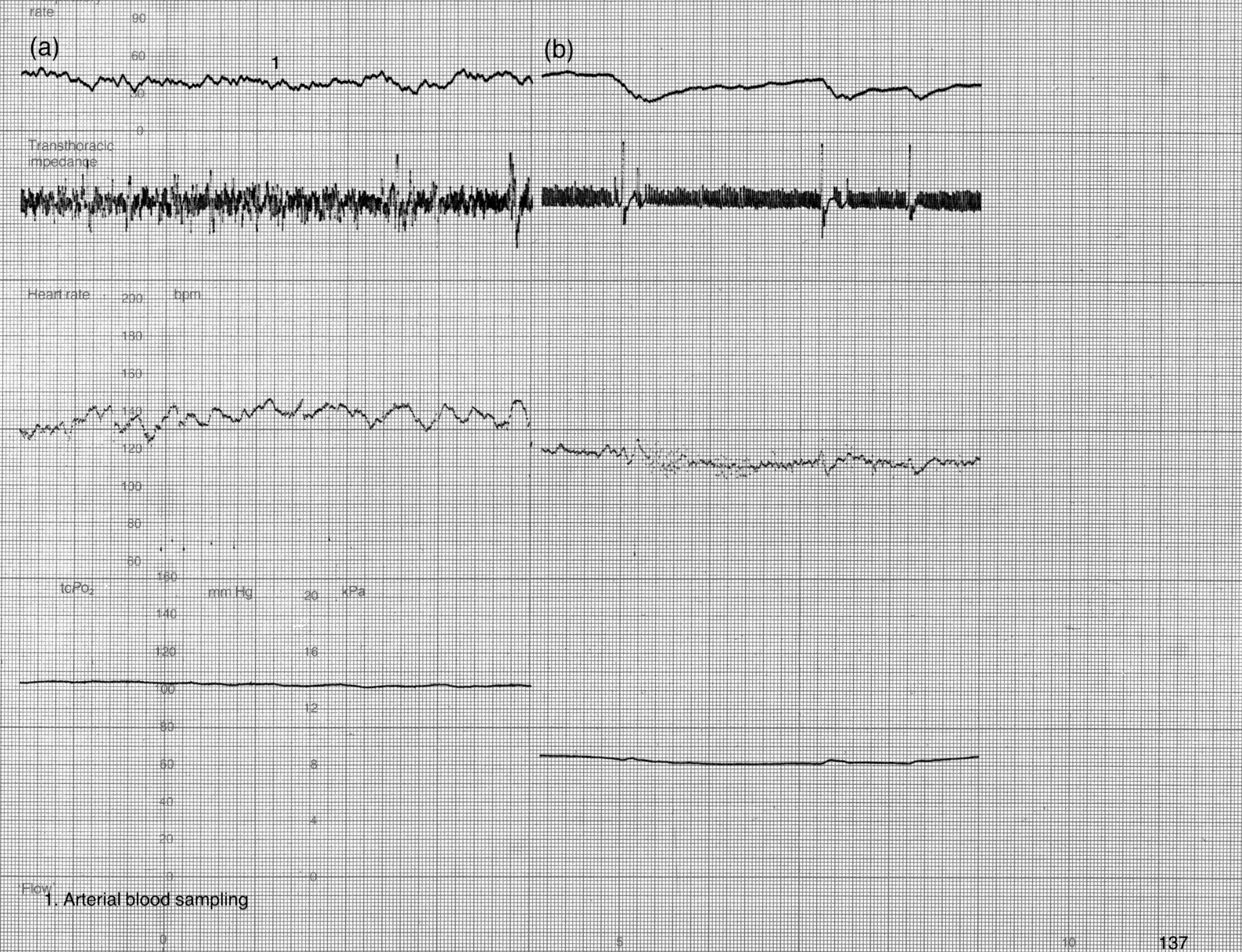

1. Arterial blood sampling

Fig. 6.1.4.c

Age (in hours) at recording:	20

Activity state	Active sleep.
Respiratory rate	Between 30 and 45 breaths/min (Monitor II).
Transthoracic impedance	Short periods of regular excursions intercepted by larger irregular excursions.
Heart rate	Baseline heart rate about 115 bpm with an amplitude of long-term variability $\leq$ 15 bpm; marked accelerations during the large breaths. Artifacts.
tcP_{O_2}	Between 52 and 64 mm Hg (6.9 and 8.5 kPa).

For neonatal data see Fig. 6.1.4.a.

Comments (a – c) There is nothing to distinguish this series of oxygen-cardio-respirograms from those of normal uncomplicated deliveries as shown in Chapter 5 in spite of the Caesarean section and particularly in spite of the extremely low pH of the umbilical blood.

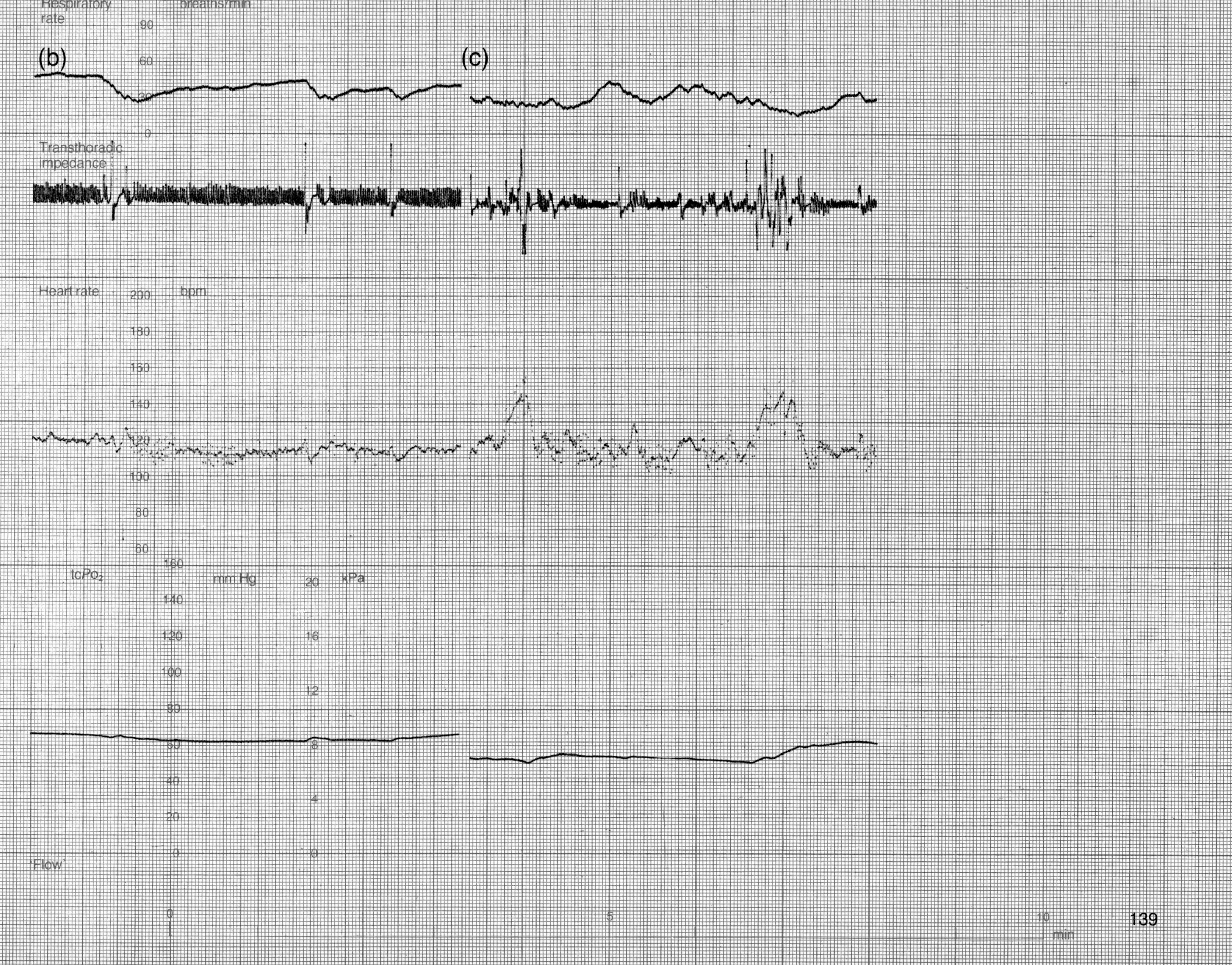
Respiratory rate
breaths/min
90
60
30
0
(b)
(c)
Transthoracic impedance
Heart rate
bpm
200
180
160
140
120
100
80
60
tcPo2
mm Hg
kPa
160
140
120
100
80
60
40
20
0
20
16
12
8
4
0
'Flow'
0
5
10
min

Fig. 6.1.5.a

Birthweight: 2930 g

Apgar score: 4/8/10

Age (in hours) at recording: 1

Delivery: Caesarean section

Cord blood acid – base and blood gases							
	pH	$P\text{CO}_2$ mm Hg	kPa	$P\text{O}_2$ mm Hg	kPa	Base deficit mmol/l
Umbilical artery	7.23	49	6.5	23	3.1	6.6
Umbilical vein	7.26	42	5.6			7.6

Activity state	Active sleep.
Respiratory rate	Between 35 and 50 breaths/min (Monitor II).
Transthoracic impedance	Mostly regular excursions, occasional larger, irregular ones.
Heart rate	Baseline heart rate was about 135 bpm with an amplitude of long-term variability $\leqslant$ 15 bpm and accelerations during the deep breaths.
tc$P\text{O}_2$	The level of tc$P\text{O}_2$ was very stable close to 90 mm Hg (12.0 kPa). Simultaneous arterial $P\text{O}_2$ and transcutaneous $P\text{O}_2$ were 78 and 88 mm Hg (10.4 and 11.7 kPa), respectively.
	Neonatal arterial acid–base and blood gases: pH, 7.26; $P\text{CO}_2$, 41 mm Hg (5.5 kPa); $P\text{O}_2$, 78 mm Hg (10.4 kPa); base deficit, 7.6 mmol/l.

Fig. 6.1.5.b

Age (in hours) at recording: 2

Activity state	Quiet sleep.
Respiratory rate	About 40 breaths/min (Monitor II).
Transthoracic impedance	Very regular excursions with occasional deep breaths.
Heart rate	Baseline heart rate about 145 bpm with an amplitude of long-term variability $\leqslant$ 5 bpm and decelerations synchronous to the deep breaths.
tc$P\text{O}_2$	The level of tc$P\text{O}_2$ was close to 74 mm Hg (9.9 kPa).

For neonatal data see Fig. 6.1.5.a.

For comments see Fig. 6.1.5.d.

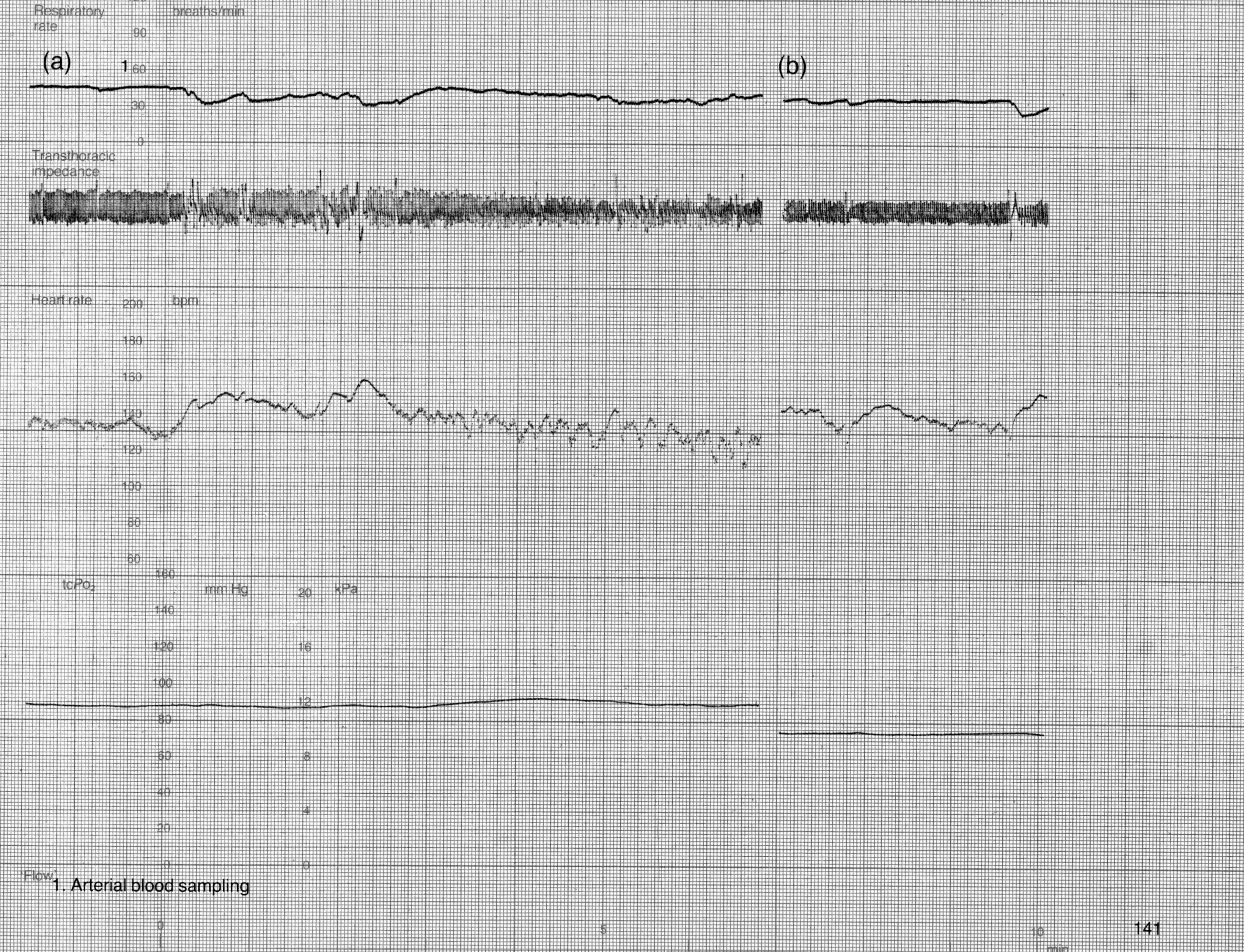
Respiratory rate
breaths/min
120
90
60
30
0
(a)
1
(b)
Transthoracic impedance
Heart rate
bpm
200
180
160
140
120
100
80
60
tcPo2
mm Hg
160
140
120
100
80
60
40
20
0
kPa
20
16
12
8
4
0
'Flow'
1. Arterial blood sampling
0
5
10
min

Fig. 6.1.5.c

Age (in hours) at recording:	4

Activity state	Active sleep.
Respiratory rate	About 40 breaths/min but there was an apnoea lasting 40 sec. Note how little of this is revealed in respiratory rate with Monitor II.
Transthoracic impedance	Mainly regular, partly irregular excursions and one long apnoea.
Heart rate	Baseline heart rate was about 150 bpm with an amplitude of long-term variability $\leqslant$ 15 bpm. There were frequent decelerations coupled with changes in the respiration. The longest apnoea period and the broad and deep deceleration coincide.
tc$P\text{O}_2$	From a level of 75 mm Hg (10.0 kPa) tc$P\text{O}_2$ began to fall seconds after the onset of the long apnoea down to 52 mm Hg (6.9 kPa).

For neonatal data see Fig. 6.1.5.a.

Fig. 6.1.5.d

Age at recording:	10 days

Activity state	Active and quiet sleep.
Respiratory rate	About 40 breaths/min (Monitor II).
Transthoracic impedance	Rather regular excursions but with larger ones in between. More regular excursions during the quiet sleep.
Heart rate	Baseline heart rate about 150 bpm with an amplitude of long-term variability $\leqslant$ 5 bpm and frequent decelerations during active sleep. These decelerations are as in **c** associated with deeper breaths.
tc$P\text{O}_2$	Between 78 and 83 mm Hg (10.4 and 11.1 kPa) in both sleep states.

For neonatal data see Fig. 6.1.5.a.

Comments (a–d) Except for one long apnoea and the simultaneous deceleration and fall in tc$P\text{O}_2$ in **c** there is nothing noteworthy in this series of four oxygen-cardiorespirograms from the same infant born after Caesarean section with a low 1 min Apgar score but normal cord blood pH. The clinical course was uneventful.

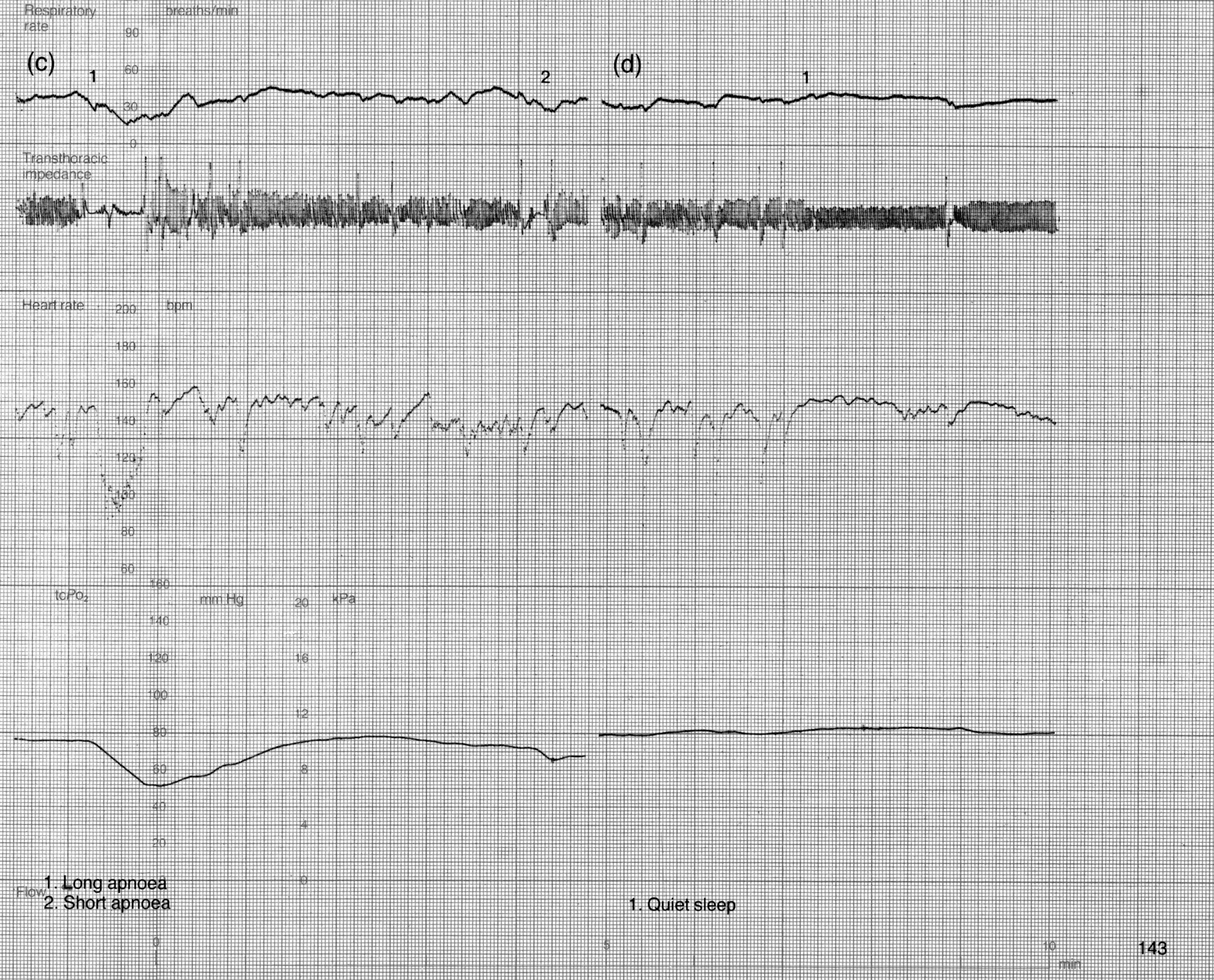
Respiratory rate
breaths/min
120
90
60
30
0
(c)
1
2
(d)
1
Transthoracic impedance
Heart rate
bpm
200
180
160
140
120
100
80
60
tcP_{O_2}
mm Hg
kPa
160
140
120
100
80
60
40
20
20
16
12
8
4
0
Flow
1. Long apnoea
2. Short apnoea
1. Quiet sleep
0
5
10
min

Fig. 6.1.6.a

Birthweight: 2320 g

Apgar score: 2/6/10

Age (in hours) at recording: 1

Delivery: Caesarean section

Cord blood acid – base and blood gases

	pH	PCO$_2$ mm Hg	kPa	PO$_2$ mm Hg	kPa	Base deficit mmol/l
Umbilical artery	7.16	64	8.5	4	0.5	5.9
Umbilical vein	7.20	52	6.9	16	2.1	7.2

Activity state	Awake, unquiet with a period of crying in between.
Respiratory rate	Cyclic changes about 60 breaths/min before crying and between 5 and 75 breaths/min during crying.
Transthoracic impedance	Mainly regular excursions, but some with larger amplitude. Irregular excursions during crying.
Heart rate	Baseline heart rate was about 155 bpm with an amplitude of long-term variability $\leqslant$ 10 bpm in the unquiet phase. During crying heart rate was 170 bpm and the amplitude of the long-term variability was about the same as before.
tc$P$O$_2$	Undulating between 60 mm Hg (8.0 kPa) and 68 mm Hg (9.1 kPa). Simultaneous arterial blood PO$_2$ and transcutaneous PO$_2$ were 55 and 60 mm Hg (7.3 and 8.0 kPa) respectively.
	Neonatal arterial acid–base and blood gases: pH, 7.31; PCO$_2$, 41 mm Hg (5.5 kPa); PO$_2$, 55 mm Hg (7.3 kPa); base deficit, 5.2 mmol/l.

Comments This is an example where tc$P$O$_2$ did not fall during crying.

Fig. 6.1.6.b

Age (in hours) at recording: 1½

Activity state	Awake, quiet.
Respiratory rate	Irregular cyclic changes between 45 and 50 breaths/min and during the oxygen test 60 to 75 breaths/min.
Transthoracic impedance	Mostly regular excursions intercepted at irregular intervals by larger breaths.
Heart rate	Baseline heart rate about 150 bpm with an amplitude of long-term variability 5 to 10 bpm.
tc$P$O$_2$	From 70 mm Hg (9.3 kPa) tc$P$O$_2$ increased to a peak of 134 mm Hg (17.9 kPa) during oxygen breathing. From this a shunt of 32 per cent is calculated. The increase in tc$P$O$_2$ was slow.

For comment see Fig. 6.1.6.d.

For neonatal data see Fig. 6.1.6.a.

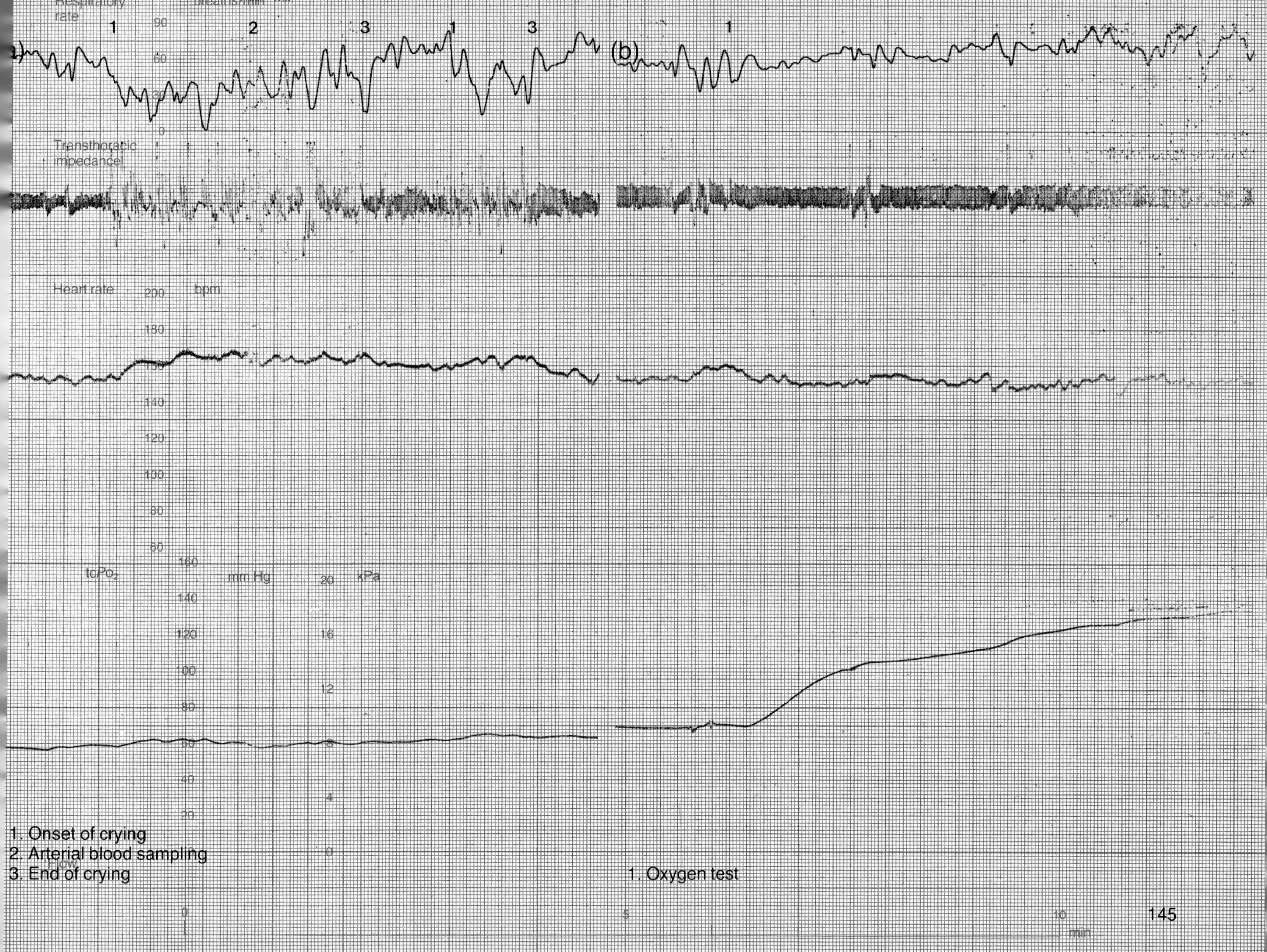
Respiratory rate
breaths/min
90
60
30
0
(a)
(b)
1
2
3
1
3
1
Transthoracic impedance
Heart rate
bpm
200
180
140
120
100
80
60
tcPo$_2$
mm Hg
kPa
160
140
120
100
80
60
40
20
20
16
12
8
4
0
1. Onset of crying
2. Arterial blood sampling
3. End of crying
1. Oxygen test
0
5
10
min

Fig. 6.1.6.c

Age (in hours) at recording:	3

Activity state	Active sleep.
Respiratory rate	Cyclic changes between 40 and 80 breaths/min in air and between 60 and 110 breaths/min in oxygen.
Transthoracic impedance	Partly regular, partly irregular excursions.
Heart rate	Baseline heart rate varied between 155 and 170 bpm with an amplitude of long-term variability $\leq$ 10 bpm.
tcP_{O_2}	From a level of 57 mm Hg (7.6 kPa) tcP_{O_2} increased to 200 mm Hg (26.7 kPa) during the oxygen test. From this a shunt of 29 per cent is calculated. The increase was slow.

For neonatal data see Fig. 6.1.6.a.

Fig. 6.1.6.d

Age (in hours) at recording:	19

Activity state	Awake, unquiet.
Respiratory rate	Cyclic changes mainly between 40 and 110 breaths/min.
Transthoracic impedance	Mainly regular excursions but frequently larger irregular ones.
Heart rate	Baseline heart rate was about 145 bpm with an amplitude of long-term variability $\leq$ 15 bpm.
tcP_{O_2}	From an initial level of 80 mm Hg (10.7 kPa) tcP_{O_2} increased to 270 mm Hg (36.0 kPa) during oxygen breathing. From this a shunt of 26 per cent is calculated. The increase was rather fast and 100 mm Hg (13.3 kPa) was reached in about 1 min.

For neonatal data see Fig. 6.1.6.a.

Comments (a – d) This premature, low birthweight infant from which a series of four oxygen-cardiorespirograms were recorded was delivered by Caesarean section and had a low Apgar score and low umbilical cord pH values. However, except for the persistent tachycardia the clinical course was uneventful. The sequential evaluation of the oxygen-cardiorespirograms shows consistent increase in the amplitude of long-term variability and in the rate of tcP_{O_2} increase as well as the peak plateau of tcP_{O_2} during the oxygen test.

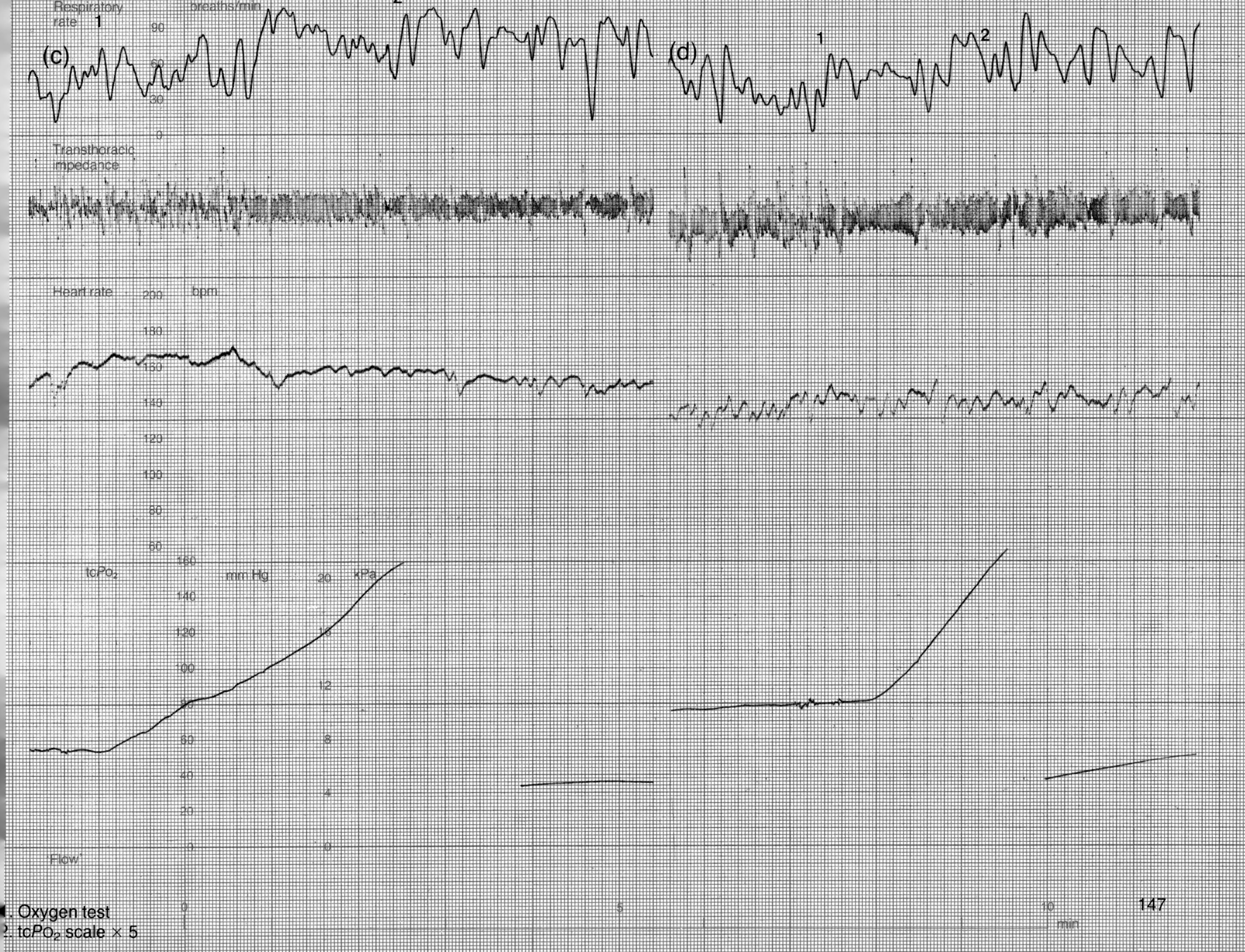

1. Oxygen test
2. $tcPo_2$ scale × 5

Fig. 6.2.1.a

Birthweight: 2000 g

Apgar score: 7/9/10

Age (in hours) at recording: 2

Delivery: vaginal

Cord blood acid – base and blood gases							
	pH	$P\text{CO}_2$ mm Hg	kPa	$P\text{O}_2$ mm Hg	kPa	Base deficit mmol/l
Umbilical vein	7.17	54	7.2	13	1.7	8.6

Activity state	Awake, unquiet or crying.
Respiratory rate	Cyclic changes between 12 and 100 breaths/min.
Transthoracic impedance	Irregular excursions.
Heart rate	Baseline heart rate about 160 bpm with an amplitude of long-term variability ≤ 15 bpm. The details are difficult to ascertain because of the artifacts.
tc$P\text{O}_2$	About 80 mm Hg (10.6 kPa) when the infant breathed air and a fast increase during the oxygen test to 290 mm Hg (38.7 kPa). From this a shunt of 25 per cent is calculated.

Fig. 6.2.1.b

Birthweight: 3470 g

Apgar score: 9/10/10

Age (in hours) at recording: 2

Delivery: vaginal

Cord blood acid – base and blood gases						
	pH	$P\text{CO}_2$ mm Hg	kPa	$P\text{O}_2$ mm Hg	kPa	Base deficit mmol/l
Umbilical artery	7.21	58	7.7	11	1.5	4.4
Umbilical vein	7.30	44	5.9	18	2.4	4.5

Activity state	Crying then awake, quiet.
Respiratory rate	Cyclic changes mainly between 10 and 30 breaths/min.
Transthoracic impedance	Irregular excursions.
Heart rate	After acceleration to 165 bpm during crying baseline heart rate was about 135 bpm with an amplitude of long-term variability ≤ 10 bpm.
tc$P\text{O}_2$	During crying tc$P\text{O}_2$ fell to 64 mm Hg (8.5 kPa) then tc$P\text{O}_2$ gradually increased to 87 mm Hg (11.6 kPa).

Comments (a and b) Oxygen-cardiorespirograms from two newborn infants whose mothers received in **a** 150 mg pethidine 1 hour before delivery and in **b** 100 mg 6 hours and 100 mg 3 hours before delivery.

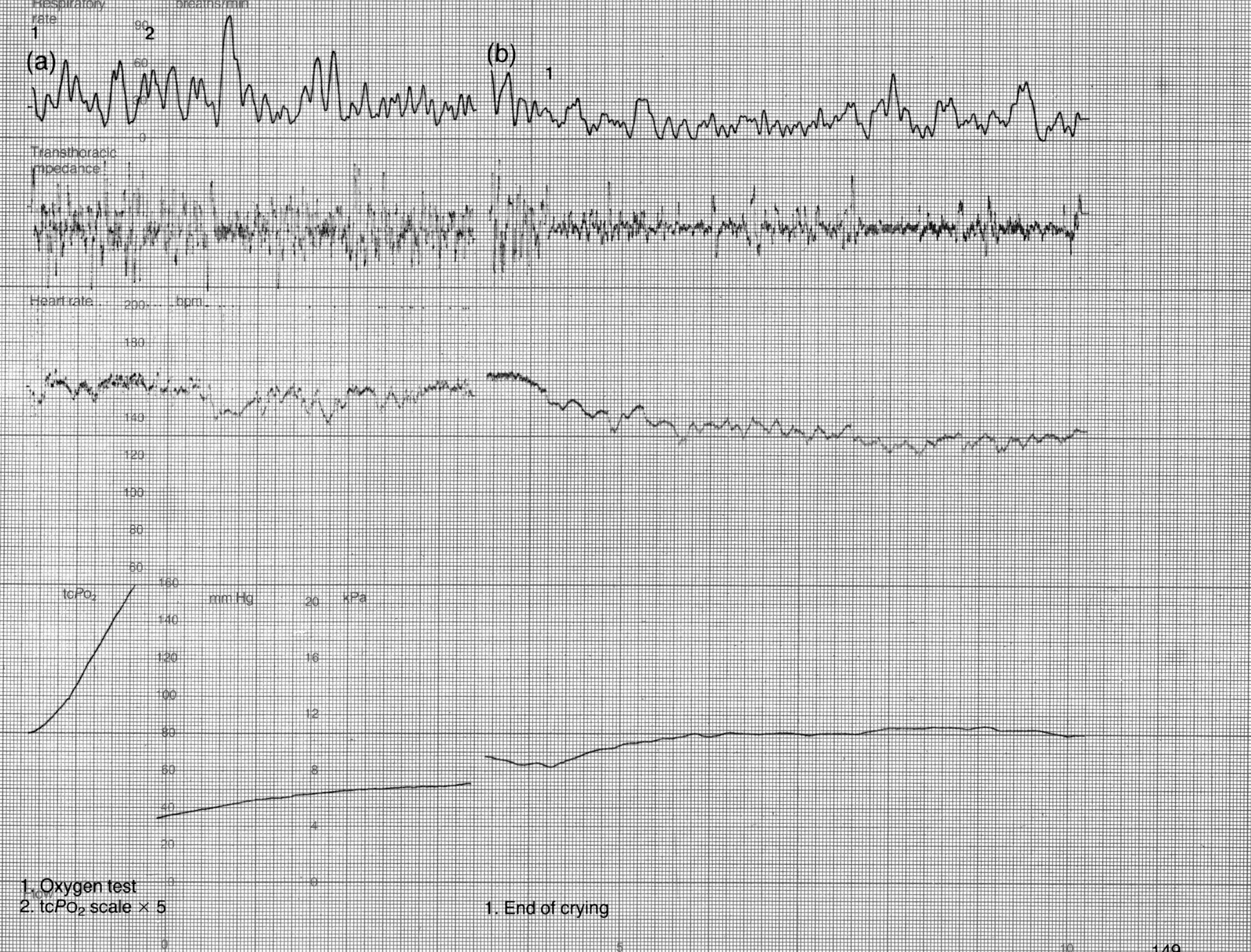

Respiratory rate
breaths/min
1
2
(a)
(b)
1
Transthoracic impedance
Heart rate
bpm
tcPo2
mm Hg
kPa
1. Oxygen test
2. tcPo2 scale × 5
1. End of crying
min

Fig. 6.2.2.a

Birthweight: 2400 g

Apgar score: 8/10/10

Age (in hours) at recording: 1

Delivery: vaginal

Cord blood acid – base and blood gases							
	pH	PCO_2 mm Hg	kPa	PO_2 mm Hg	kPa	Base deficit mmol/l
Umbilical artery	7.38	30	4.0	22	2.9	7.0
Umbilical vein	7.40	25	3.3	26	3.4	8.4

Activity state	Awake, quiet.
Respiratory rate	Cyclic changes mainly between 30 and 60 breaths/min.
Transthoracic impedance	Some regular excursions but periods of larger, irregular excursions as well.
Heart rate	Baseline heart rate was about 150 bpm with an amplitude of long-term variability ≤ 5 bpm.
tcPO_2	Between 75 and 84 mm Hg (10.0 and 11.2 kPa).

Fig. 6.2.2.b

Birthweight: 2560 g

Apgar score: 9/10/10

Age (in hours) at recording: 1

Delivery: vaginal

Cord blood acid – base and blood gases						
	pH	PCO_2 mm Hg	kPa	PO_2 mm Hg	kPa	Base deficit mmol/l
Umbilical artery	7.24	43	5.7	19	2.5	8.6
Umbilical vein	7.30	34	4.5	33	4.4	8.9

Activity state	Awake, quiet.
Respiratory rate	Undulation between 30 and 50 breaths/min (Monitor II).
Transthoracic impedance	Mostly regular excursions interrupted by larger ones.
Heart rate	Baseline heart rate was about 125 bpm and the amplitude of long-term variability ≤ 15 bpm. There were some narrow decelerations.
tcPO_2	Between 74 and 87 mm Hg (9.9 and 11.6 kPa).

Comments (a and b) Oxygen-cardiorespirograms from newborn infants whose mothers received in **a** 50 mg pethidine 4 hours before delivery and in **b** 100 mg 3½ hours before delivery.

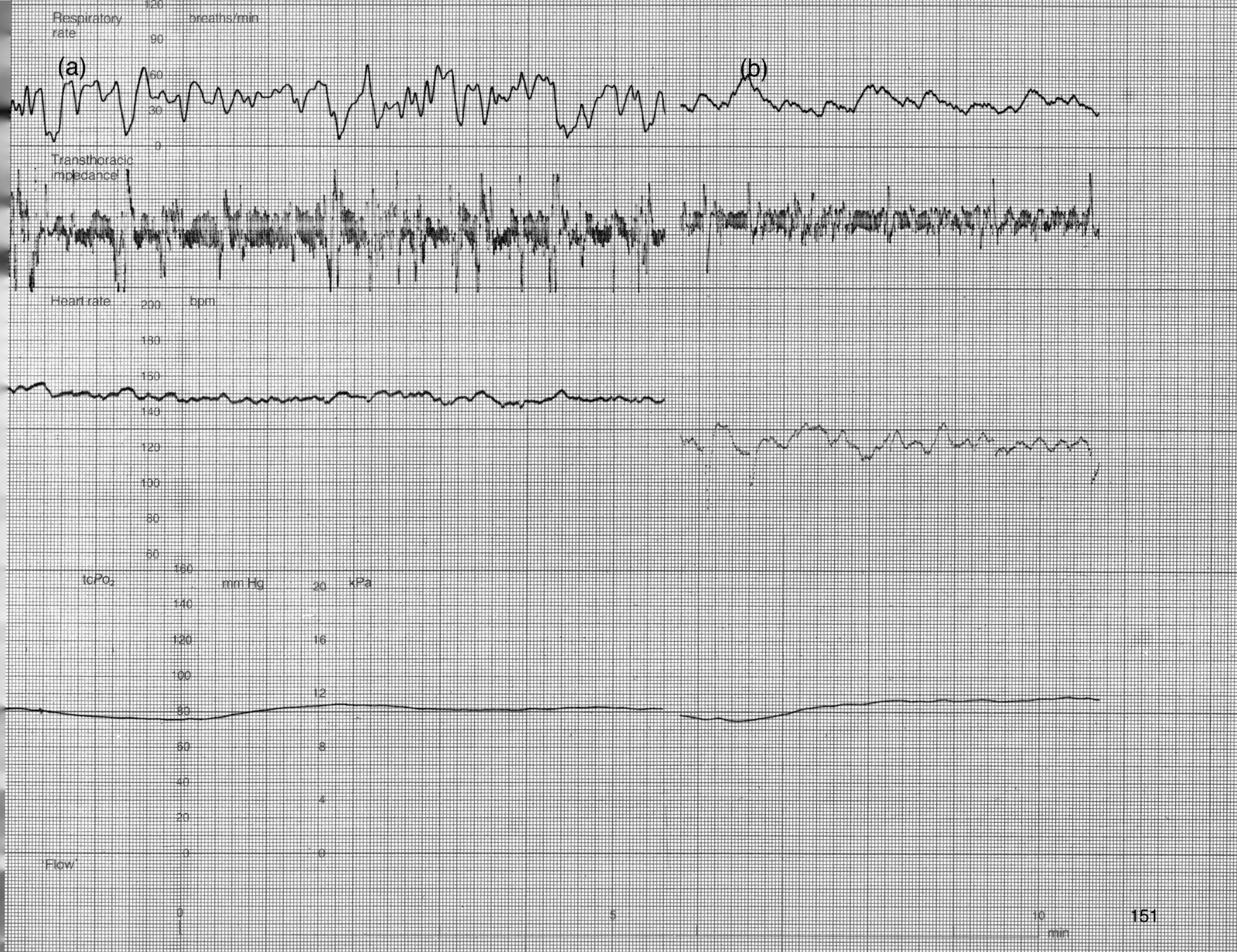
Respiratory rate
breaths/min
120
90
60
30
0
(a)
(b)
Transthoracic impedance
Heart rate
bpm
200
180
160
140
120
100
80
60
$tcPo_2$
mm Hg
kPa
160
140
120
100
80
60
40
20
0
20
16
12
8
4
0
Flow
0
5
10
min

Fig. 6.2.2.c

Birthweight: 3140 g

Apgar score: 9/10/10

Age (in hours) at recording: 1

Delivery: vaginal

Cord blood acid – base and blood gases							
	pH	P_{CO_2}	mm Hg	kPa	P_{O_2}	mm Hg	kPa	Base deficit mmol/l
Umbilical artery	7.32		39	5.2		16	2.1	5.8
Umbilical vein	7.34		34	4.5		22	2.9	6.7

Activity state	Awake, quiet.
Respiratory rate	Somewhat irregular cyclic changes between 15 and 75 breaths/min.
Transthoracic impedance	Mostly rather regular excursions.
Heart rate	Baseline heart rate was about 125 bpm with an amplitude of long-term variability ≤ 10 bpm. Some small decelerations.
tcP_{O_2}	The level increased from 92 to 101 mm Hg (12.3 to 13.5 kPa). Simultaneous arterial and transcutaneous P_{O_2} were 97 and 101 mm Hg (12.9 and 13.5 kPa) respectively.
	Neonatal arterial acid–base and blood gases: pH, 7.32; P_{CO_2}, 38 mm Hg (5.1 kPa); P_{O_2}, 97 mm Hg (12.9 kPa); base deficit, 5.2 mmol/l.

Fig. 6.2.2.d

Birthweight: 3310 g

Apgar score: 9/10

Age (in hours) at recording: 1

Delivery: vaginal

Cord blood acid – base and blood gases								
	pH	P_{CO_2}	mm Hg	kPa	P_{O_2}	mm Hg	kPa	Base deficit mmol/l
Umbilical artery	7.29		41	5.5		21	2.8	6.3
Umbilical vein	7.38		33	4.4		29	3.9	5.4

Activity state	Awake, quiet.
Respiratory rate	Cyclic changes between 15 and 60 breaths/min.
Transthoracic impedance	Partly regular, partly irregular excursions.
Heart rate	Baseline heart rate was about 135 bpm with an amplitude of long-term variability ≤ 15 bpm and occasional narrow decelerations.
tcP_{O_2}	Close to 68 mm Hg (9.1 kPa).

Comments See Fig. 6.2.2.e.

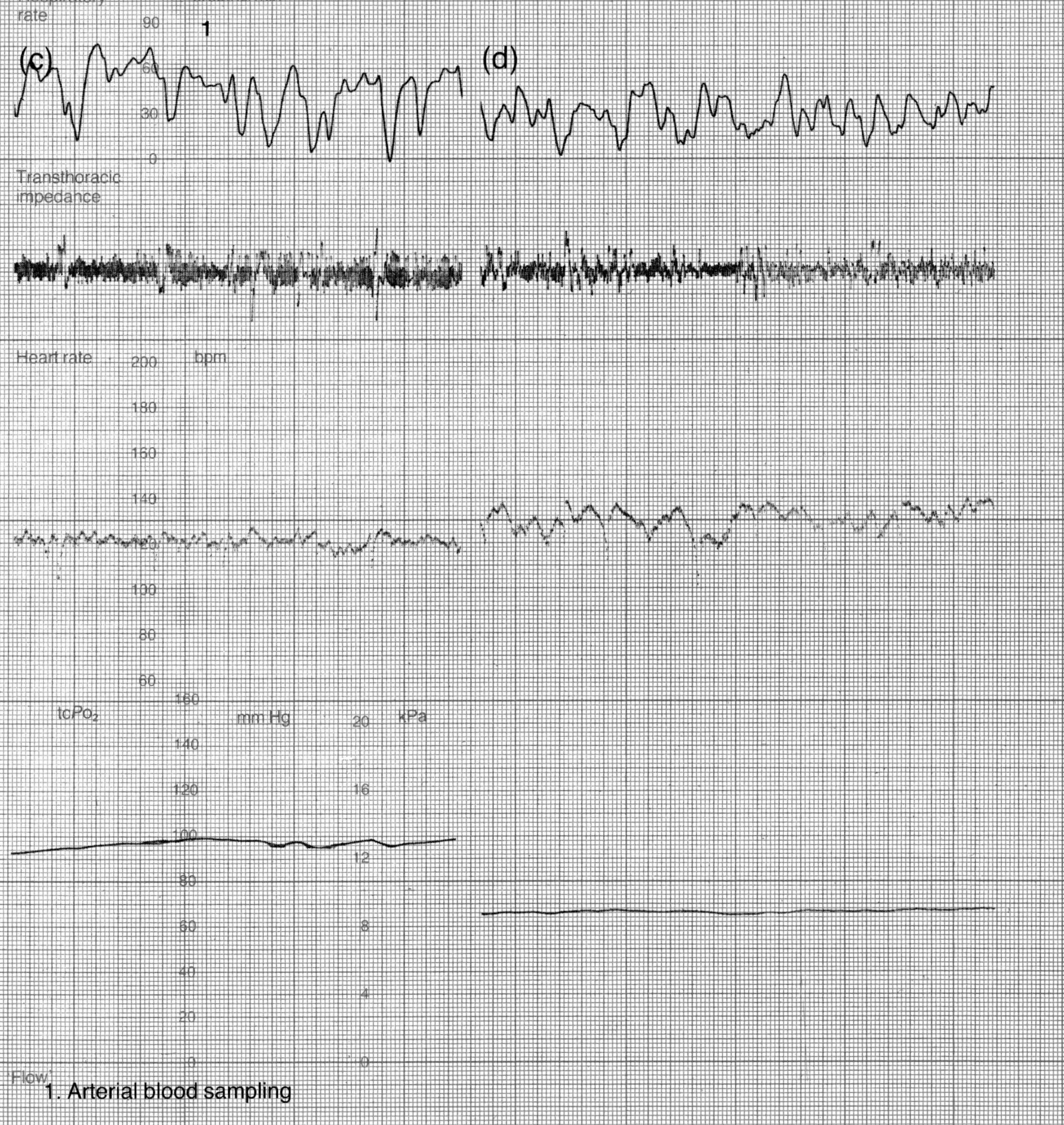
Respiratory rate
breaths/min
120
90
60
30
0
1
(c)
(d)
Transthoracic impedance
Heart rate
bpm
200
180
160
140
120
100
80
60
tcPo_2
mm Hg
kPa
160
140
120
100
80
60
40
20
0
20
16
12
8
4
0
Flow
1. Arterial blood sampling
0
5
10
min

Fig. 6.2.2.e

Birthweight: 3480 g

Apgar score: 10/10

Age (in hours) at recording:	1

Delivery: vaginal

Activity state	Active sleep.
Respiratory rate	Cyclic changes around 60 breaths/min.
Transthoracic impedance	Fairly regular excursions, a few larger ones and occasionally apnoea lasting 3–4 seconds.
Heart rate	Baseline heart rate was 150 bpm with an amplitude of long-term variability ⩽ 5 bpm.
tc$P$O$_2$	The level increased slowly from 80 to 101 mm Hg (10.7 to 13.5 kPa).

Comments (c–e) Oxygen-cardiorespirograms from newborn infants whose mothers received 100 mg pethidine 2½, 3, and 3 hours respectively before delivery.

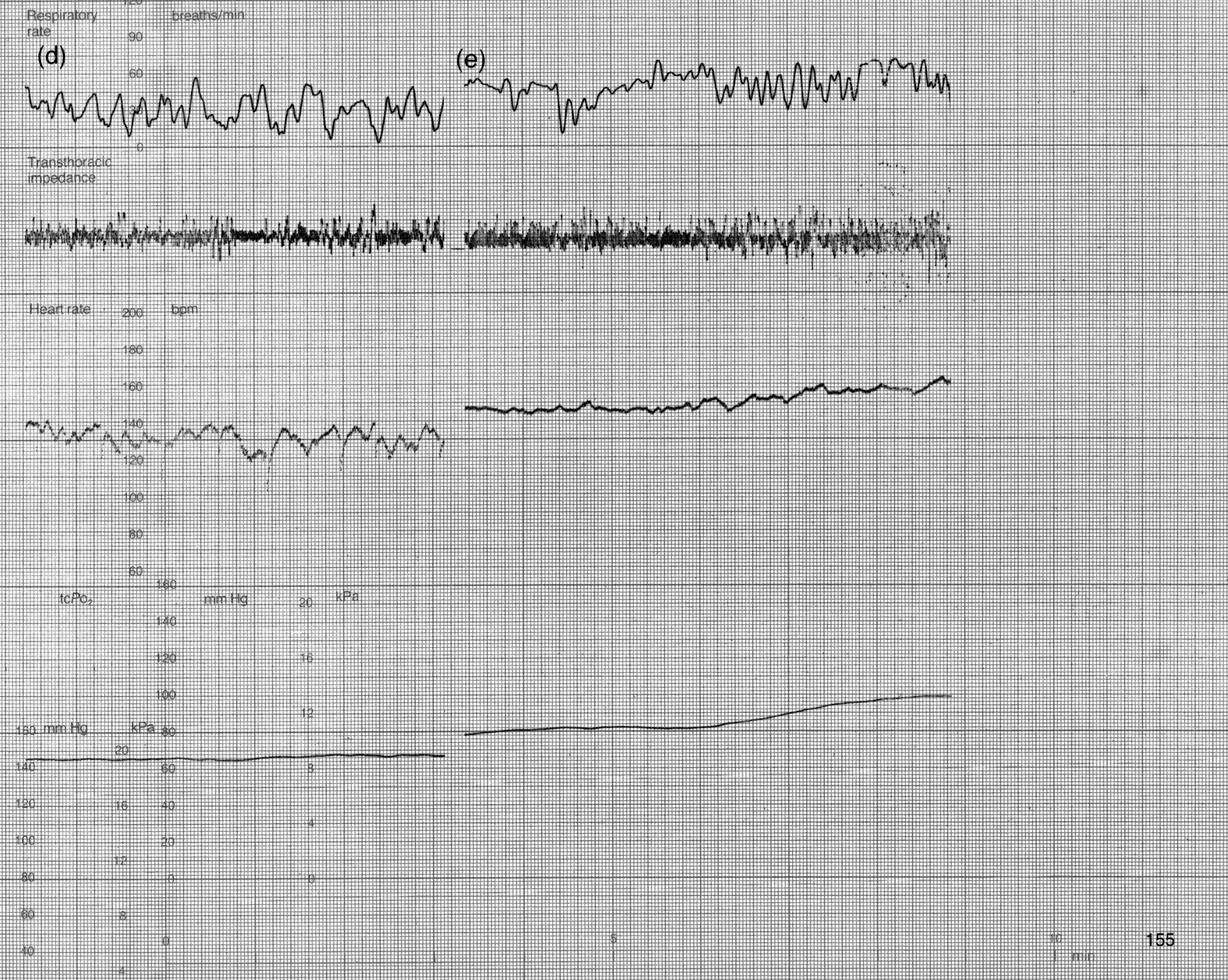
Respiratory rate
breaths/min
(d)
(e)
Transthoracic impedance
Heart rate
bpm
tcPo₂
mm Hg
kPa
5
10
min

Fig. 6.2.3.a

Birthweight: 3300 g

Apgar score: 10

Age (in hours) at recording: 2

Delivery: vaginal

Cord blood acid – base and blood gases							
	pH	$P\text{CO}_2$	mm Hg	kPa	$P\text{O}_2$ mm Hg	kPa	Base deficit mmol/l
Umbilical artery	7.30		43	5.7	18	2.4	4.9
Umbilical vein	7.34		33	4.4	26	3.5	7.1

Activity state	Awake, quiet and crying.
Respiratory rate	Initially between 20 and 80 breaths/min then mainly cyclic changes about 70 breaths/min.
Transthoracic impedance	Initially periodicity then regular excursions but large irregular ones during crying.
Heart rate	Baseline heart rate about 115 bpm with an amplitude of long-term variability $\leqslant$ 20 bpm.
tc$P\text{O}_2$	During the oxygen test a plateau of 365 mm Hg (48.7 kPa) was reached from which a shunt of 21 per cent is calculated.

Comments (a and b) Oxygen-cardiorespirograms from newborn infants (**b** was a breech delivery) whose mothers received 100 mg pethidine 1 and 7 hours respectively before delivery.

Fig. 6.2.3.b

Birthweight: 3240 g

Apgar score: 7/10/10

Age (in hours) at recording: 2

Delivery: vaginal (breech)

Cord blood acid – base and blood gases							
	pH	$P\text{CO}_2$	mm Hg	kPa	$P\text{O}_2$ mm Hg	kPa	Base deficit mmol/l
Umbilical artery	7.23		49	6.5	19	2.5	6.5
Umbilical vein	7.25		36	4.8	29	3.9	10.7

Activity state	Awake, quiet and crying.
Respiratory rate	At first close to 80 breaths/min then irregular cycles with respiratory rate between 30 and 80 breaths/min.
Transthoracic impedance	Somewhat regular excursions in the quiet period then larger more irregular ones during crying.
Heart rate	Baseline heart rate when quiet about 135 bpm with an amplitude of long-term variability $\leqslant$ 10 bpm and some small decelerations.
tc$P\text{O}_2$	A slow increase from 94 to 100 mm Hg (12.3 to 13.3 kPa) and then a decrease to 80 mm Hg (10.7 kPa) during crying.

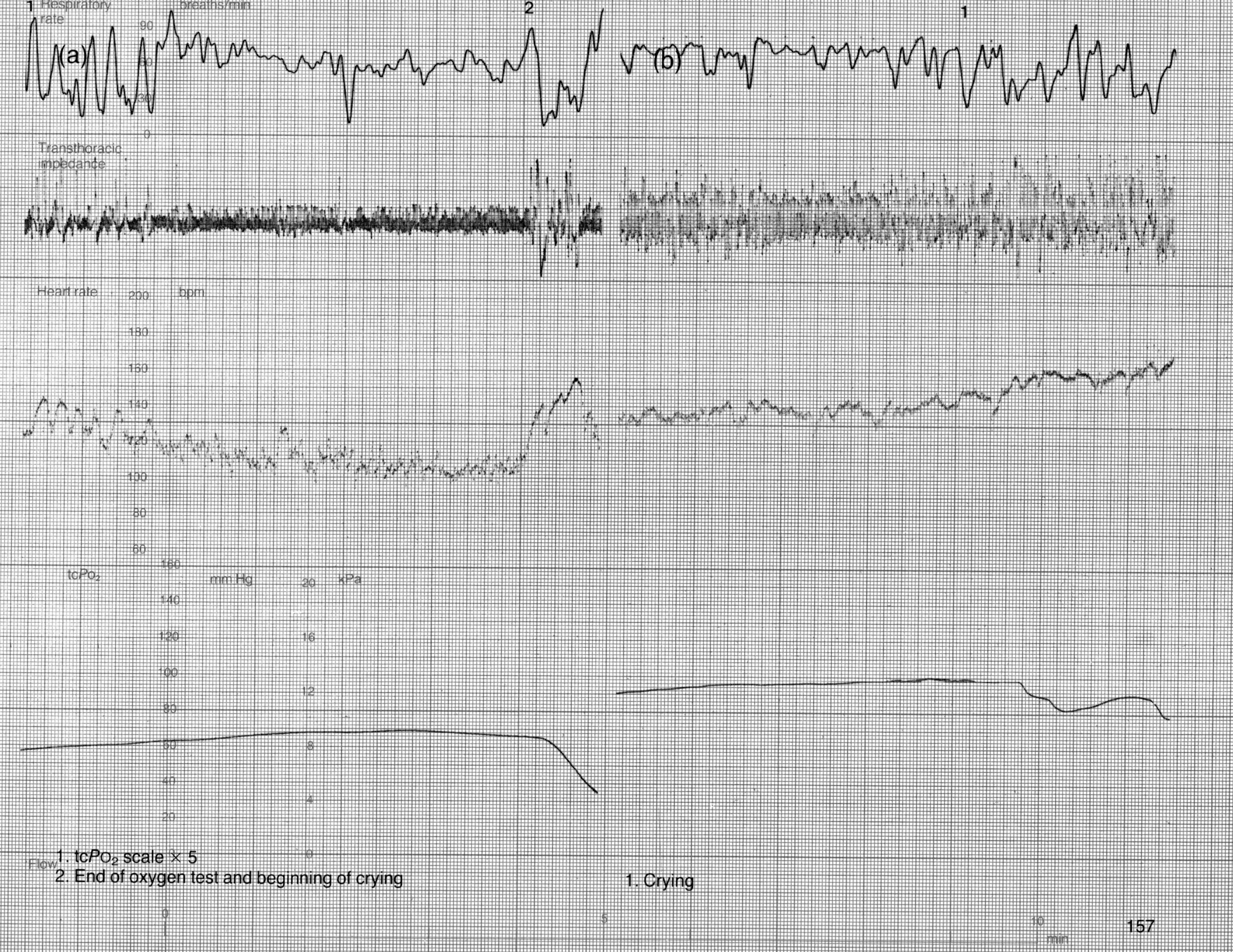

1
Respiratory rate
breaths/min
90
60
30
0
2
1
(a)
(b)
Transthoracic impedance
Heart rate
200
bpm
180
160
140
120
100
80
60
tcPo2
160
mm Hg
20
kPa
140
120
16
100
12
80
60
8
40
4
20
0
Flow
1. tcPO2 scale × 5
2. End of oxygen test and beginning of crying
1. Crying
0
5
10
min

Fig. 6.2.4

Birthweight: 2930 g

Apgar score: 9/10/10

Age (in hours) at recording: 2

Delivery: vaginal

Cord blood acid – base and blood gases							
	pH	$P\text{CO}_2$	mm Hg	kPa	$P\text{O}_2$	mm Hg	kPa	Base deficit mmol/l
Umbilical artery	7.30		37	4.9		22	2.9	7.9
Umbilical vein	7.34		33	4.4		25	3.3	7.2

Activity state	Awake, quiet and crying.
Respiratory rate	Cyclic changes with different amplitudes from 15 to 100 breaths/min.
Transthoracic impedance	Larger irregular excursions during crying and smaller somewhat irregular ones during the quiet periods.
Heart rate	Baseline heart rate about 135 bpm when quiet with an amplitude of long-term variability $\leqslant$ 10 bpm and occasional decelerations.
tc$P\text{O}_2$	About 90 mm Hg (12.0 kPa) and fell to 82 mm Hg (10.9 kPa) after crying.

Comments Oxygen-cardiorespirogram from an infant whose mother was not given pethidine included for direct comparison with the other recordings shown in Figs 6.2.

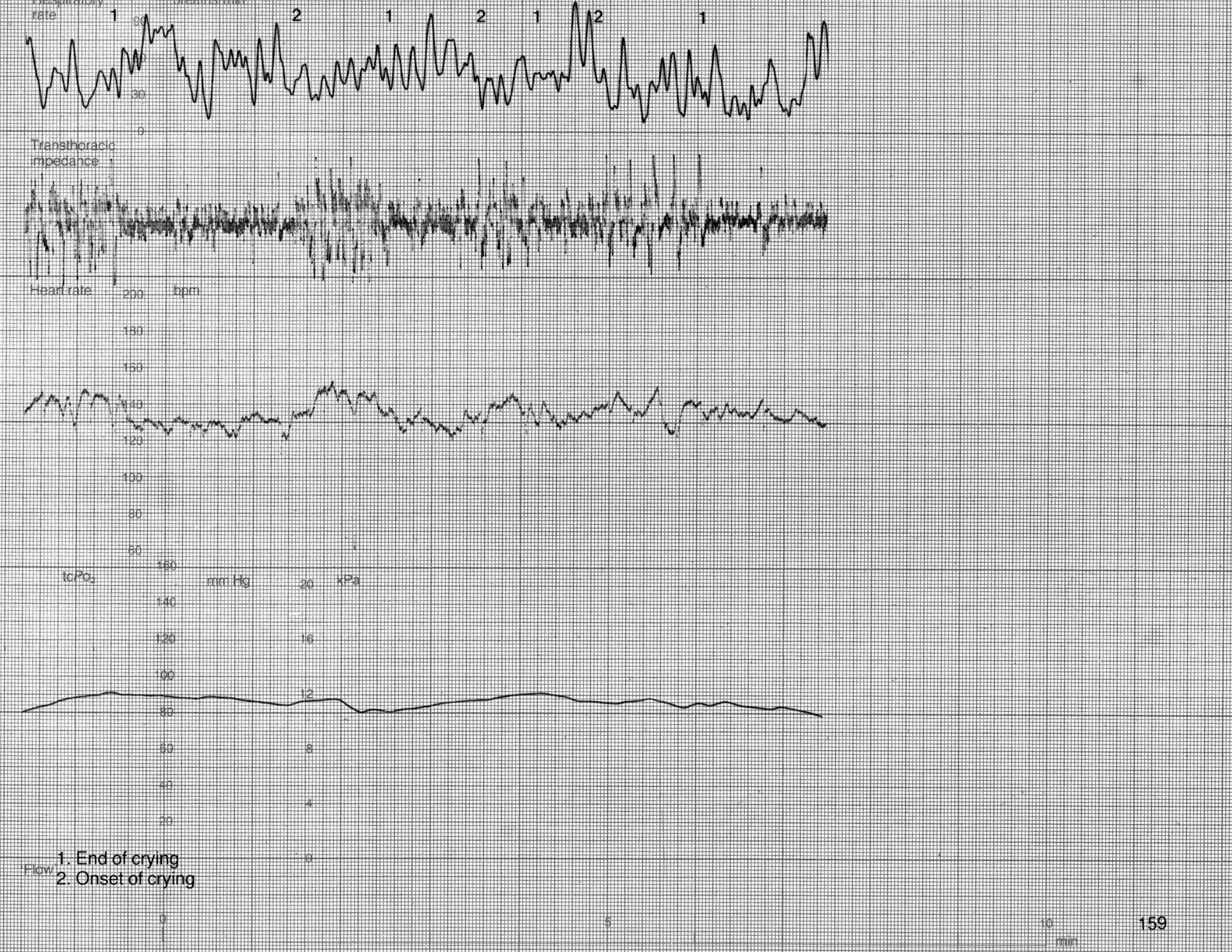
Respiratory rate
breaths/min
1
2
1
2
1
2
1
90
30
0
Transthoracic impedance
Heart rate
200
bpm
180
160
140
120
100
80
60
tcPo₂
160
mm Hg
20
kPa
140
120
16
100
12
80
60
8
40
4
20
0
Flow
1. End of crying
2. Onset of crying
0
5
10
min

7 Oxygen-cardiorespirograms in the first hours of life in relation to different clinical findings

Fig. 7.1.1

Birthweight: 3600 g

Apgar score: 8/9/10

Age (in hours) at recording: 4

Delivery: vaginal

Cord blood acid – base and blood gases							
	pH	$P\text{CO}_2$	mm Hg	kPa	$P\text{O}_2$	mm Hg	kPa	Base deficit mmol/l
Umbilical artery	7.07		70	9.3		9	1.2	9.7
Umbilical vein	7.13		56	7.5		17	2.3	9.8

Activity state	Awake, quiet and active sleep.
Respiratory rate	Cyclic changes at first between 0 and 50 breaths/min (trigger error cannot be excluded) and when sleeping about 35 breaths/min.
Transthoracic impedance	Almost regular but with occasional larger excursions, which became very regular during sleep.
Heart rate	Baseline heart rate about 100 bpm with an amplitude of long-term variability $\leqslant$ 15 bpm and accelerations during the large breaths. During sleep the amplitude was reduced to $\leqslant$ 10 bpm.
tc$P\text{O}_2$	About 65 mm Hg (8.7 kPa) and increasing towards 80 mm Hg (10.7 kPa) when the infant was sleeping.

Comments In spite of the umbilical artery blood pH of 7.066 this oxygen-cardiorespirogram in no way differs from that of infants born with normal pH values. However, it should be noted that this registration was not obtained immediately after birth but 4 hours later.

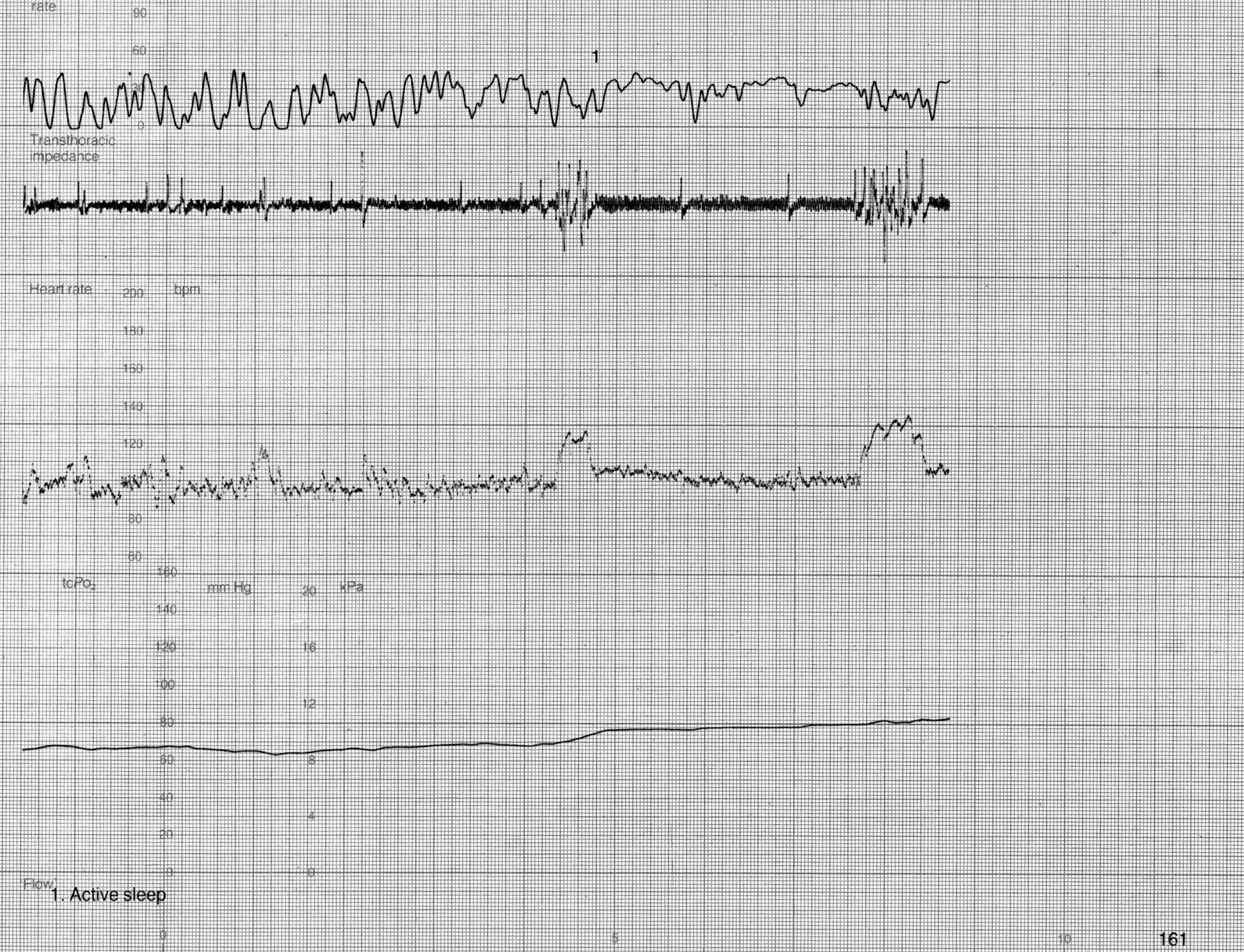
Respiratory rate
breaths/min
90
60
30
0
1
Transthoracic impedance
Heart rate
200
bpm
180
160
140
120
80
60
tcPo$_2$
160
mm Hg
20
kPa
140
120
16
100
12
80
60
8
40
4
20
0
0
Flow
1. Active sleep
0
5
10
min

Fig. 7.1.2

Birthweight: 3200 g

Apgar score: 9/10

Age (in hours) at recording: 3

Delivery: vaginal

Cord blood acid – base and blood gases							
	pH	$P\text{CO}_2$	mm Hg	kPa	$P\text{O}_2$ mm Hg	kPa	Base deficit mmol/l
Umbilical artery	7.06		61	8.1	15	2.0	12.5
Umbilical vein	7.14		48	6.4	26	3.5	11.7

Activity state	Awake, quiet and active sleep.
Respiratory rate	Cyclic changes between 0 and 50 breaths/min (frequent trigger errors).
Transthoracic impedance	Long spells of regular excursions, but intercepted by larger irregular excursions.
Heart rate	Baseline heart rate about 130 bpm with an amplitude of long-term variability $\leqslant$ 10 bpm and accelerations coinciding with the deep breaths. The amplitude of the long-term variability tended to decrease when the infant went to sleep.
$\text{tc}P\text{O}_2$	Between 82 and 70 mm Hg (10.9 and 9.3 kPa).

Comments As in Fig. 7.1.1 this oxygen-cardiorespirogram from an infant with low umbilical artery blood pH does not differ from that of an infant born with normal pH.

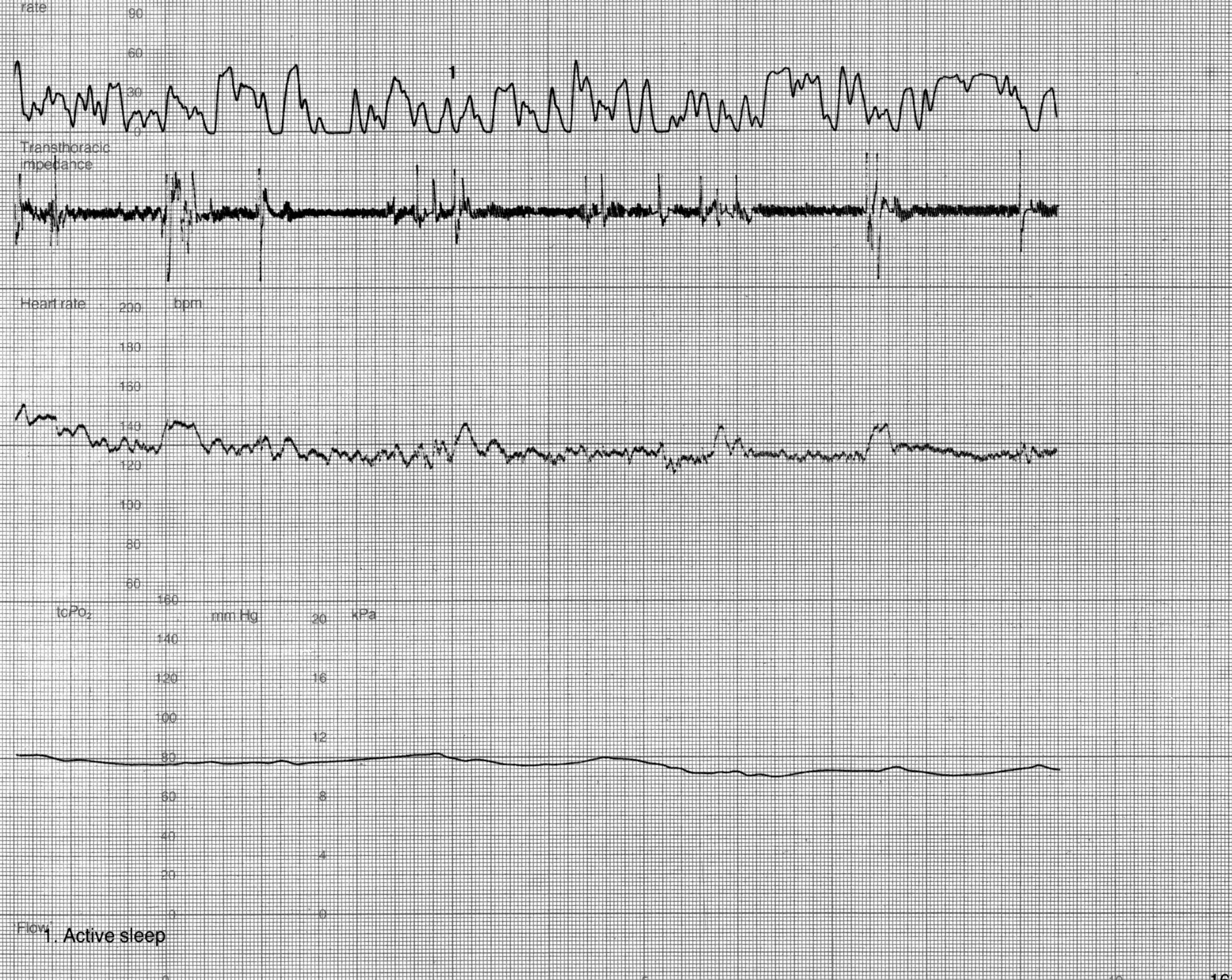

1. Active sleep

Fig. 7.1.3

Birthweight: 2910 g

Apgar score: 7/10/10

Age (in hours) at recording: 1

Delivery: vaginal

Cord blood acid – base and blood gases							
	pH	$P\text{CO}_2$ mm Hg	kPa	$P\text{O}_2$ mm Hg	kPa	Base deficit mmol/l
Umbilical artery	7.03	83	11.1	14	1.9	9.3
Umbilical vein	7.10	64	8.5	20	2.7	9.4

Activity state	Crying, awake, quiet and unquiet.
Respiratory rate	During the active periods cyclic variations from 30 to > 100 breaths/min. In the quiet period smaller variations around 90 breaths/min.
Transthoracic impedance	Regular excursions in the quiet phases, large irregular excursions during the unquiet phases and during crying.
Heart rate	Baseline heart rate was 160 – 170 bpm with an amplitude of long-term variability ≤ 10 bpm in the quiet phase. During the active phases there were accelerations and decelerations. During crying heart rate reached 200 bpm.
tc$P\text{O}_2$	Fell from 97 mm Hg (12.9 kPa) to 70 mm Hg (9.3 kPa) during crying. Activity without crying only resulted in minor decreases in tc$P\text{O}_2$. Simultaneous arterial and transcutaneous $P\text{O}_2$ were 61 and 69 mm Hg (8.1 and 9.2 kPa) respectively.
	Neonatal arterial acid–base and blood gases: pH, 7.34; $P\text{CO}_2$, 28 mm Hg (7.3 kPa); $P\text{O}_2$, 61 mm Hg (8.1 kPa); base deficit, 9.7 mmol/l.

Comments This oxygen-cardiorespirogram from an infant born with very low cord blood pH values shows more tachycardia and tachypnoea than usually seen in the first hour of life.

Two hours before delivery 100 mg pethidine was given to the mother. In spite of this and the acidosis the amplitude of the long-term variability was not affected.

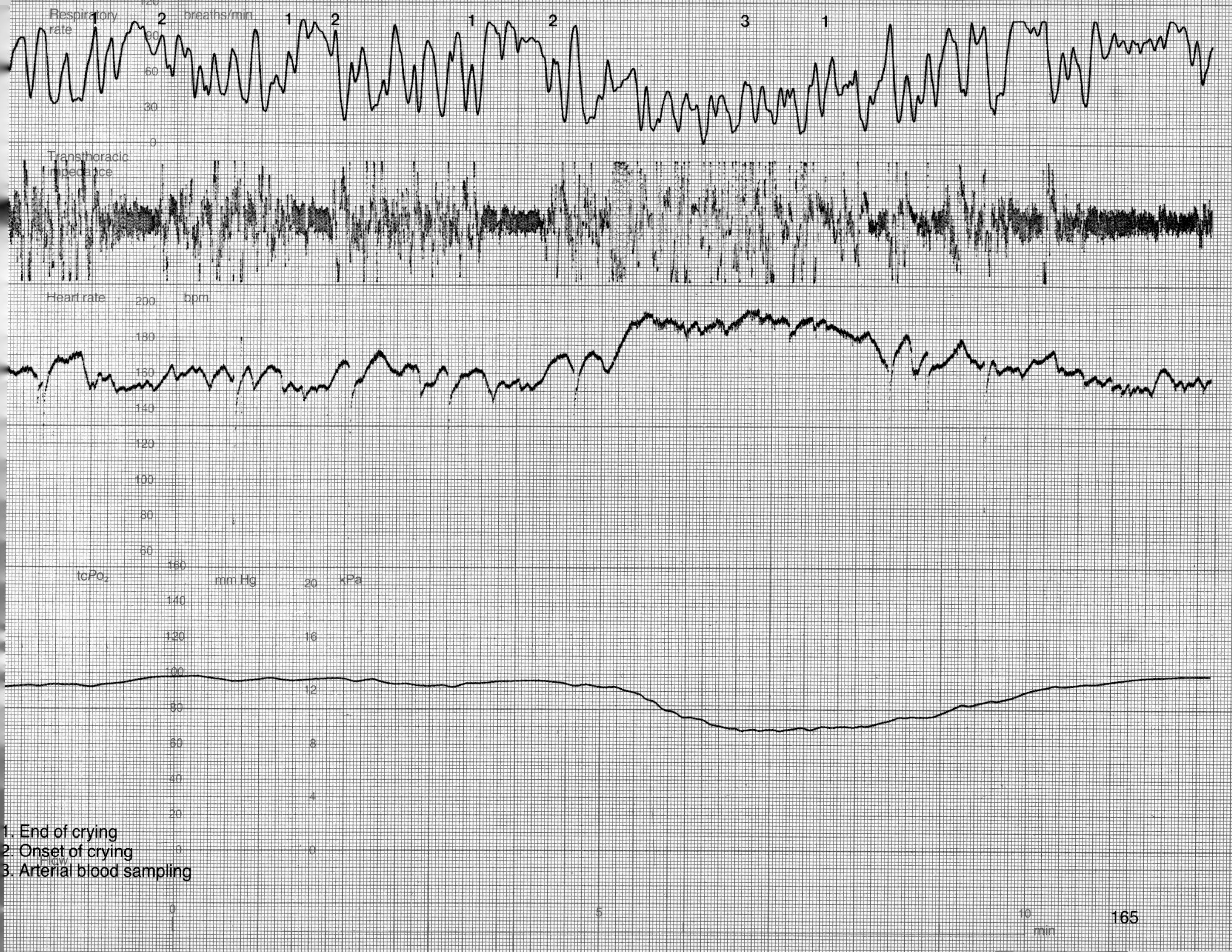
Respiratory rate
breaths/min
120
90
60
30
0
1
2
1
2
1
2
3
1
Transthoracic impedance
Heart rate
bpm
200
180
160
140
120
100
80
60
tcPo2
mm Hg
kPa
160
140
120
100
80
60
40
20
0
20
16
12
8
4
0
1. End of crying
2. Onset of crying
3. Arterial blood sampling
Flow
0
5
10
min

Fig. 7.1.4

Birthweight: 3020 g

Apgar score: 9/10

Age (in hours) at recording: 1

Delivery: vaginal (breech)

Cord blood acid – base and blood gases							
	pH	PCO$_2$ mm Hg	kPa	PO$_2$ mm Hg	kPa	Base deficit mmol/l
Umbilical artery	7.18	65	8.7	5	0.7	3.0
Umbilical vein	7.24	50	6.7	13	1.7	4.4

Activity state	Awake, unquiet.
Respiratory rate	Cyclic changes between 30 and 40 breaths/min (Monitor II).
Transthoracic impedance	Irregular excursions.
Heart rate	Heart rate is so variable that no baseline heart rate can be given. For a few minutes the amplitude of long-term variability is $\leq$ 15 bpm, but otherwise it is $\leq$ 40. There are frequently short decelerations.
tc$P$O$_2$	Before the oxygen test tc$P$O$_2$ was slightly below 80 mm Hg (10.7 kPa) and after slightly above this value. The peak value during the oxygen test was 400 mm Hg (53.3 kPa) from which a shunt of 19 per cent is calculated.

Comments Oxygen-cardiorespirogram from an infant delivered by the breech with low cord blood pH mainly due to high PCO$_2$. Heart rate long-term variability was quite marked.

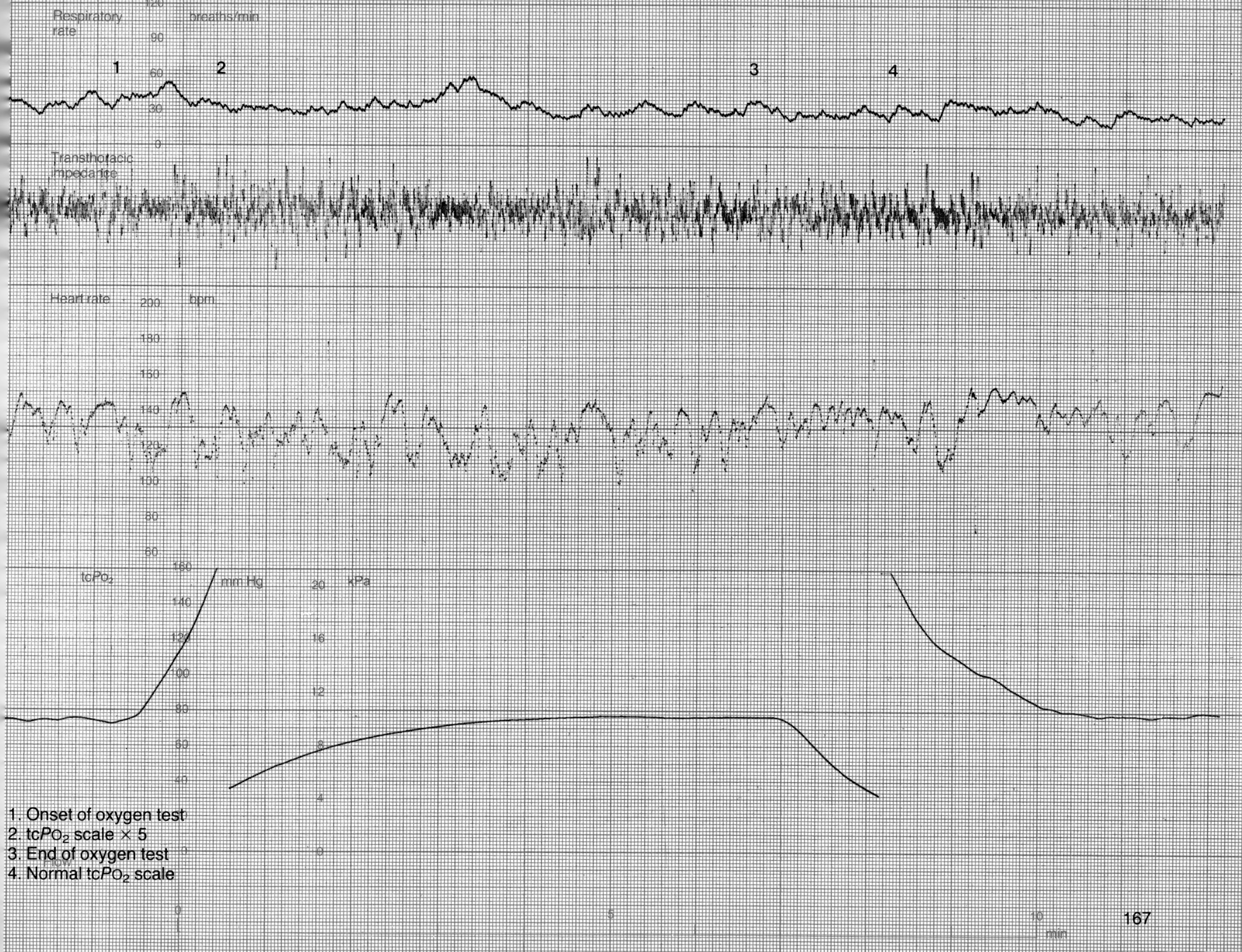

Respiratory rate
breaths/min
120
90
60
30
0
1
2
3
4
Transthoracic impedance
Heart rate
bpm
200
180
160
140
120
100
80
60
$tcPo_2$
mm Hg
160
140
120
100
80
60
40
kPa
20
16
12
8
4
0
Flow
0
5
10
min
1. Onset of oxygen test
2. $tcPo_2$ scale × 5
3. End of oxygen test
4. Normal $tcPo_2$ scale

Fig. 7.2.1

Birthweight: 3200 g

Apgar score: 3/10/10

Age (in hours) at recording: 1

Delivery: vaginal

Cord blood acid – base and blood gases								
	pH	$P\text{CO}_2$	mm Hg	kPa	$P\text{O}_2$	mm Hg	kPa	Base deficit mmol/l
Umbilical artery	7.13		70	9.3		5	0.7	5.8
Umbilical vein	7.20		55	7.3		14	1.9	6.5

Activity state	Awake, quiet.
Respiratory rate	About 40 breaths/min (Monitor II).
Transthoracic impedance	Mostly regular excursions but occasionally some larger excursions.
Heart rate	Baseline heart rate 110–120 bpm and the amplitude of long-term variability < 5 bpm. There were small decelerations related to the deep breaths.
tc$P\text{O}_2$	During the oxygen test tc$P\text{O}_2$ reached 300 mm Hg (40.0 kPa) from which a shunt of 25 per cent is calculated. Thereafter tc$P\text{O}_2$ level was at 88 mm Hg (11.7 kPa).

Comments This oxygen-cardiorespirogram, from an infant born with low Apgar score and rather low cord blood pH values (mainly attributable to high $P\text{CO}_2$ levels), showed a reduced amplitude of the long-term variability as well as some small decelerations. Six hours before delivery the mother was given 100 mg pethidine.

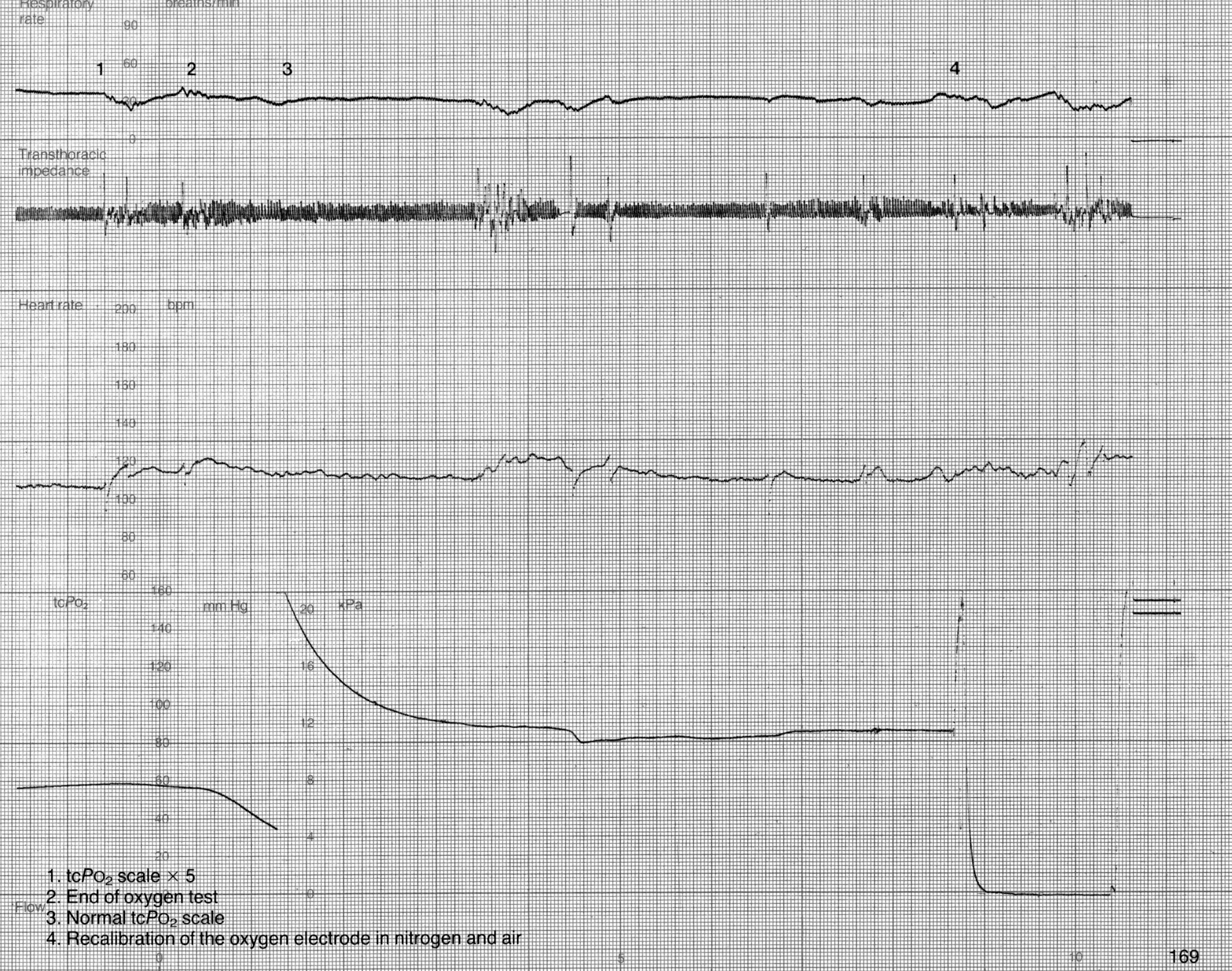
Respiratory rate
breaths/min
120
90
60
30
0
1
2
3
4
Transthoracic impedance
Heart rate
bpm
200
180
160
140
120
100
80
60
tcPo₂
mm Hg
kPa
160
140
120
100
80
60
40
20
20
16
12
8
4
0
Flow
0
5
10
min
1. tcPO₂ scale × 5
2. End of oxygen test
3. Normal tcPO₂ scale
4. Recalibration of the oxygen electrode in nitrogen and air

Fig. 7.3.1

Birthweight: 2400 g

Apgar score: 8/10/10

Age (in hours) at recording: 1

Delivery: vaginal

Cord blood acid – base and blood gases							
	pH	$P\text{CO}_2$ mm Hg	kPa	$P\text{O}_2$ mm Hg	kPa	Base deficit mmol/l
Umbilical artery	7.37	30	4.0	22	2.9	7.1
Umbilical vein	7.40	25	3.3	26	3.5	8.4

Activity state	Awake, unquiet.
Respiratory rate	Cyclic changes mainly between 30 and 60 breaths/min.
Transthoracic impedance	Short periods of regular excursions interrupted by larger breaths.
Heart rate	Baseline heart rate was about 150 bpm with an amplitude of long-term variability $\leq$ 5 bpm.
$\text{tc}P\text{O}_2$	75 to 84 mm Hg (10.0 to 11.2 kPa).

Comments See Figs 7.3.2 a and b.

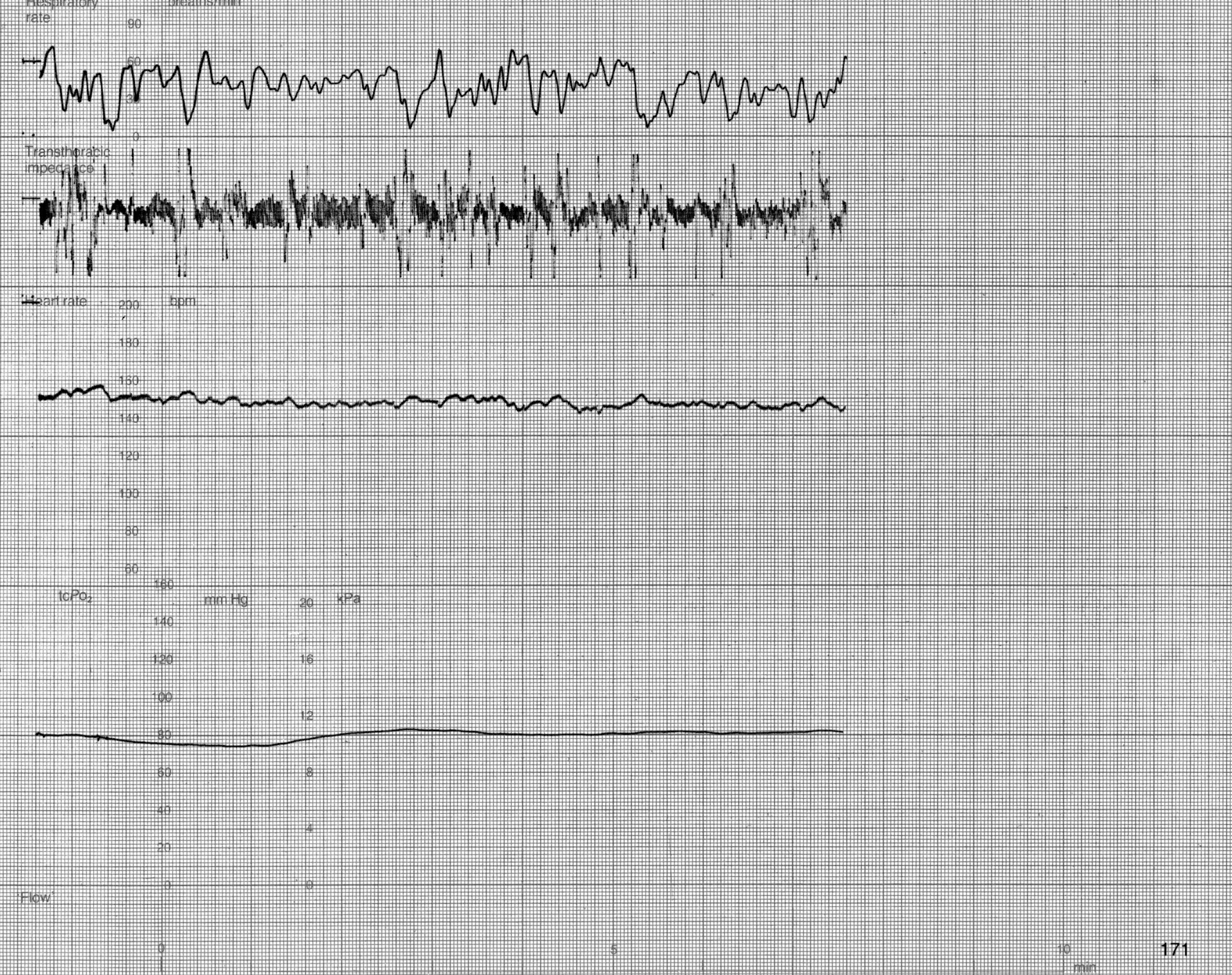

Respiratory rate
breaths/min
120
90
60
30
0
Transthoracic impedance
Heart rate
bpm
200
180
160
140
120
100
80
60
tcPo_2
mm Hg
kPa
160
140
120
100
80
60
40
20
0
20
16
12
8
4
0
'Flow'
0
5
10
min

Fig. 7.3.2.a

Birthweight: 2390 g

Apgar score: 9/10

Age (in hours) at recording: 1

Delivery: Caesarean section

Activity state	Awake, quiet and active sleep.
Respiratory rate	Cyclic changes between 40 and 100 breaths/min. In the quiet phase close to 60 breaths/min.
Transthoracic impedance	Smaller and larger excursions during both activity states.
Heart rate	Baseline heart rate was about 125 bpm with an amplitude of long-term variability $\leqslant$ 10 bpm, decreasing to $\leqslant$ 5 bpm in the most quiet phases.
tc$P$O$_2$	Between 95 mm Hg (12.7 kPa) and 88 mm Hg (11.7 kPa).

Comments (7.3.1, 7.3.2 a and b) These oxygen-cardiorespirograms from newborn infants with low birthweight (two delivered by Caesarean section) do not differ from the range seen after uncomplicated deliveries except that there is a tendency to reduced long-term variability.

Fig. 7.3.2.b

Birthweight: 1990 g

Apgar score: 7/10/10

Age (in hours) at recording: 1

Delivery: Caesarean section

Cord blood acid – base and blood gases							
	pH	PCO$_2$	mm Hg	kPa	PO$_2$	mm Hg	kPa	Base deficit mmol/l
Umbilical artery	7.26		51	6.8		21	2.8	4.2
Umbilical vein	7.28		45	6.0				5.3

Activity state	Awake, unquiet and frequent periods of crying.
Respiratory rate	During the intermittent crying respiratory rate varied between 5 and 70 breaths/min.
Transthoracic impedance	Irregular, small excursions in the quiet period and larger more irregular excursions during crying. A tendency to periodicity.
Heart rate	Heart rate was about 170 bpm during the intermittent crying. The amplitude of the long-term variability was $<$ 10 bpm.
tc$P$O$_2$	Because of the intermittent crying undulating tc$P$O$_2$ curve between 79 and 59 mm Hg (10.5 and 7.9 kPa).

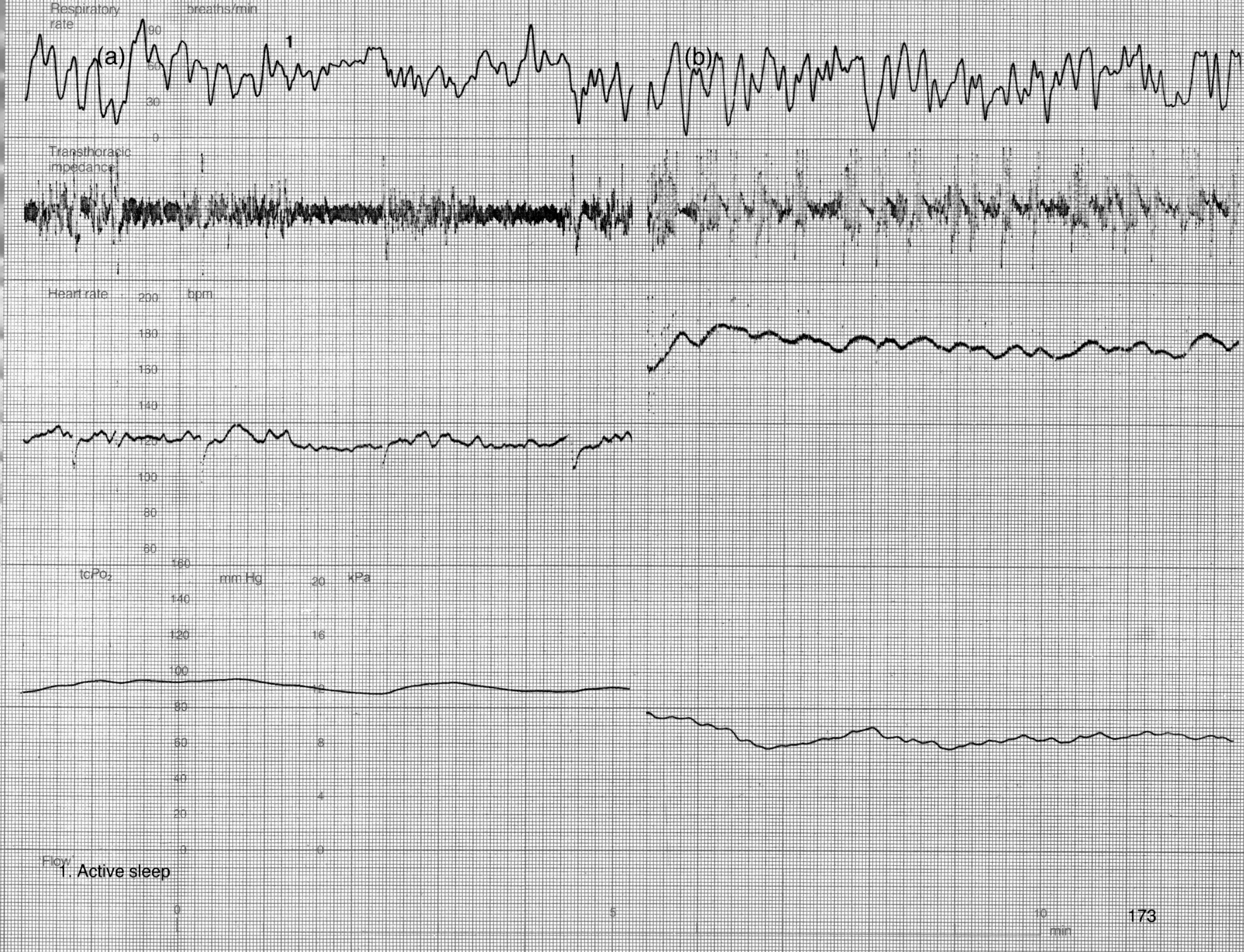

Respiratory rate
breaths/min
90
60
30
0
(a)
1
(b)
Transthoracic impedance
Heart rate
bpm
200
180
160
140
120
100
80
60
tcPo2
mm Hg
kPa
160
140
120
100
80
60
40
20
0
20
16
12
8
4
0
Flow
1. Active sleep
0
5
10
min

Fig. 7.3.3

Birthweight: 2330 g

Apgar score: 6/10/10

Age (in hours) at recording: 1

Delivery: vaginal

Activity state	Awake, unquiet.
Respiratory rate	Cyclic changes between 5 and 90 breaths/min.
Transthoracic impedance	Irregular excursions.
Heart rate	Baseline heart rate about 130 bpm with an amplitude of long-term variability $\leq$ 10 bpm and occasional spikes.
tcP_{O_2}	Between 85 and 96 mm Hg (11.3 and 12.8 kPa).

Comments This illustrates an oxygen-cardiorespirogram from an infant with low birthweight and low Apgar score. All parameters were within the normal range.

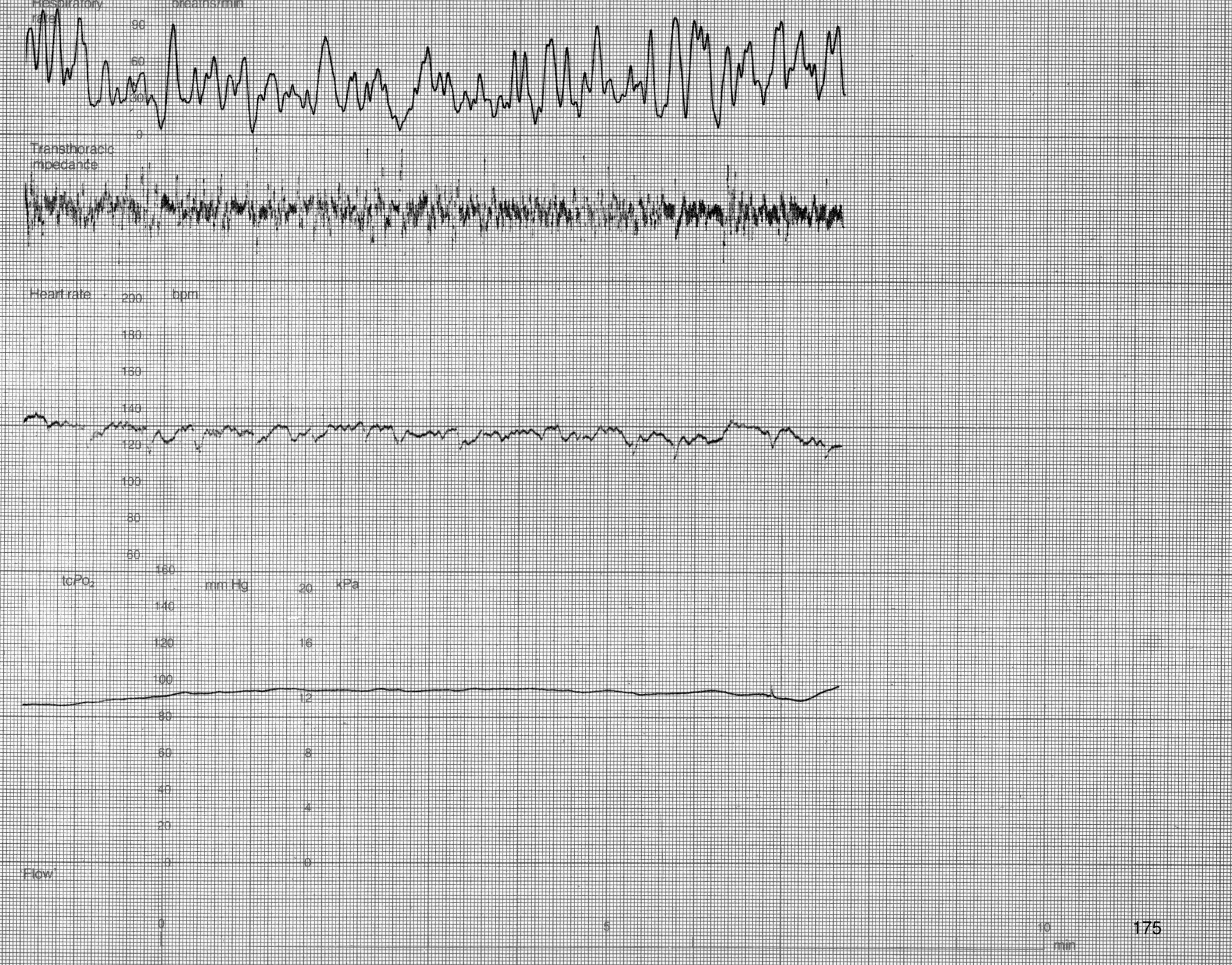

Respiratory rate
breaths/min
90
60
30
0
Transthoracic impedance
Heart rate
bpm
200
180
160
140
120
100
80
60
$tcPo_2$
mm Hg
kPa
160
140
120
100
80
60
40
20
0
20
16
12
8
4
0
Flow
0
5
10
min

Fig. 7.3.4

Birthweight: 2170 g

Apgar score: 3/9/10

Age at recording: 30 min

Delivery: vaginal

Cord blood acid – base and blood gases							
	pH	$P\text{CO}_2$	mm Hg	kPa	$P\text{O}_2$ mm Hg	kPa	Base deficit mmol/l
Umbilical artery	7.30		42	5.6	13	1.7	5.1
Umbilical vein	7.32		39	5.2	18	2.4	5.4

Activity state	Active sleep.
Respiratory rate	Cyclic changes mainly between 20 and 60 breaths/min.
Transthoracic impedance	Short periods of regular excursions intercepted by irregular ones.
Heart rate	Baseline heart rate was about 130 bpm with an amplitude of long-term variability $\leqslant$ 10 bpm. In connection with the arterial blood sampling heart rate increased to 140 bpm and the amplitude of long-term variability was $\leqslant$ 5 bpm.
tc$P\text{O}_2$	Between 64 and 80 mm Hg (8.5 and 10.7 kPa). Simultaneous arterial blood $P\text{O}_2$ and transcutaneous $P\text{O}_2$ were 60 and 65 mm Hg respectively (8.0 and 8.7 kPa).
	Neonatal arterial acid–base and blood gases: pH, 7.27; $P\text{CO}_2$, 44 mm Hg (5.9 kPa); $P\text{O}_2$, 60 mm Hg (8.0 kPa); base deficit, 6.1 mmol/l.

Comments This oxygen-cardiorespirogram does not differ from that seen from full-term infants in spite of the low birthweight and the low Apgar score.

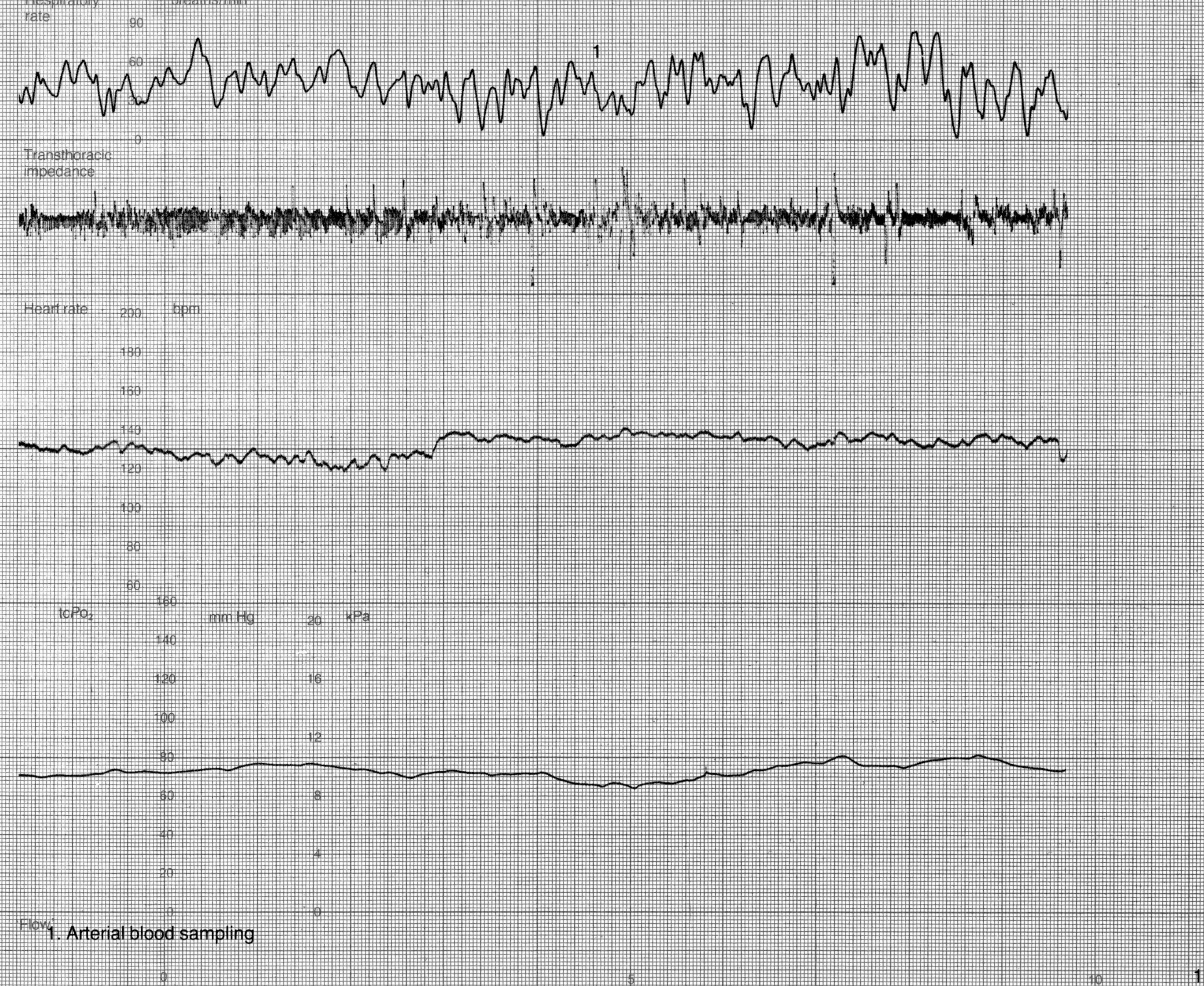

1. Arterial blood sampling

Fig. 7.3.5.a

Birthweight: 1870 g

Apgar score: 2/9/10

Age (in hours) at recording: 1

Delivery: Caesarean section

Cord blood acid – base and blood gases							
	pH	PCO$_2$	mm Hg	kPa	PO$_2$ mm Hg	kPa	Base deficit mmol/l
Umbilical artery	7.17		60	8.0	6	0.8	6.7
Umbilical vein	7.23		47	6.3	19	2.5	7.2

Activity state	Active sleep.
Respiratory rate	Between 20 and 30 breaths/min (Monitor II).
Transthoracic impedance	Irregular excursions.
Heart rate	Baseline heart rate 140–150 bpm with an amplitude of long-term variability usually $\leq$ 5 bpm.
tc$P$O$_2$	Stable level at 96 mm Hg (12.8 kPa).

Comments (a and b) Both the two infants had small heart rate variability, but not different from the range within the normal population in spite of the combined factors here of low Apgar score, low birthweight and Caesarean section. In Fig. 7.3.5.b heart rate variability was initially low because the infant was asleep.

Fig. 7.3.5.b

Birthweight: 2320 g

Apgar score: 2/6/10

Age (in hours) at recording: 1

Delivery: Caesarean section

Cord blood acid – base and blood gases							
	pH	PCO$_2$	mm Hg	kPa	PO$_2$ mm Hg	kPa	Base deficit mmol/l
Umbilical artery	7.16		64	8.5	4	0.5	5.5
Umbilical vein	7.20		52	6.9	16	2.1	7.2

Activity state	Quiet sleep and crying.
Respiratory rate	In the quiet phase about 60 breaths/min, during crying between 5 and 75 breaths/min.
Transthoracic impedance	Mainly small regular excursions in the quiet phase, large irregular excursions during crying.
Heart rate	Baseline heart rate was 155 bpm with an amplitude of long-term variability $\leq$ 5 bpm. During crying heart rate increased to 170 bpm.
tc$P$O$_2$	There was a gradual increase from 55 to 68 mm Hg (7.3 to 9.1 kPa) with no change that can be attributed to the crying. Simultaneous arterial and transcutaneous PO$_2$ were 55 and 60 mm Hg respectively (7.3 and 8.0 kPa).
	Neonatal arterial acid–base and blood gases: pH, 7.31; PCO$_2$, 41 mm Hg (5.5 kPa); PO$_2$, 55 mm Hg (7.3 kPa); base deficit, 5.2 mmol/l.

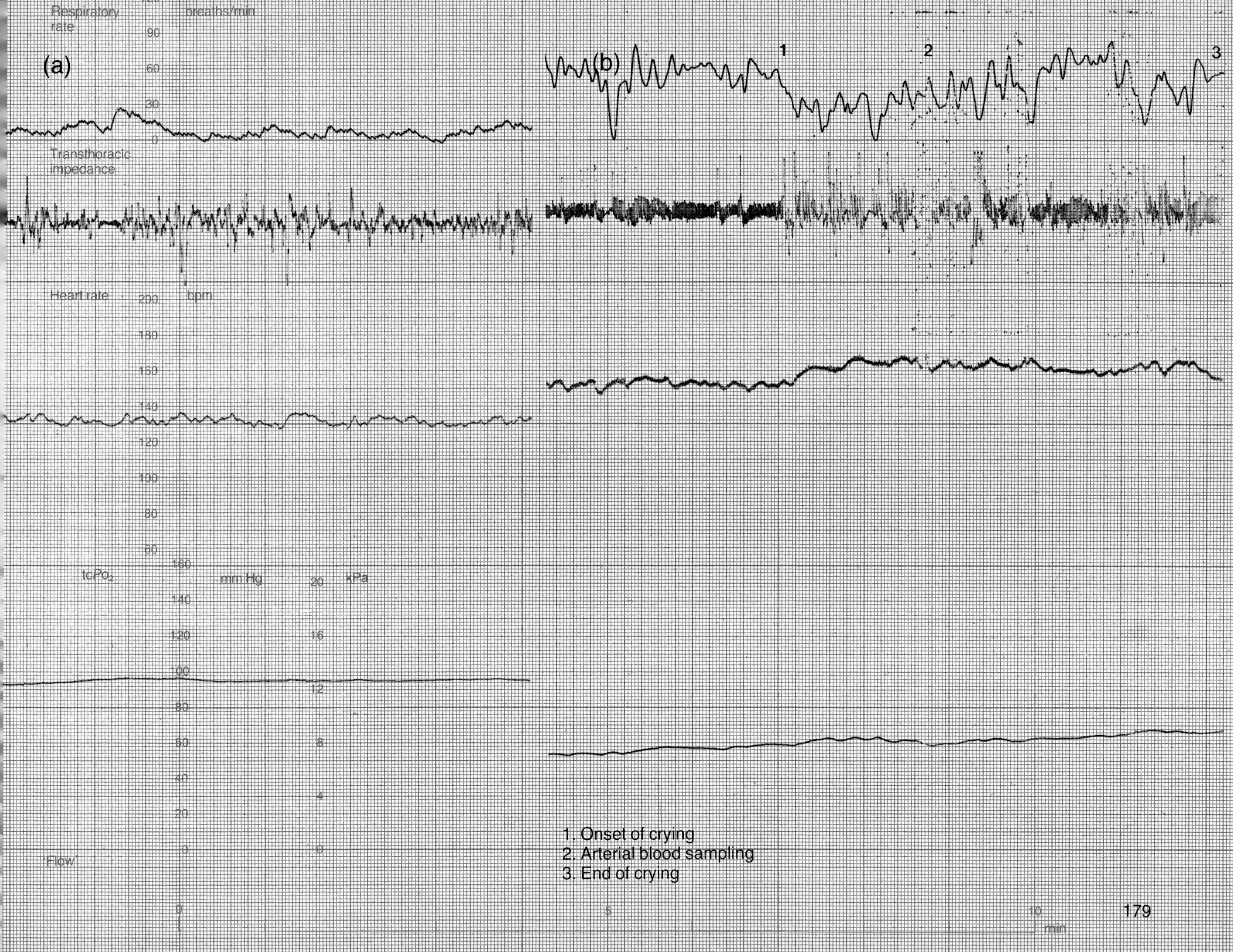
Respiratory rate
breaths/min
90
60
30
0
(a)
(b)
1
2
3
Transthoracic impedance
Heart rate
bpm
200
180
160
140
120
100
80
60
$tcPo_2$
mm Hg
kPa
160
140
120
100
80
60
40
20
0
20
16
12
8
4
0
Flow
0
5
10
min
1. Onset of crying
2. Arterial blood sampling
3. End of crying

8 Miscellaneous observations

Fig. 8.1.1

Birthweight: 3380 g
Apgar score: 9/10
Age (in hours) at recording: 4
Delivery: vaginal

Activity state	Awake, quiet.
Respiratory rate	Cyclic changes between 5 and 55 breaths/min. During oxygen breathing the excursions became so small that the rate meter was not triggered any more.
Transthoracic impedance	Fairly regular excursions frequently intercepted by larger ones.
Heart rate	Baseline heart rate was about 95 bpm falling to 90 bpm during the oxygen test. The amplitude of long-term variability was $\leq$ 15 bpm. Coinciding with the deeper respirations there were decelerations. Artifacts from the respiration obscure the heart rate tracing during the oxygen test.
tcP_{O_2}	About 60 mm Hg (8.0 kPa) increasing to 222 mm Hg (29.6 kPa) during the oxygen test. From this a shunt of 28 per cent is calculated.

Comments This was a normal uncomplicated delivery and clinically uneventful adaptation period. The only abnormality found was the low heart rate. This figure illustrates some of the difficulties sometimes encountered in the registration of the respiration and the heart rate. See also Chapter 2.6.

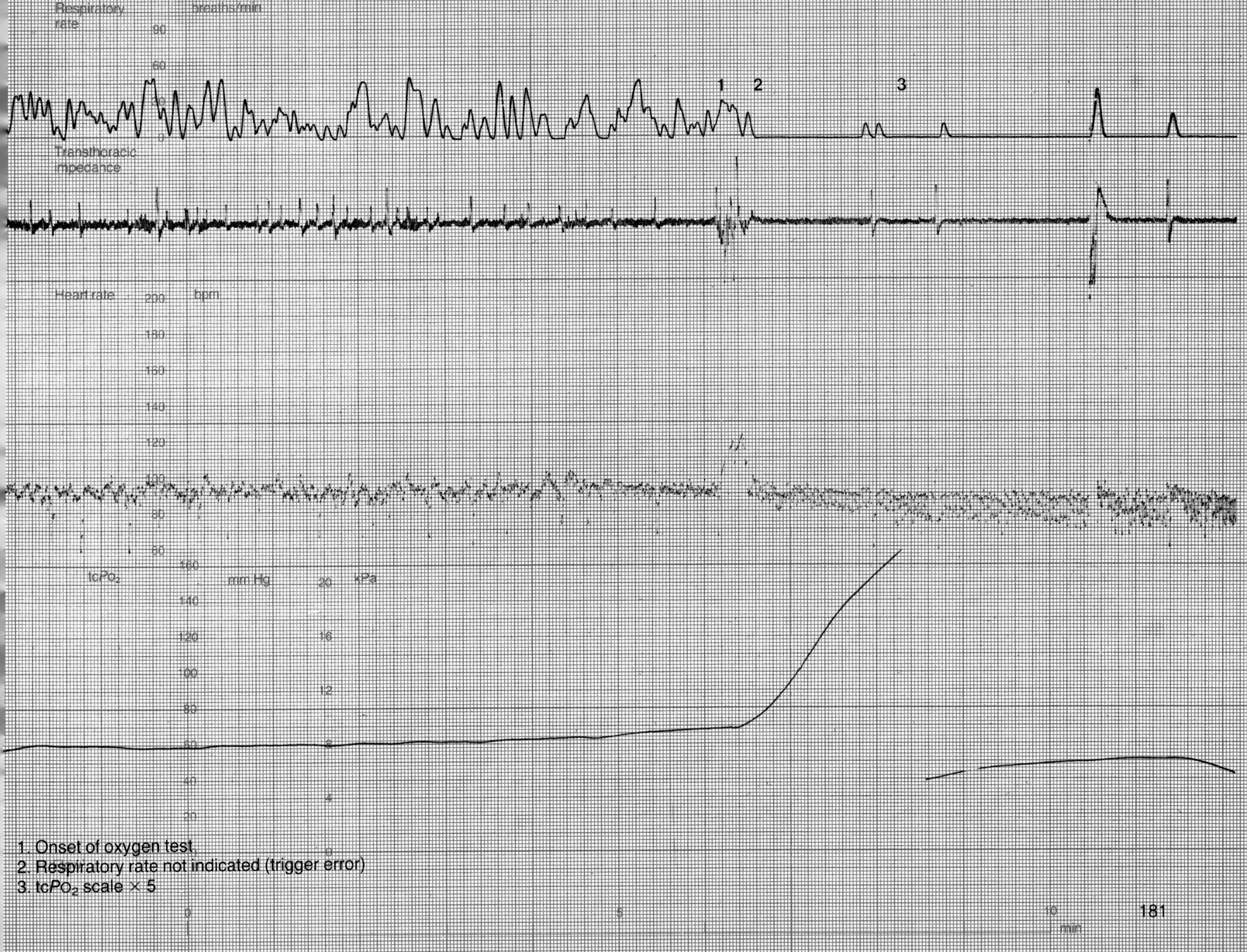

1. Onset of oxygen test
2. Respiratory rate not indicated (trigger error)
3. tcPo_2 scale × 5

Fig. 8.1.2

Birthweight: 3890 g

Apgar score: 9/10

Age (in hours) at recording: 48

Delivery: vaginal

Activity state	Quiet sleep.
Respiratory rate	Between 50 and 60 breaths/min (Monitor II).
Transthoracic impedance	Mainly regular excursions with occasional deeper breaths.
Heart rate	Baseline heart rate about 95 bpm with an amplitude of long-term variability $\leq$ 20 bpm. Marked, short accelerations during the deeper breaths.
tcP_{O_2}	Remained close to 70 mm Hg (9.3 kPa).

Comments As in the example in Fig. 8.1.1 this oxygen-cardiorespirogram was from an infant born after an uncomplicated pregnancy and delivery and, apart from the bradycardia, no clinical abnormalities were noted.

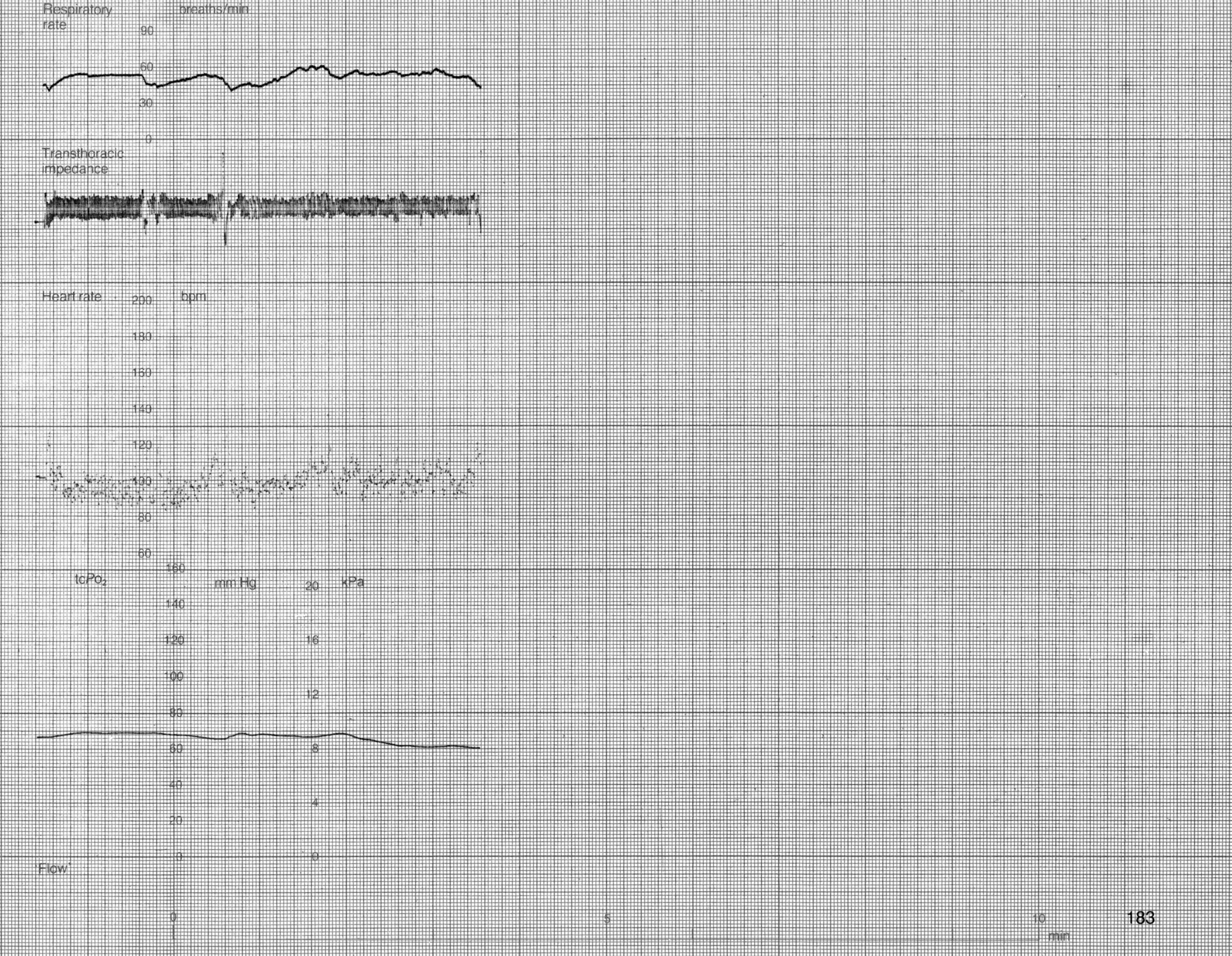
Respiratory rate
breaths/min
90
60
30
0
Transthoracic impedance
Heart rate
200
bpm
180
160
140
120
100
80
60
tcP_{O_2}
160
mm Hg
20
kPa
140
120
16
100
12
80
60
8
40
4
20
0
0
'Flow'
0
5
10
min

Fig. 8.2.1

Birthweight: 2420 g

Apgar score: 8/10/10

Age (in hours) at recording: 18

Delivery: vaginal

Cord blood acid – base and blood gases							
	pH	$P\text{CO}_2$ mm Hg	kPa	$P\text{O}_2$ mm Hg	kPa	Base deficit mmol/l
Umbilical artery	7.30	39	5.2	16	2.1	5.4
Umbilical vein	7.38	41	5.5			0.6

Activity state	Quiet sleep.
Respiratory rate	About 45 breaths/min.
Transthoracic impedance	Regular excursions interrupted by deep breaths and periods of apnoea lasting 10 – 15 seconds.
Heart rate	Baseline heart rate about 160 bpm with an amplitude of long-term variability <5 bpm.
tc$P\text{O}_2$	About 90 mm Hg (12.0 kPa). Subsequent to the apnoeas tc$P\text{O}_2$ fell about 5 mm Hg (0.7 kPa).

Comments This was the first born of a pair of twins. The only abnormality was the high heart rate. The small amplitude of long-term variability is partly attributable to the activity state, i.e. sleep, partly to the high heart rate. The subsequent clinical course was uneventful.

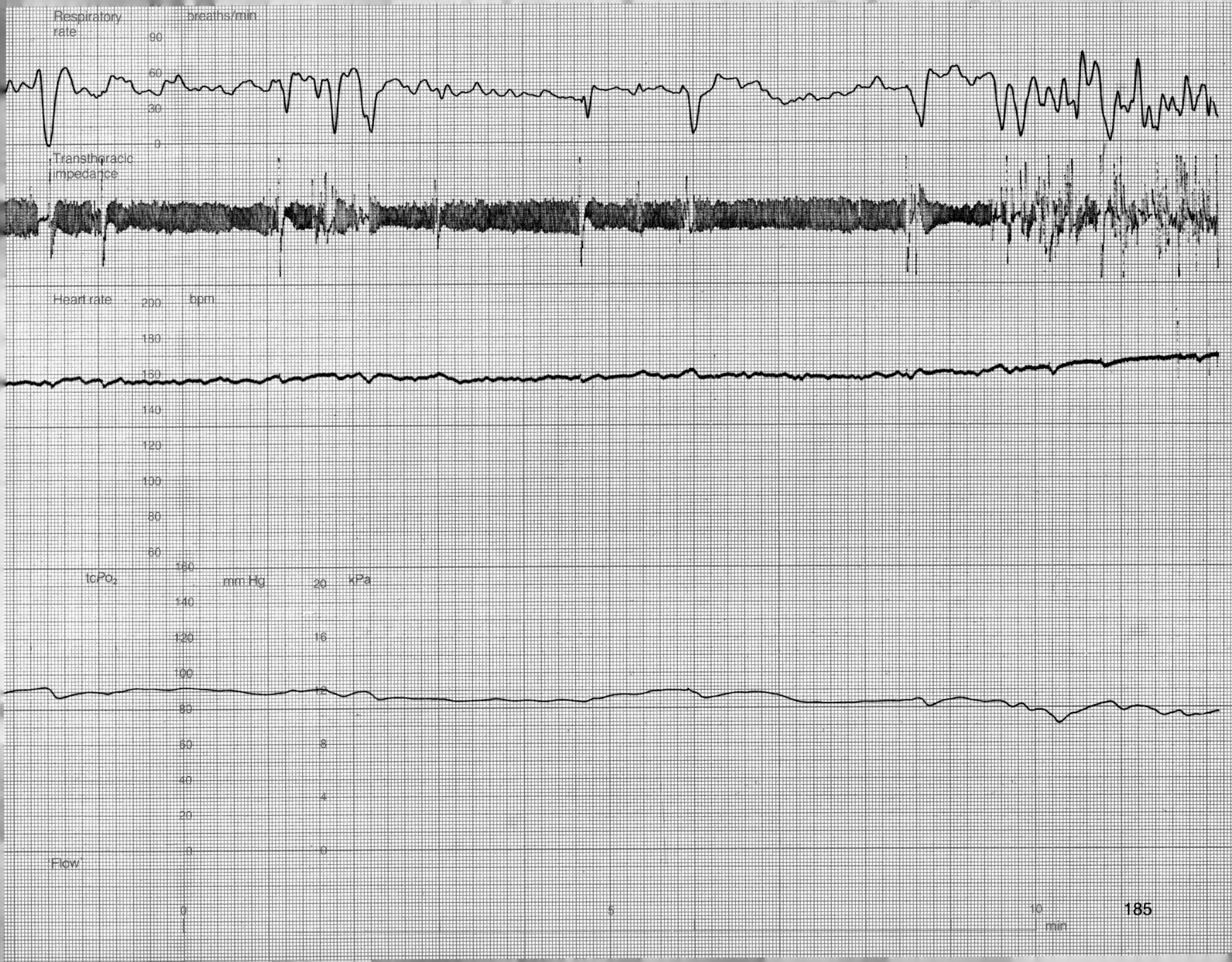
Respiratory rate
breaths/min
90
60
30
0
Transthoracic impedance
Heart rate
bpm
200
180
160
140
120
100
80
60
$tcPo_2$
mm Hg
160
140
120
100
80
60
40
20
0
kPa
20
16
12
8
4
0
Flow
0
5
10
min

Fig. 8.2.2

Birthweight: 3480 g

Apgar score: 10/10

Age (in hours) at recording: 1

Delivery: vaginal

Activity state	Awake, quiet.
Respiratory rate	Cyclic changes mainly between 40 and 90 breaths/min.
Transthoracic impedance	Short periods of almost regular excursions intercepted by phases of irregular, larger excursions.
Heart rate	Baseline heart rate was between 150 and 170 bpm with an amplitude of long-term variability $\leqslant$ 10 bpm. During oxygen breathing baseline heart rate fell to 140 bpm.
tcP_{O_2}	At first 83 mm Hg (11.1 kPa) but with some small change in the respiratory pattern tcP_{O_2} increased to 101 mm Hg (13.5 kPa). During the oxygen test a peak of 350 mm Hg (46.7 kPa) was reached. From this a shunt of 22 per cent is calculated.

Comments In this infant with normal birthweight and a good Apgar score heart rate was high with a distinct long-term variability. The clinical course was uneventful.

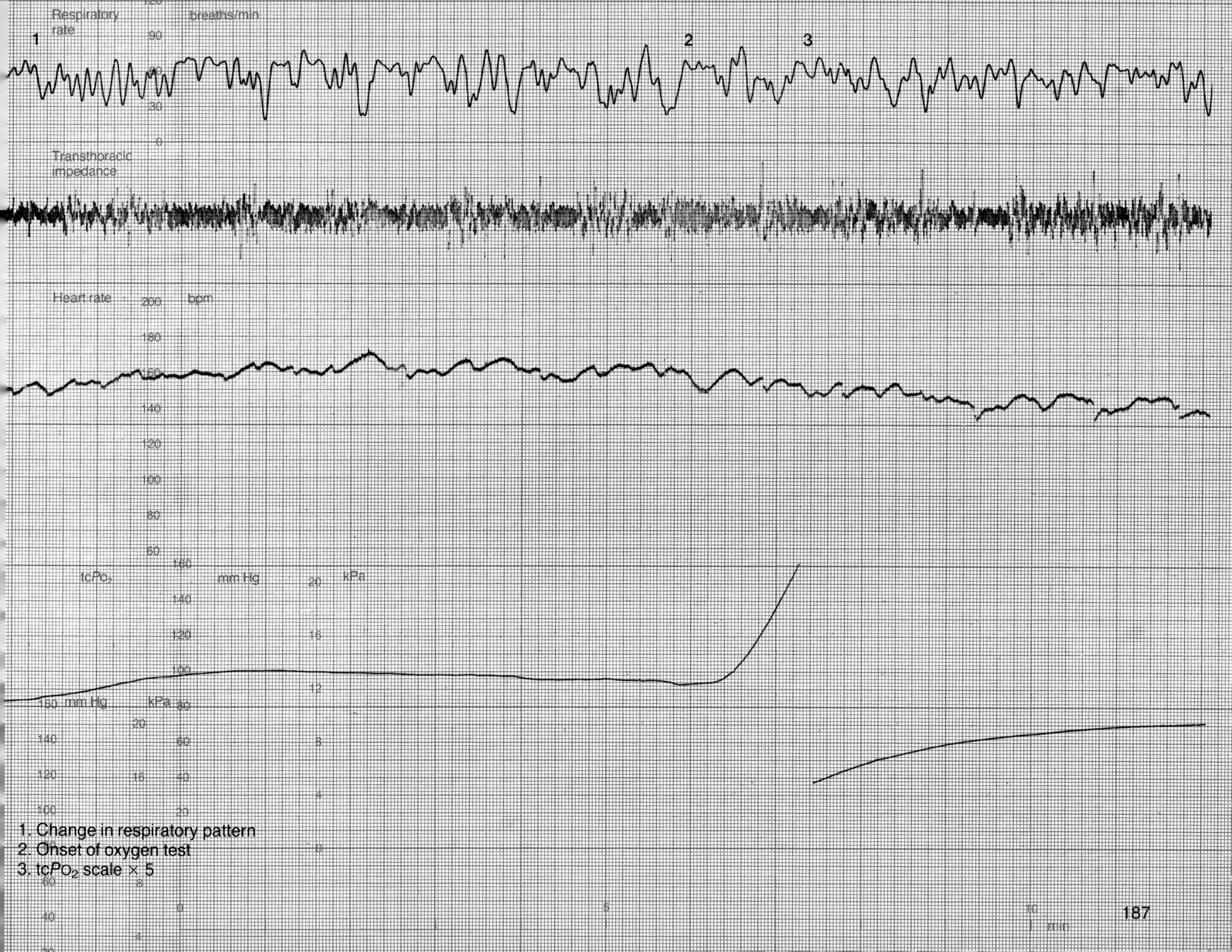
Respiratory rate
breaths/min
Transthoracic impedance
Heart rate
bpm
tcPo_2
mm Hg
kPa
mm Hg
kPa
min
1. Change in respiratory pattern
2. Onset of oxygen test
3. tcPo_2 scale × 5

Fig. 8.2.3

Birthweight: 2550 g

Apgar score: 8/9/10

Age (in hours) at recording: 10

Delivery: vaginal (breech)

Activity state	Awake, unquiet.
Respiratory rate	Mostly between 40 and 50 breaths/min but occasionally 80 breaths/min (Monitor II).
Transthoracic impedance	Fairly regular excursions often interrupted by larger ones.
Heart rate	Baseline heart rate between 190 and 200 bpm with an amplitude of long-term variability $\leqslant$ 20 bpm. One or two decelerations.
tc$P\text{O}_2$	Between 60 and 72 mm Hg (8.0 and 9.6 kPa). Simultaneous arterial and transcutaneous $P\text{O}_2$ were 56 and 60 mm Hg respectively (7.5 and 8.0 kPa).
	Neonatal arterial acid–base and blood gases: pH, 7.29; $P\text{CO}_2$, 38 mm Hg (5.1 kPa); $P\text{O}_2$, 56 mm Hg (7.5 kPa); base deficit, 7.2 mmol/l.

Comments This oxygen-cardiorespirogram shows a pronounced tachycardia but nothing conspicuous in the other variables. The subsequent clinical course was uneventful.

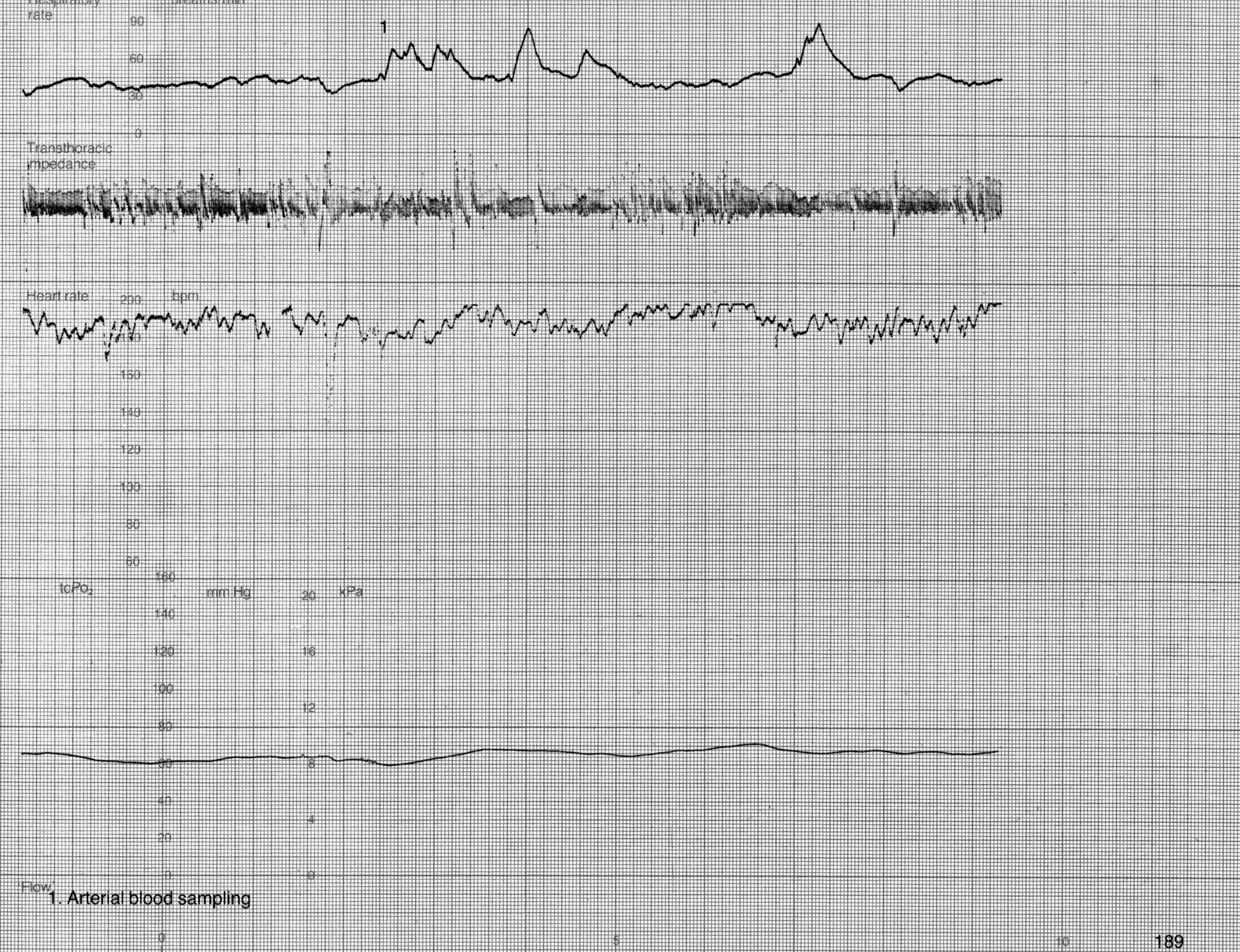
Respiratory rate
breaths/min
90
60
30
0
1
Transthoracic impedance
Heart rate
bpm
200
160
140
120
100
80
60
tcPo2
mm Hg
kPa
160
140
120
100
80
60
40
20
0
20
16
12
8
4
0
Flow
1. Arterial blood sampling
0
5
10
min

Fig. 8.3.1

Birthweight: 3930 g
Apgar score: 8/10/10
Age (in hours) at recording: 30
Delivery: vaginal

Activity state	Active sleep.
Respiratory rate	Cyclic changes mainly between 30 and 90 breaths/min.
Transthoracic impedance	During the more quiet phases fairly regular excursions, otherwise irregular ones.
Heart rate	Baseline heart rate was probably about 105 bpm with an amplitude of long-term variability $\leqslant$ 10 bpm. During activity there were marked accelerations up to 150 bpm. All the time there were frequent spikes in both directions corresponding to the extrasystoles in the electrocardiogram. The 5 seconds excerpt from the ECG shows sinus rhythm intercepted by supraventricular and by ventricular extrasystoles.
tcP_{O_2}	From a level of 87 mm Hg (11.6 kPa) tcP_{O_2} increased to 370 mm Hg (49.3 kPa) during the oxygen test. From this a shunt of 21 per cent is calculated.

Comments The case history as well as the clinical findings of this infant were uneventful and no abnormality was noted except the extrasystoles (see below). This oxygen-cardiorespirogram shows the typical pattern of active sleep including a distinct heart rate reactivity.

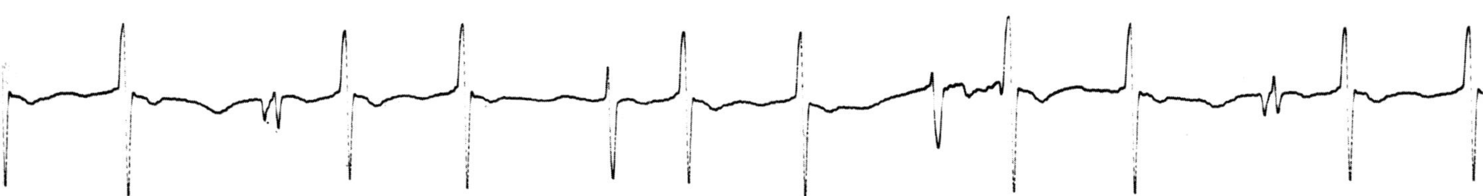

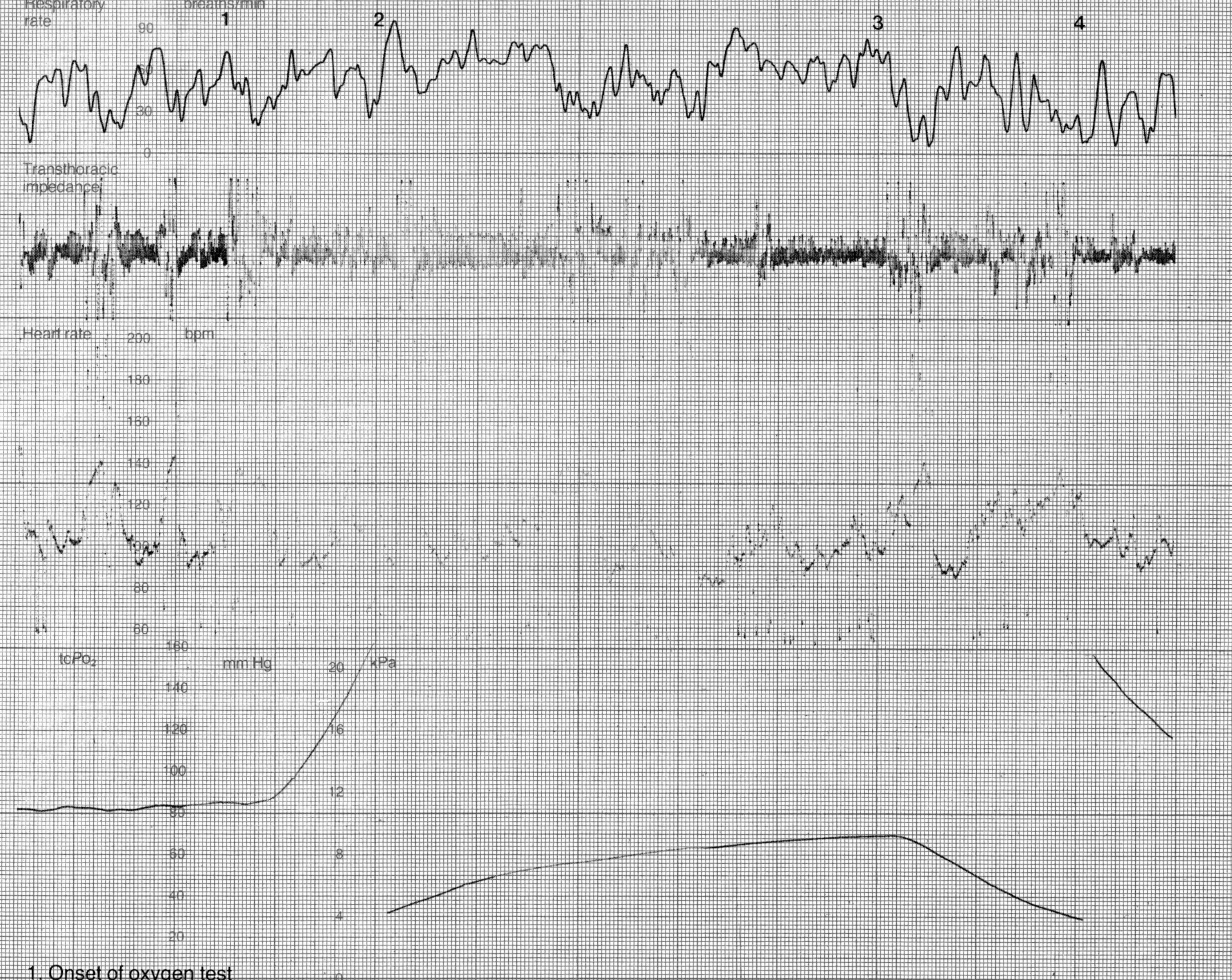

1. Onset of oxygen test
2. tcPo_2 scale × 5, 5 seconds excerpt from the ECG
3. End of oxygen test
4. Normal tcPo_2 scale

Fig. 8.4.1

Birthweight: 3420 g

Apgar score: 8/10

Age (in hours) at recording: 3

Delivery: vaginal

Cord blood acid – base and blood gases							
	pH	$P\text{CO}_2$	mm Hg	kPa	$P\text{O}_2$	mm Hg	kPa	Base deficit mmol/l
Umbilical artery	7.32		43	5.7		21	2.8	3.8
Umbilical vein	7.35		34	4.5		30	4.0	6.4

Activity state	Awake, quiet and vomiting.
Respiratory rate	Apnoea during vomiting, otherwise cyclic changes between 15 and 70 breaths/min.
Transthoracic impedance	As stated, apnoea during vomiting, otherwise intermittently large, irregular excursions and smaller, more regular ones.
Heart rate	Baseline heart rate 160–170 bpm with an amplitude of long-term variability $\leqslant$ 10 bpm. Concomitant with the vomiting and the apnoea there were marked decelerations.
tc$P\text{O}_2$	From a peak of 90 mm Hg (12.0 kPa) tc$P\text{O}_2$ fell to 40 mm Hg (5.3 kPa) after the vomiting and apnoea.

Comments In this example vomiting was accompanied by apnoea and marked decelerations. In Fig. 6.1.2.b the findings during vomiting were less dramatic.

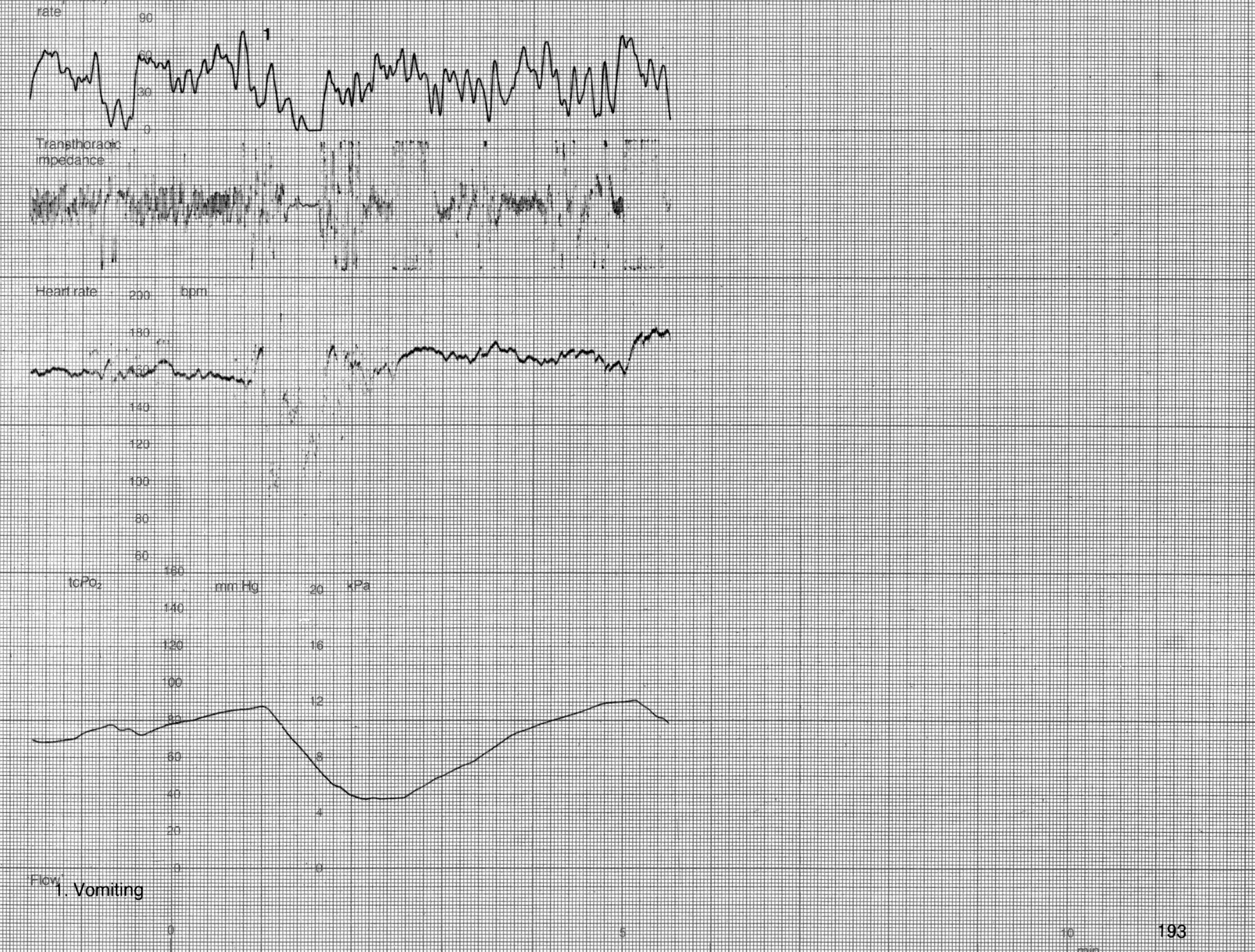
Respiratory rate
breaths/min
120
90
60
30
0
1
Transthoracic impedance
Heart rate
bpm
200
180
160
140
120
100
80
60
tcPo2
mm Hg
kPa
160
140
120
100
80
60
40
20
0
20
16
12
8
4
0
Flow
1. Vomiting
0
5
10
min

9 Cardiorespiratory problems

Fig. 9.1.1

Birthweight: 3020 g

Apgar score: 9/4/7

Age at recording: 30 min

Delivery: vaginal

Cord blood acid – base and blood gases							
	pH	P_{CO_2}	mm Hg	kPa	P_{O_2}	mm Hg	kPa	Base deficit mmol/l
Umbilical artery	7.32		48	6.4		16	2.1	1.7
Umbilical vein	7.44		29	3.9		34	4.5	4.0

Activity state	Awake, unquiet and awake, quiet.
Respiratory rate	About 25 breaths/min in the unquiet period and 35 breaths/min in the quiet period and when given oxygen (Monitor II).
Transthoracic impedance	Cycles of large irregular excursions and short periods of apnoea in the unquiet period, smaller, but still irregular excursions in the quiet phase. A tendency to periodic breathing.
Heart rate	Baseline heart rate about 165 bpm with an amplitude of long-term variability of about 10 bpm in the unquiet phase. Decrease to 140 bpm in the quiet phase and when breathing oxygen. Frequent minute decelerations became even more frequent during the oxygen breathing.
tcP_{O_2}	The level of tcP_{O_2} was 14 mm Hg (1.9 kPa) when the infant breathed air and gradually increased to 88 mm Hg (11.7 kPa) when given oxygen. From this a shunt of 45 per cent is calculated.

Case history The umbilical cord was wound twice round the neck. Amniotic fluid was heavily stained by meconium. The girl was cyanotic in the first minute of life and developed retractions and periodic breathing which was reduced after oxygen administration. Clinical diagnosis: aspiration.

Comments The abnormality in this oxygen-cardiorespirogram from an infant with aspiration is the low tcP_{O_2} value of 14 mm Hg (1.9 kPa), the slow increase after oxygen was given and the low peak value. The repeated decelerations in heart rate during oxygen administration draw attention to themselves but their interpretation is uncertain.

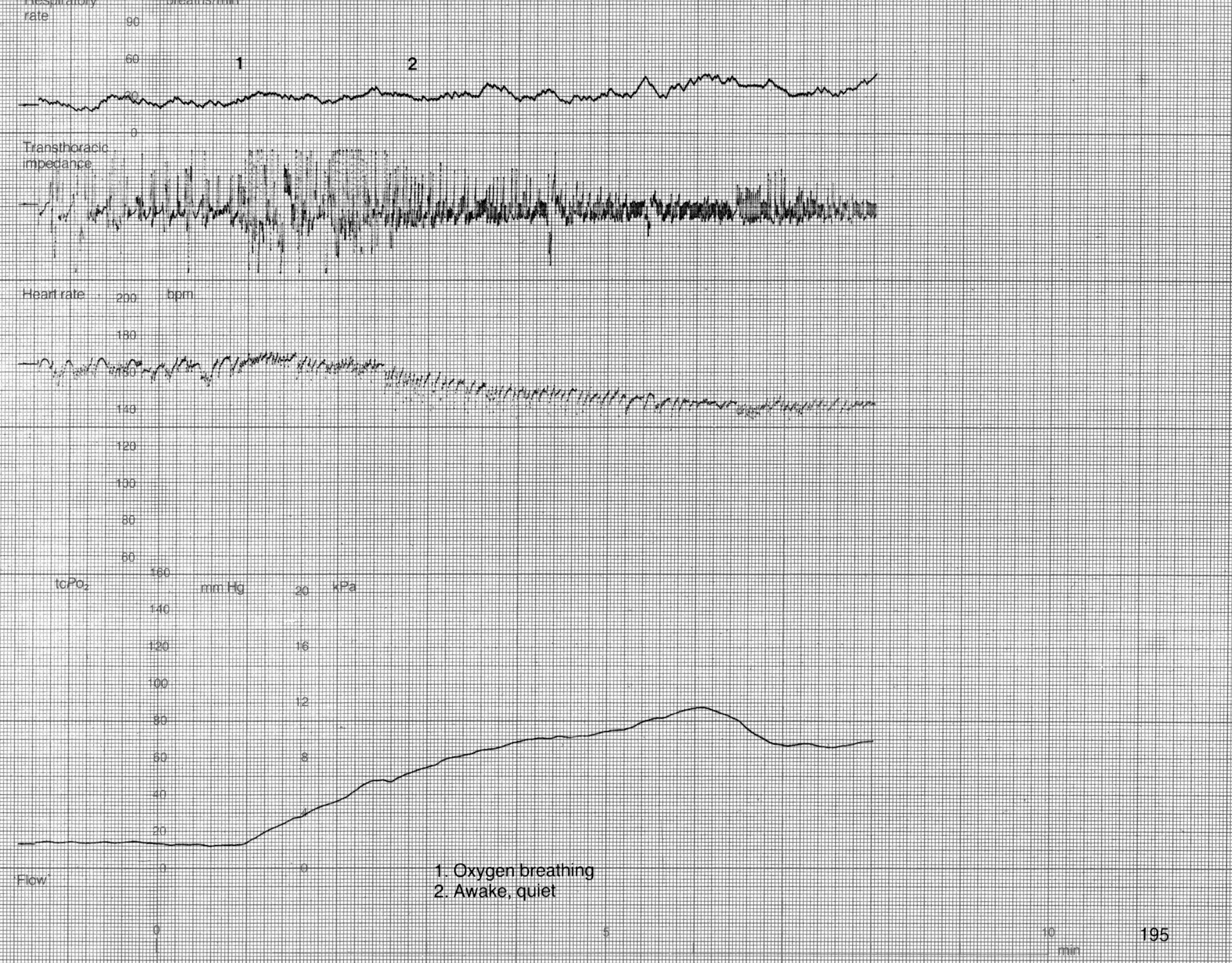

Respiratory rate
breaths/min
90
60
30
0
1
2
Transthoracic impedance
Heart rate
200
bpm
180
160
140
120
100
80
60
tcPo_2
160
mm Hg
20
kPa
140
120
16
100
12
80
60
8
40
4
20
0
0
Flow
1. Oxygen breathing
2. Awake, quiet
0
5
10
min

Fig. 9.1.2.a

Birthweight: 2550 g
Apgar score: 8/9/10
Age (in hours) at recording: 11
Delivery: vaginal (breech)

Activity state	Awake, unquiet (grunting).
Respiratory rate	Mostly between 45 and 60 breaths/min (Monitor II).
Transthoracic impedance	Mainly regular excursions but frequent deeper and irregular ones, sometimes associated with apnoea.
Heart rate	Baseline heart rate was about 180 bpm with an amplitude of long-term variability $\leqslant$ 15 bpm. No decrease in heart rate was seen when oxygen was given. There were occasional decelerations synchronous to the deeper breaths.
tc$P\text{O}_2$	From a plateau of 56 mm Hg (7.5 kPa) tc$P\text{O}_2$ fell to 51 mm Hg (6.8 kPa) after a short apnoea. During the oxygen test there was a rapid increase in tc$P\text{O}_2$ to a peak value of 280 mm Hg (37.3 kPa). From this a shunt of 26 per cent is calculated.

Comments See Fig. 9.1.2.b.

Case history Spontaneous onset of labour in the 34th week of gestation. Breech delivery with the cord once around the neck. Initially no clinical symptoms but during the first day the infant developed gruntings and retractions and was referred to the Children's Hospital. Clinical diagnosis: respiratory distress syndrome.

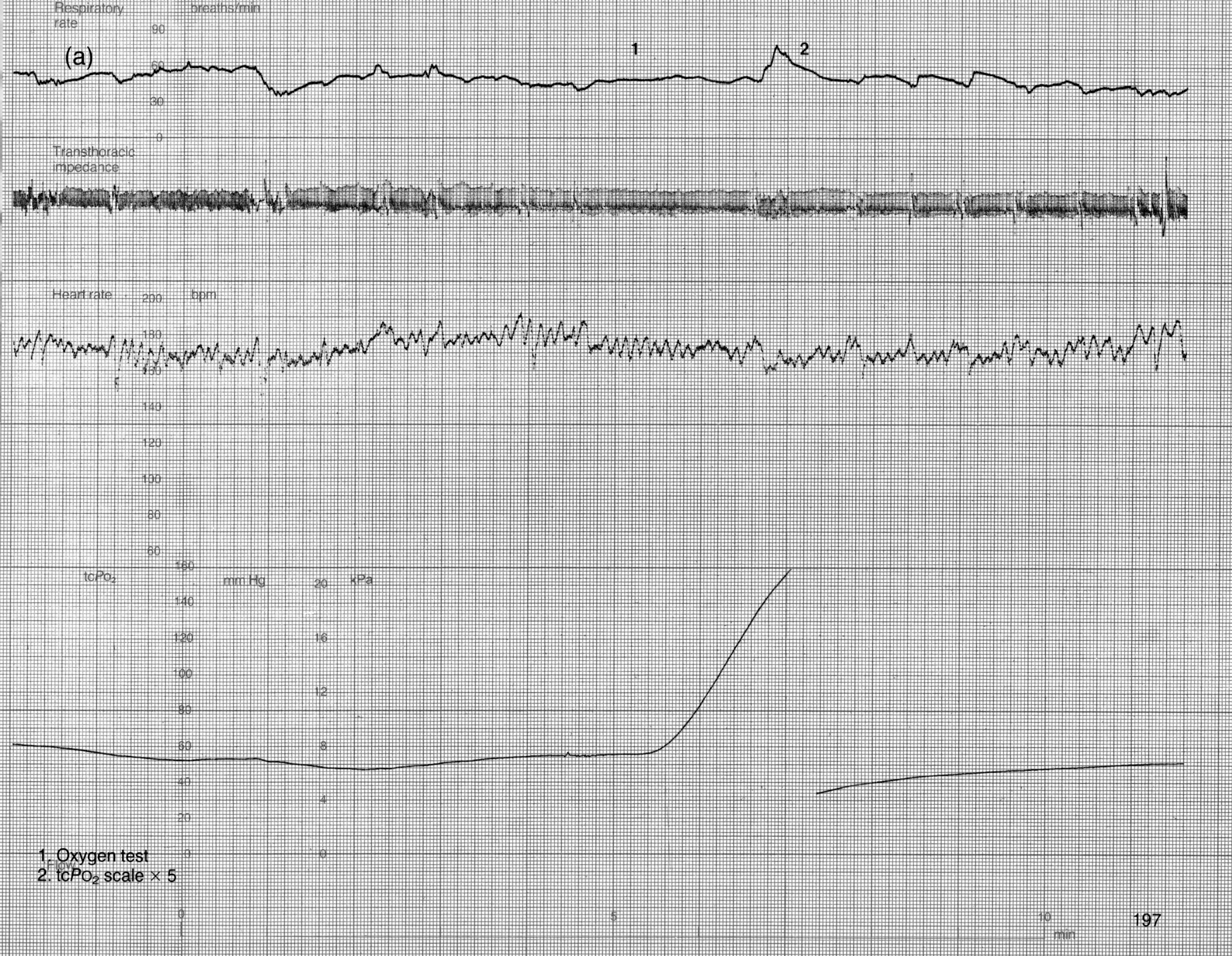

Respiratory rate
breaths/min
90
(a)
1
2
60
30
0
Transthoracic impedance
Heart rate
200
bpm
180
160
140
120
100
80
60
160
tc$P$o$_2$
mm Hg
20
kPa
140
120
16
100
12
80
60
8
40
4
20
0
0
1. Oxygen test
2. tc$P$o$_2$ scale × 5
0
5
10
min

Fig. 9.1.2.b

a continuation of the record in Fig. 9.1.2.a.

Age (in hours) at recording:	11

Activity state	Awake, unquiet (grunting).
Respiratory rate	Mostly about 45 breaths/min, but occasionally as fast as 90 breaths/min. (Monitor II.)
Transthoracic impedance	Partly regular, partly irregular.
Heart rate	Baseline heart rate 190 bpm with an amplitude of long-term variability $\leqslant$ 15 bpm.
tc$P\text{O}_2$	Between 60 and 72 mm Hg (8.0 and 9.6 kPa). Simultaneous arterial and transcutaneous $P\text{O}_2$ were 56 and 60 mm Hg (7.5 and 8.0 kPa) respectively.
	Neonatal arterial acid–base and blood gases: pH, 7.29; $P\text{CO}_2$, 38 mm Hg (5.1 kPa); $P\text{O}_2$, 56 mm Hg (7.5 kPa); base deficit, 7.2 mmol/l.

For neonatal data see Fig. 9.1.2.a.

Comments (a and b) These two oxygen-cardiorespirograms from the same infant are shown in order to illustrate both the oxygen test and the simultaneous arterial and transcutaneous $P\text{O}_2$ measurements.

This infant had clinical symptoms of respiratory distress syndrome, but both transcutaneous and arterial $P\text{O}_2$ were within normal limits. The high heart rate was the only conspicuous finding in these oxygen-cardiorespirograms. In view of the high heart rate the amplitude of the variability was larger than expected.

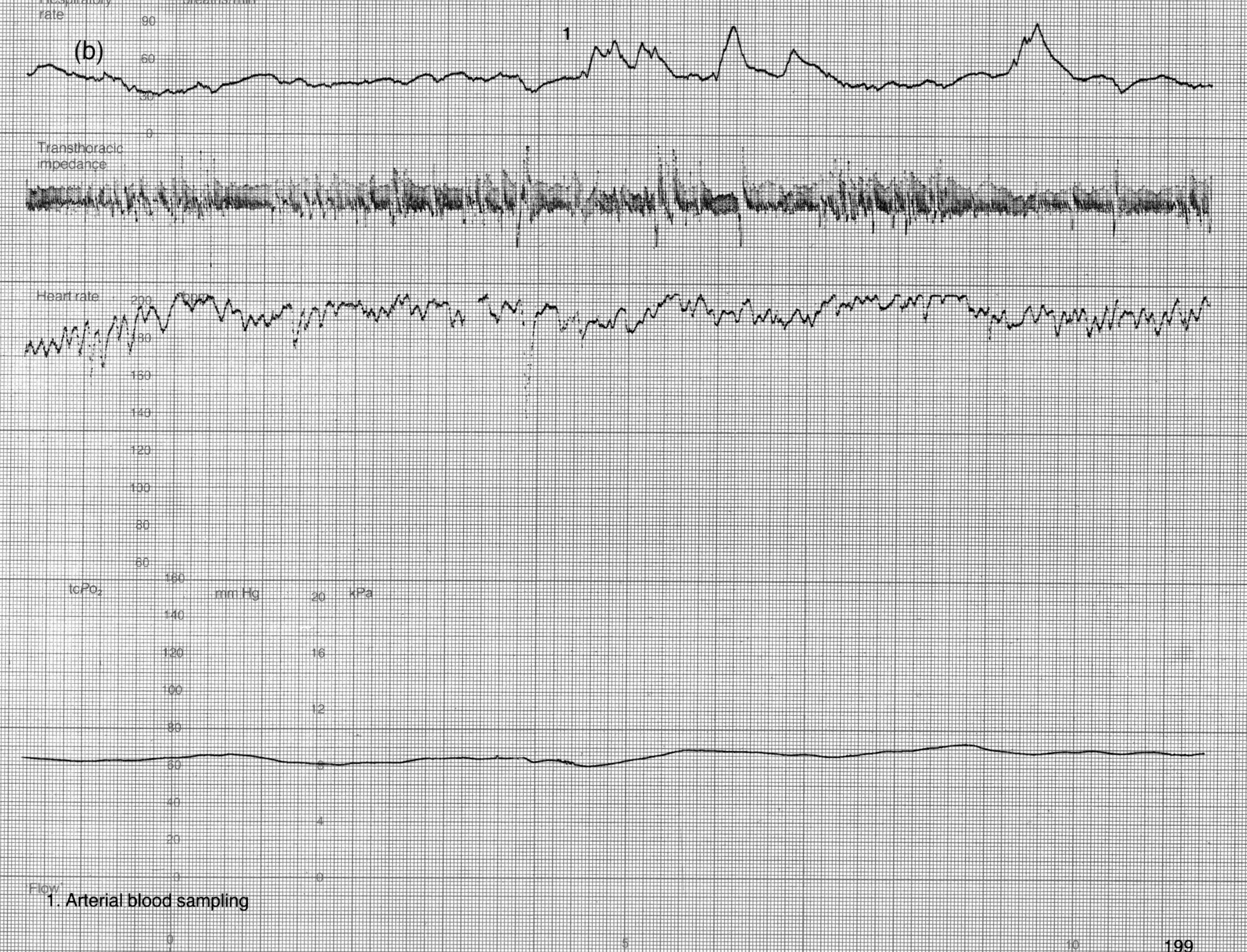

Respiratory rate
breaths/min
(b)
1
90
60
30
0
Transthoracic impedance
Heart rate
200
180
160
140
120
100
80
60
tcPo2
mm Hg
kPa
160
140
120
100
80
60
40
20
0
20
16
12
8
4
0
Flow
1. Arterial blood sampling
0
5
10
min

Fig. 9.1.3

Birthweight: 2800 g

Apgar score: 10/9/10

Age (in hours) at recording: 1

Delivery: vaginal

Cord blood acid – base and blood gases

	pH	P_{CO_2} mm Hg	kPa	P_{O_2} mm Hg	kPa	Base deficit mmol/l
Umbilical artery	7.32	40	5.3	20	2.7	5.1
Umbilical vein	7.40	27	3.6	25	3.3	7.5

Activity state	Awake, unquiet (grunting).
Respiratory rate	About 45 breaths/min in the quiet phase and cyclic changes between 15 and 55 breaths/min during grunting.
Transthoracic impedance	Periodic changes in the amplitude of the excursions.
Heart rate	Baseline heart rate was about 160 bpm with shallow decelerations down to 150 bpm during the grunting. The amplitude of the long-term variability $\leqslant$ 10 bpm.
tcP_{O_2}	There was a gradual fall in the level of tcP_{O_2} from 60 to 50 mm Hg (8.0 to 6.7 kPa). Simultaneous arterial blood P_{O_2} and transcutaneous P_{O_2} were 42 and 51 mm Hg (5.6 and 6.8 kPa) respectively.

Neonatal arterial acid–base and blood gases

Age (in hours)	pH	P_{CO_2} mm Hg	kPa	P_{O_2} mm Hg	kPa	Base deficit mmol/l
1	7.18	64	8.5	42	5.6 (in air)	4.6
2	7.20	63	8.4	87	11.6 (in 100% O_2)	3.7

Case history The mother of this infant had a cervical incompetence and premature labour could not be prevented by tocolysis. Delivery was in the 36th week of gestation. The neonatal status was normal but within one hour grunting and retractions appeared.

Comments This recording was from a case of respiratory distress syndrome at the onset of the symptoms. The grunting was indicated in the transthoracic impedance, but was of course much more evident clinically. The oxygen level was low and the oxygen test in particular indicated a large functional right–left shunt calculated as 43 per cent from the blood gas values given above.

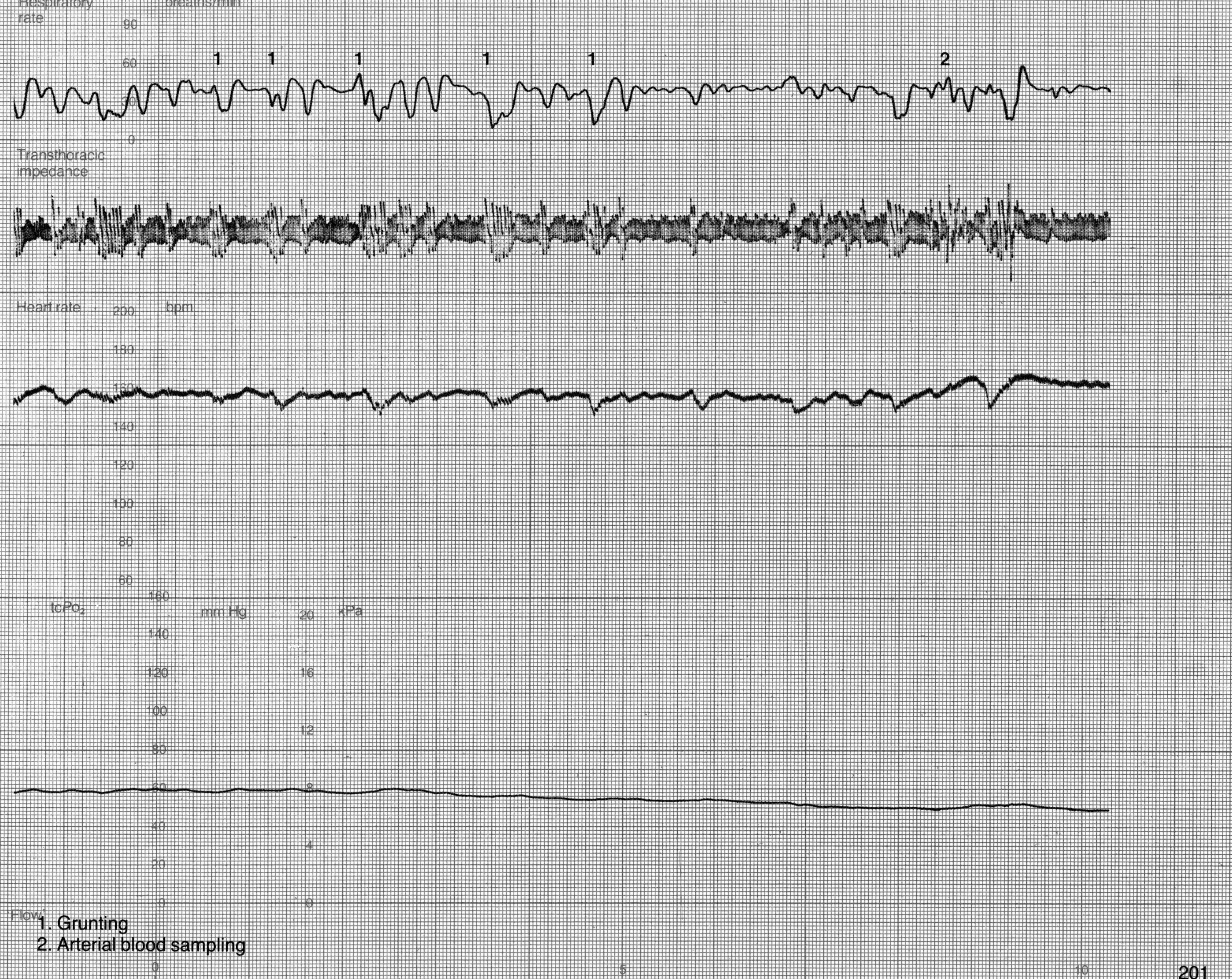

1. Grunting
2. Arterial blood sampling

Fig. 9.1.4

Birthweight: 2249 g

Apgar score: 7/9/9

Age (in hours) at recording: 1

Delivery: vaginal

Cord blood acid – base and blood gases

	pH	PCO$_2$ mm Hg	kPa	PO$_2$ mm Hg	kPa	Base deficit mmol/l
Umbilical artery	7.22	52	6.9	19	2.5	6.1
Umbilical vein	7.26	46	6.1	20	2.7	6.2

Activity state	Asleep (grunting).
Respiratory rate	About 40 breaths/min, occasionally slower.
Transthoracic impedance	The pattern was regular but with occasional larger, irregular excursions.
Heart rate	Baseline heart rate was about 150 bpm before and 140 bpm during the oxygen test and the amplitude of the long-term variability was 5 to 10 bpm.
tc$P$O$_2$	Between 67 and 60 mm Hg (8.9 and 8.0 kPa) and rapid increase during the oxygen test to a peak value of 285 mm Hg (38.0 kPa). From this a shunt of 26 per cent is calculated. Simultaneous arterial blood PO$_2$ and transcutaneous PO$_2$, 57 and 61 mm Hg (7.6 and 8.1 kPa) respectively.
	Neonatal arterial acid–base and blood gases: pH, 7.11; PCO$_2$, 73 mm Hg (9.7 kPa); PO$_2$, 57 mm Hg (7.6 kPa); base deficit, 5.4 mmol/l.

Case history This boy was born prematurely in the 36th week of gestation. Within one hour he developed grunting, retractions and was hypotonic. He was referred to the Children's Hospital. Clinical diagnosis: respiratory distress syndrome.

Comments The amplitude of long-term variability was small and there was a tachycardia but there were no gross pathological findings in this oxygen-cardiorespirogram from an infant which clinically had respiratory distress syndrome.

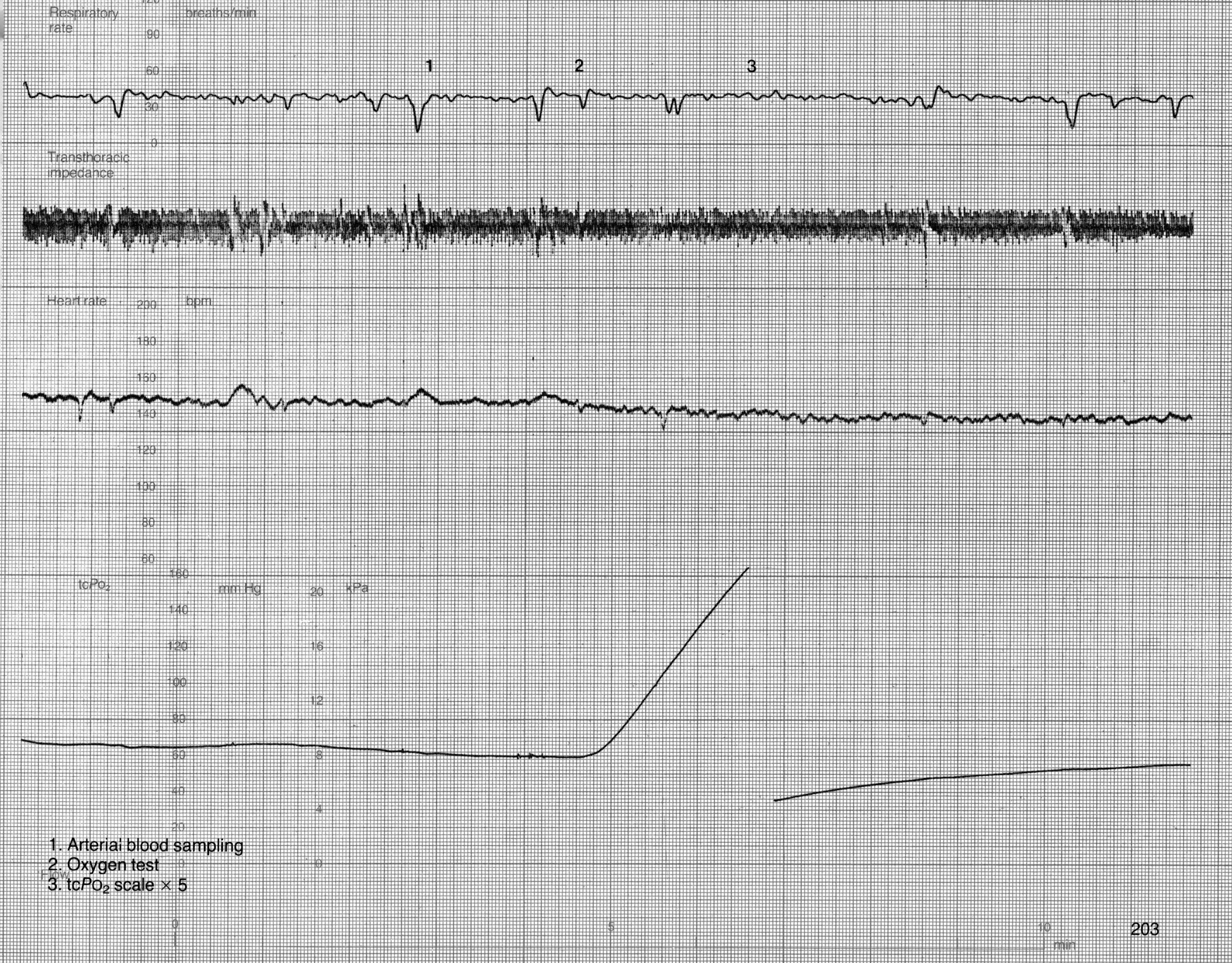
Respiratory rate
breaths/min
90
60
30
0
1
2
3
Transthoracic impedance
Heart rate
bpm
200
180
160
140
120
100
80
60
tcPo2
mm Hg
kPa
160
140
120
100
80
60
40
20
0
20
16
12
8
4
0
1. Arterial blood sampling
2. Oxygen test
3. tcPo2 scale × 5
0
5
10
min

Fig. 9.1.5

Birthweight: 3030 g

Apgar score: 4/8/10

Age (in hours) at recording: 1

Delivery: Caesarean section

Cord blood acid – base and blood gases							
	pH	P_{CO_2}	mm Hg	kPa	P_{O_2}	mm Hg	kPa	Base deficit mmol/l
Umbilical artery	7.28		60	8.0		25	3.3	−1.5

Activity state	Awake, unquiet, crying and grunting.
Respiratory rate	Cyclic changes mainly between 30 and > 100 breaths/min, slower during crying.
Transthoracic impedance	Short periods of rather regular excursions intercepted by larger, irregular ones. Distinct periodicity. During crying only irregular excursions.
Heart rate	Baseline heart rate about 135 bpm with an amplitude of long-term variability ≤ 10 bpm in the quiet periods. Accelerations to 150 bpm during crying. During oxygen breathing baseline heart rate was about 125 bpm.
tcP_{O_2}	About 40 mm Hg (5.3 kPa) and increased to 225 mm Hg (30.0 kPa) during the oxygen test. From this a shunt of 28 per cent is calculated.
	Neonatal arterial acid–base and blood gases (sampling subsequent to figure): pH, 7.26; P_{CO_2}, 46 mm Hg (6.1 kPa); P_{O_2}, 25 mm Hg (3.3 kPa); base deficit, 5.1 mmol/l.

Case history This boy was born in the 37th week of gestation because of spontaneous onset of labour. A repeat Caesarean section was performed. In the first hour of life grunting and retractions developed. He was referred to the Children's Hospital. Clinical diagnosis: respiratory distress syndrome.

Comments Oxygen-cardiorespirogram from a prematurely born infant with clinical symptoms of respiratory distress syndrome. There was a periodicity in the respiration with tachypnoea. The tcP_{O_2} level was only 40 mm Hg (5.3 kPa) and the small increase during the oxygen test indicated a large functional shunt.

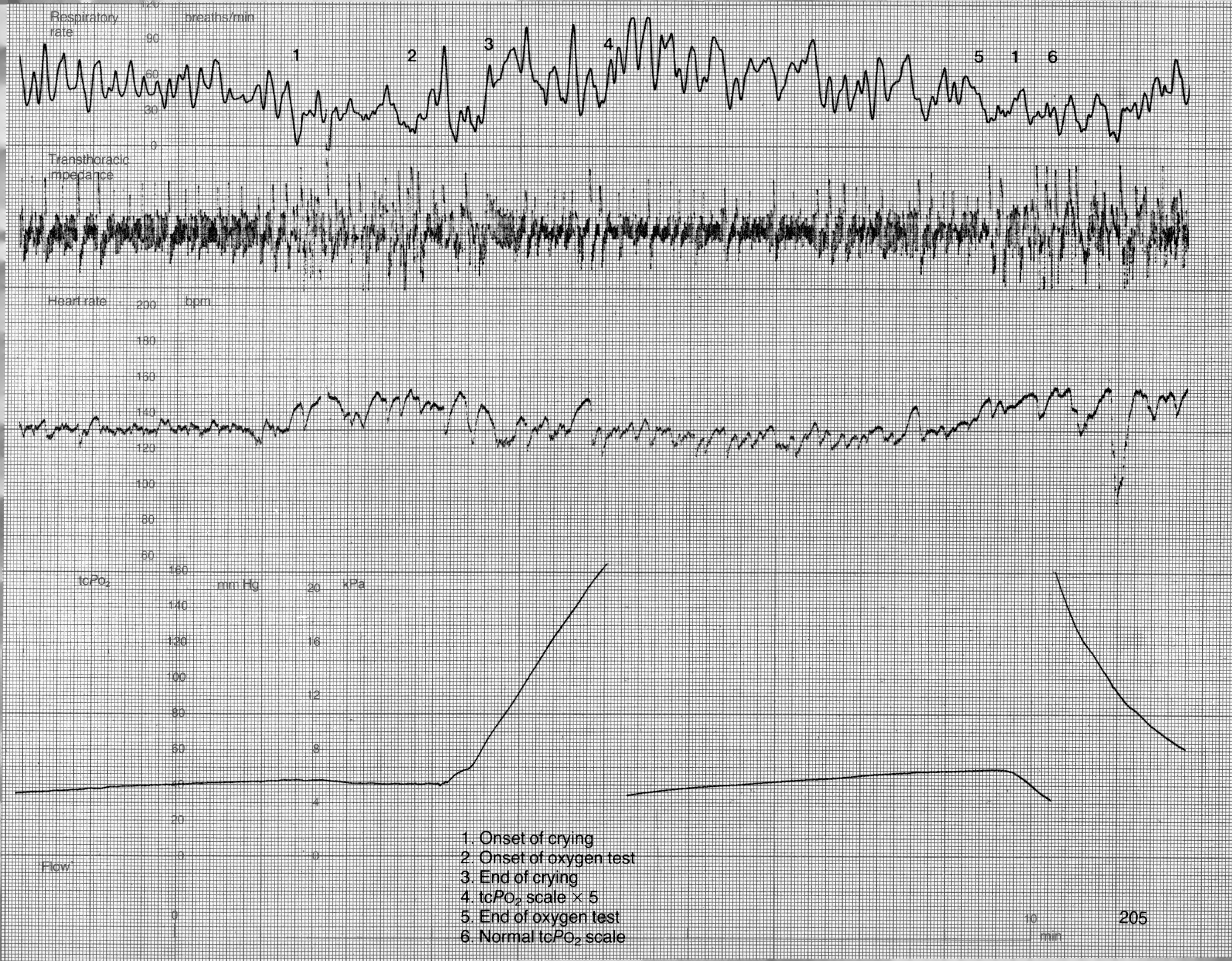

Respiratory rate
breaths/min
120
90
60
30
0
1
2
3
4
5
1
6
Transthoracic impedance
Heart rate
bpm
200
180
160
140
120
100
80
60
$tcPo_2$
mm Hg
kPa
160
140
120
100
80
60
40
20
0
20
16
12
8
4
0
'Flow'
0
10
min
1. Onset of crying
2. Onset of oxygen test
3. End of crying
4. $tcPo_2$ scale × 5
5. End of oxygen test
6. Normal $tcPo_2$ scale

Fig. 9.1.6

Birthweight: 2880 g

Apgar score: 9/10

Age (in hours) at recording:	3

Delivery: vaginal

Cord blood acid – base and blood gases							
	pH	$P\text{CO}_2$	mm Hg	kPa	$P\text{O}_2$	mm Hg	kPa	Base deficit mmol/l
Umbilical artery	7.28		38	5.1		32	4.1	8.2
Umbilical vein	7.34		30	4.0		35	4.7	8.8

Activity state	Quiet sleep, grunting.
Respiratory rate	About 45 breaths/min in air and 55 breaths/min during the oxygen test.
Transthoracic impedance	Very regular excursions except for some periods of larger excursions and short periods of apnoea.
Heart rate	Baseline heart rate was about 165 bpm with an amplitude of long-term variability $\leqslant 10$. One long and deep deceleration occurred as well as some smaller ones together with apnoea.
tc$P\text{O}_2$	After the onset of the electrode tc$P\text{O}_2$ stabilized initially at a level of 58 mm Hg (7.7 kPa). After the repeated small apnoea tc$P\text{O}_2$ fell to 50 mm Hg (6.7 kPa). During the oxygen test tc$P\text{O}_2$ increased to 275 mm Hg (36.7 kPa). From this a shunt of 26 per cent is calculated.
	Arterial blood sampling was done following the record shown here. Neonatal arterial acid–base and blood gases: pH, 7.23; $P\text{CO}_2$, 57 mm Hg (7.6 kPa); $P\text{O}_2$, 52 mm Hg (6.9 kPa); base deficit, 3.9 mmol/l.

Case history Spontaneous labour began in the 38th week of gestation. Soon after birth the infant developed grunting and retractions.

Comments Oxygen-cardiorespirogram 3 hours after birth from an infant with respiratory distress syndrome. Abnormal tc$P\text{O}_2$ level as well as tachycardia during quiet sleep.

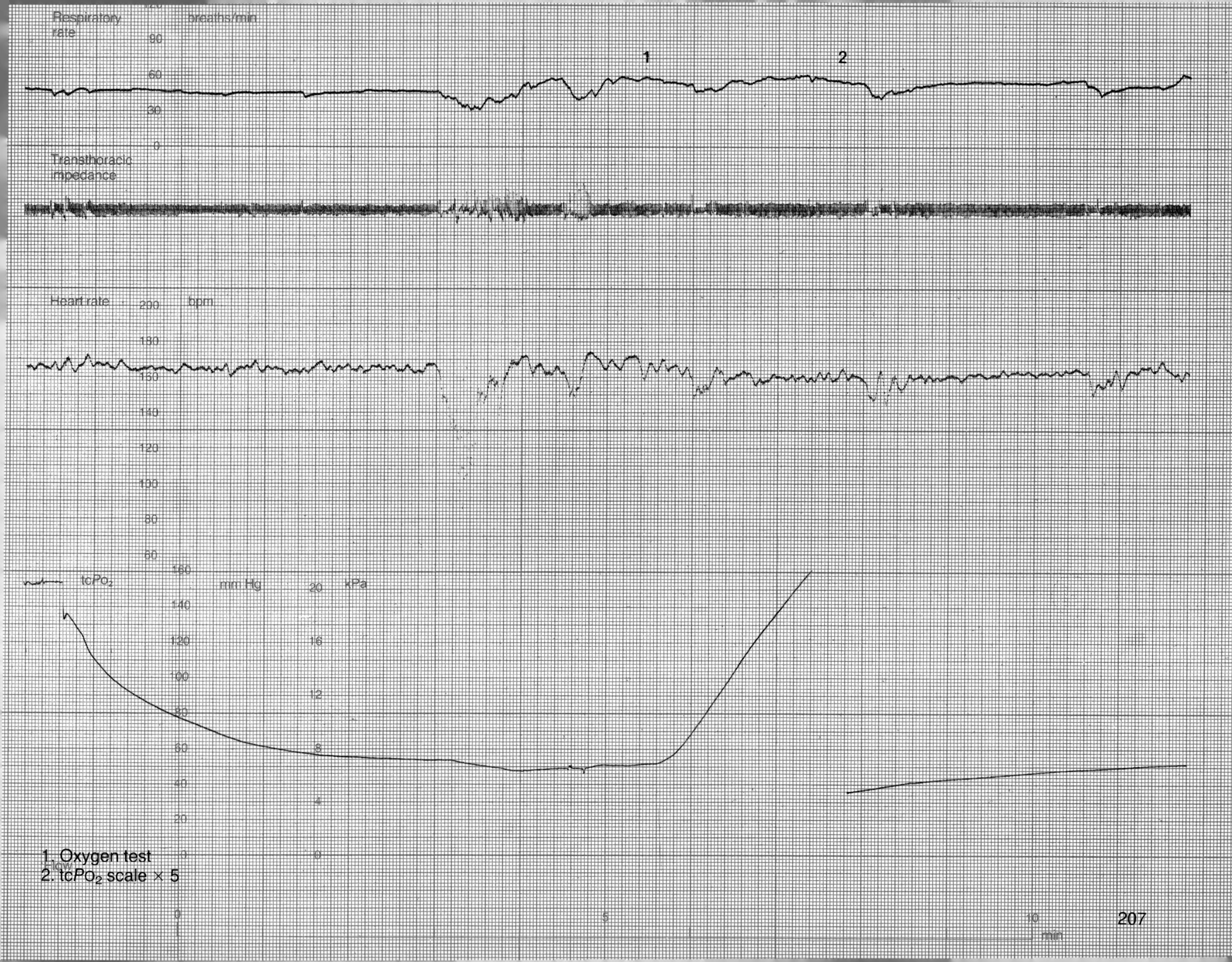
Respiratory rate
breaths/min
90
60
30
0
1
2
Transthoracic impedance
Heart rate
200
bpm
180
160
140
120
100
80
60
tcPo2
160
mm Hg
20
kPa
140
120
16
100
12
80
60
8
40
4
20
0
0
1. Oxygen test
2. tcPo2 scale × 5
0
5
10
min

Fig. 9.2.1.a

Birthweight: 2280 g

Apgar score: 6/8/10

Age (in hours) at recording: 1

Delivery: Caesarean section

Cord blood acid – base and blood gases							
	pH	$P\text{CO}_2$	mm Hg	kPa	$P\text{O}_2$	mm Hg	kPa	Base deficit mmol/l
Umbilical artery	7.27		52	6.9		24	3.2	3.0
Umbilical vein	7.29		45	6.0		38	5.1	4.7

Activity state	Crying and awake, unquiet.
Respiratory rate	About 40 breaths/min during crying and up to 50 breaths/min when not crying (Monitor II).
Transthoracic impedance	Irregular excursions all the time and with large amplitude during crying intercepted by short periods of apnoea.
Heart rate	When not crying baseline heart rate was about 100 bpm with an amplitude of long-term variability $\leqslant$ 25 bpm. During crying heart rate was 135 bpm and with accelerations coinciding with periods of apnoea in between the intense crying.
tc$P\text{O}_2$	The level of tc$P\text{O}_2$ was between 35 and 50 mm Hg (4.7 and 6.7 kPa). During the oxygen test there was a slow increase up to 84 mm Hg (11.2 kPa). From this a shunt of 44 per cent is calculated.

Case history In the 41st week of gestation there were signs of intrauterine distress and a Caesarean section was performed. The girl was low birthweight for gestational age. Clinically no abnormality was noted in the first hour. The low tc$P\text{O}_2$ values in air and the very abnormal oxygen test were reconfirmed at 3 and 5 hours of life and the girl was referred to cardiologists at the Children's Hospital. Clinical diagnosis: tetralogy of Fallot.

Comments See Fig. 9.2.1.b.

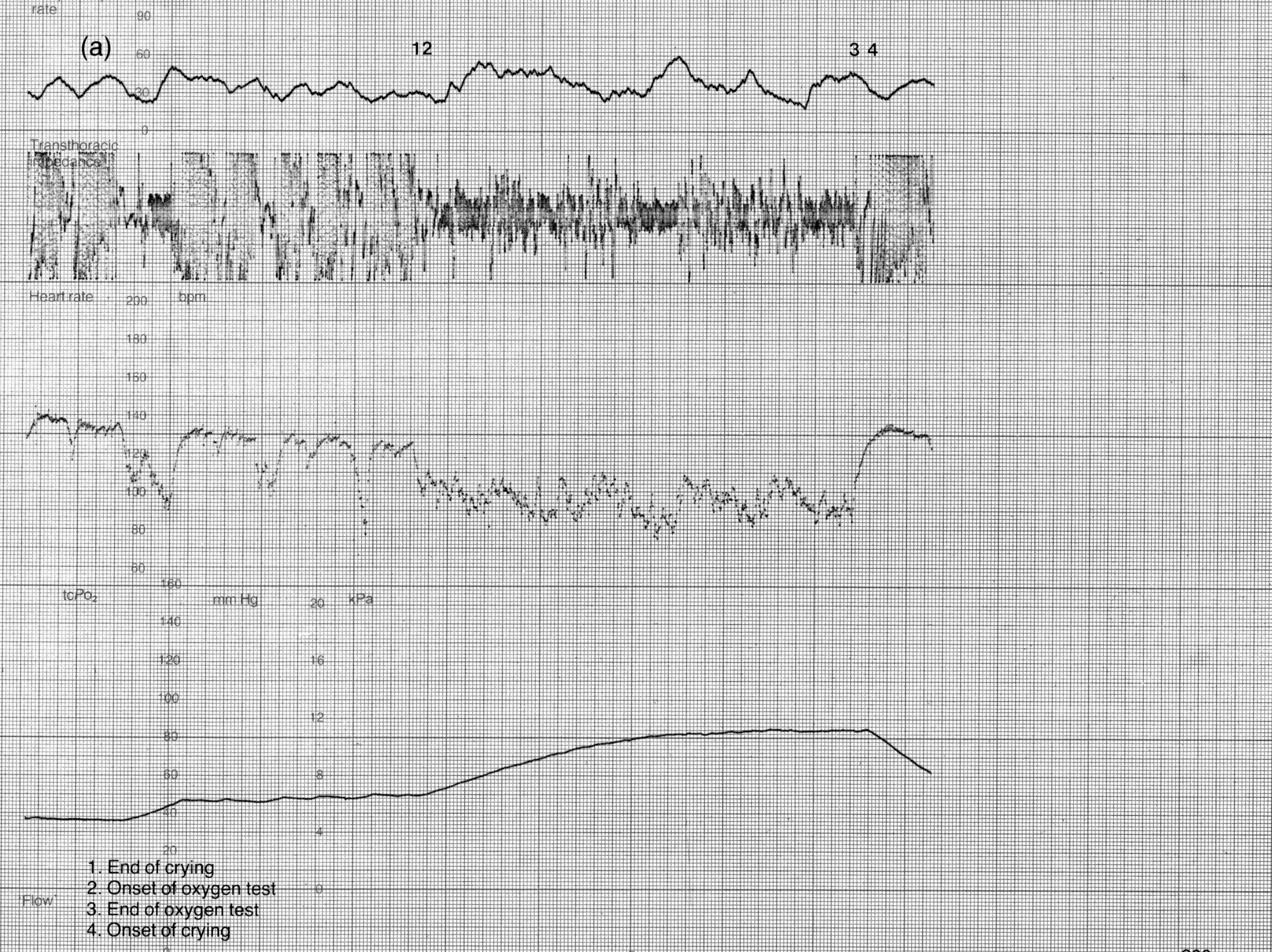

Respiratory rate
breaths/min
(a)
90
60
30
0
1 2
3 4
Transthoracic impedance
Heart rate
bpm
200
180
160
140
120
100
80
60
tcP_{O_2}
mm Hg
kPa
160
140
120
100
80
60
40
20
20
16
12
8
4
0
1. End of crying
2. Onset of oxygen test
3. End of oxygen test
4. Onset of crying
'Flow'
0
5
10
min

Fig. 9.2.1.b

obtained 10 min after Fig. 9.2.1.a.

Age (in hours) at recording:	1

Activity state	Awake, unquiet and crying.
Respiratory rate	About 35 breaths/min (Monitor II).
Transthoracic impedance	Irregular excursions, larger during crying.
Heart rate	When not crying, baseline heart rate was about 100 bpm with an amplitude of long-term variability $\leqslant$ 20 bpm. During crying heart rate attained 145 bpm.
tcP_{O_2}	From a level of 53 mm Hg (7.1 kPa) tcP_{O_2} fell to 32 mm Hg (4.1 kPa) during crying. Simultaneous arterial P_{O_2} and transcutaneous P_{O_2} were 36 and 39 mm Hg respectively (4.8 and 5.2 kPa).
	Neonatal arterial acid–base and blood gases: pH, 7.39; P_{CO_2}, 31 mm Hg (4.1 kPa); P_{O_2}, 36 mm Hg (4.8 kPa); base deficit, 5.0 mmol/l.

For neonatal data and case history see Fig. 9.2.1.a.

Comments (a and b) Two figures are shown from the same infant in order to illustrate the large right–left shunt as manifested during the oxygen test in **a** and the simultaneous arterial and transcutaneous P_{O_2} in **b**. The most important finding in both oxygen-cardiorespirograms is the low tcP_{O_2} level in air.

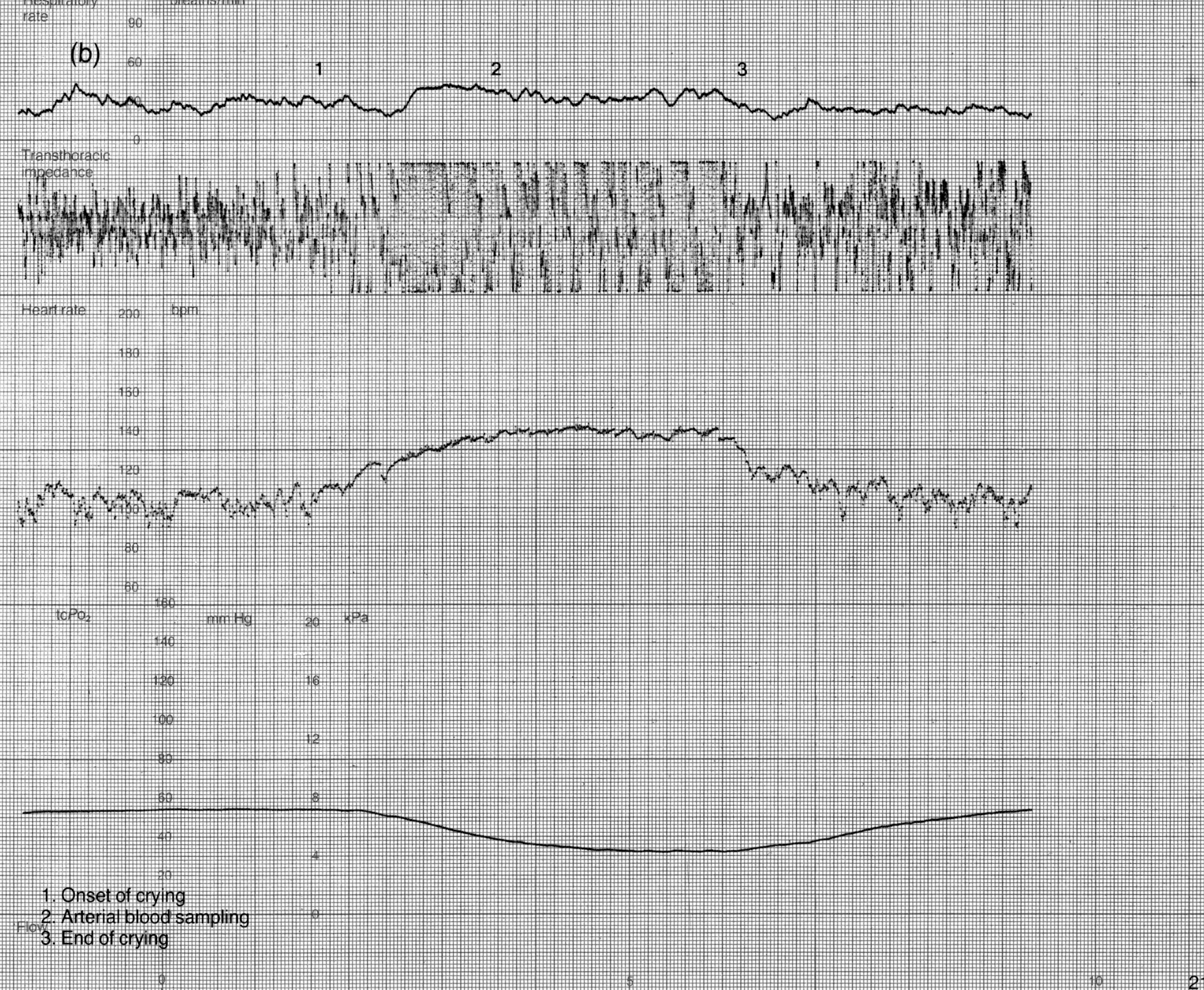

Respiratory rate
breaths/min
120
90
60
30
0
(b)
1
2
3
Transthoracic impedance
Heart rate
bpm
200
180
160
140
120
100
80
60
$tcPo_2$
mm Hg
kPa
160
140
120
100
80
60
40
20
20
16
12
8
4
0
1. Onset of crying
2. Arterial blood sampling
3. End of crying
Flow
0
5
10
min

Fig. 9.3.1

Birthweight: 3000 g
Apgar score: 9/5/8
Age (in hours) at recording: 1
Delivery: vaginal

Cord blood acid – base and blood gases							
	pH	$P\text{CO}_2$ mm Hg	kPa	$P\text{O}_2$ mm Hg	kPa	Base deficit mmol/l
Umbilical artery	7.34	44	5.9	21	2.8	2.1
Umbilical vein	7.38	36	4.8	28	3.7	3.7

Activity state	Intermittent crying, awake, quiet.
Respiratory rate	Irregular changes between 5 and 80 breaths/min.
Transthoracic impedance	Partly regular, partly irregular excursions.
Heart rate	Heart rate was about 160 bpm but fell to 135 bpm when the infant was quieter. Occasional shallow decelerations. The amplitude of long-term variability was $\leq$ 10 bpm.
tc$P\text{O}_2$	The level of tc$P\text{O}_2$ fell to 25 mm Hg (3.3 kPa) in the most unquiet phase and rose to 40 mm Hg (5.3 kPa) in the most quiet phase. Simultaneous arterial blood $P\text{O}_2$ and transcutaneous $P\text{O}_2$ were 35 and 25 mm Hg respectively (4.7 and 3.3 kPa).
	Neonatal arterial acid–base and blood gases: pH, 7.25; $P\text{CO}_2$, 51 mm Hg (6.8 kPa); $P\text{O}_2$, 35 mm Hg (4.7 kPa); base deficit, 3.8 mmol/l.

Case history Spontaneous delivery in the 36th week of gestation. Immediately after birth the infant became hypotonic. The haemoglobin concentration in the cord blood was 120 g/l and 1 hour after birth it was 116 g/l in the arterial blood.

Comments The only pathological sign in this oxygen-cardiorespirogram was the low tc$P\text{O}_2$ value when the infant breathed air. Almost as low a value was found in the arterial blood. During the oxygen test performed after the recording shown the peak value was 330 mm Hg (44.0 kPa) and from this a shunt of 23 per cent was calculated.

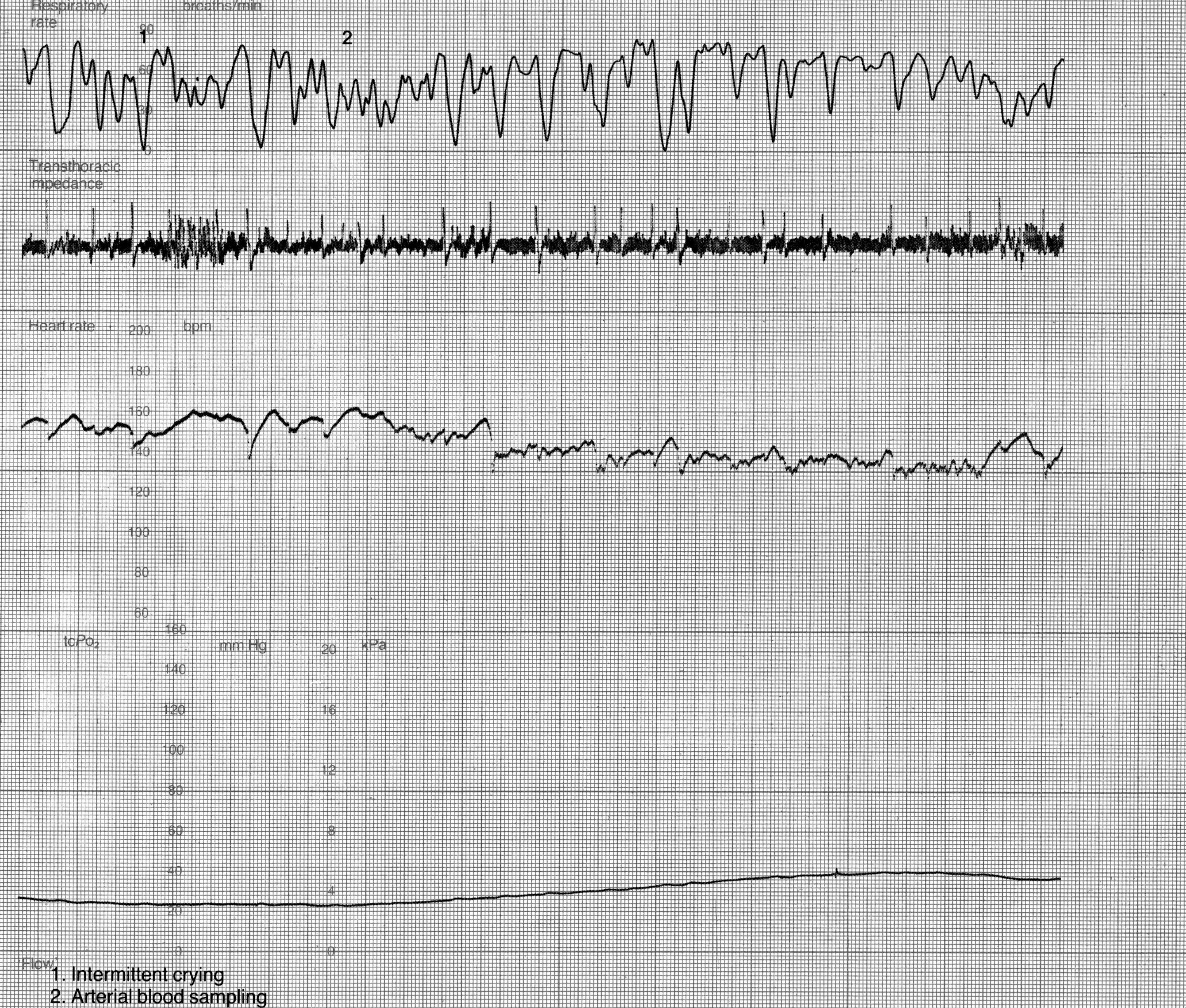
Respiratory rate
breaths/min
Transthoracic impedance
Heart rate
bpm
tcPo2
mm Hg
kPa
Flow
1. Intermittent crying
2. Arterial blood sampling
min

10 Statistical analysis

The oxygen-cardiorespiograms in Chapters 4–9 show what is encountered at different times after birth as well as in different clinical conditions.

10.1 Influence of time after birth on baseline heart rate, respiratory rate and tcP_{O_2}

In order to describe what is normal for the different variables in the oxygen-cardiorespirogram in the first week of life we shall at first present an analysis of healthy infants with the following criteria.

1. Vaginal deliveries.
2. Apgar score ⩾7 at 1 min.
3. Birthweight ⩾2500 g.

The influence of an activity on the different variables of the oxygen-cardiorespirogram was demonstrated in Chapter 4. In the subsequent analysis we have therefore only used those periods from the records in which the infants were quiet, i.e. awake, quiet and both sleep states.

The oxygen-cardiorespirograms were recorded at different times after birth. Grouping into time periods was done as exemplified in Fig. 10.1.1 and Table 10.1.1. The age group > 120 hours refers to data obtained between 5 and 7 days after birth for the vaginal deliveries and 5 and 10 days for the Caesarean sections.

When repeated measurements were made on the same infant the result was only used once for statistical comparisons of the means at different times after birth.

10.1.1 Baseline heart rate

Fig. 10.1.1 and Table 10.1.1 give the mean baseline heart rate in the different time groups. Quiet, undisturbed infants could only occasionally be monitored in the first 30 minutes after birth. Therefore the time group 0–1 hour only refers to measurements done in the second half of the first hour of life. However, in 72 infants data were obtained from between 20 and 30 minutes after birth. These are included in Figs. 10.1.1–3, 10.1.6, 10.1.9 and the appropriate tables.

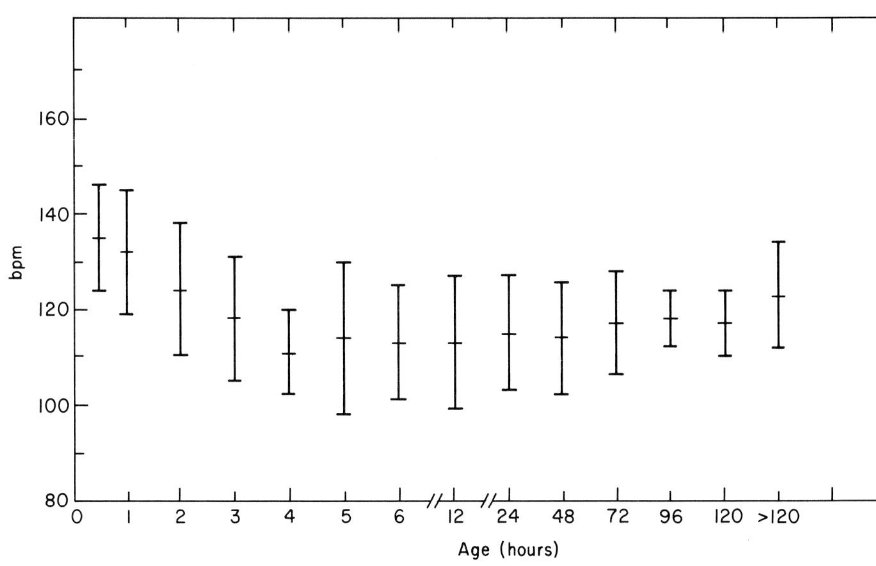

Fig. 10.1.1 Baseline heart rate.*

*If not otherwise stated the figures give mean ± s.d.

Table 10.1.1 Baseline heart rate (vaginal deliveries, Apgar score $\geqslant 7$, birthweight $\geqslant 2500$ g).

Age in hours	Heart rate mean	s.d.	No
20– 30 min	135	11	72
0– 1	132	13	679
1– 2	124	14	166
2– 3	118	13	131
3– 4	111	9	73
4– 5	114	16	99
5– 6	113	12	98
6– 12	113	14	394
12– 24	115	12	634
24– 48	114	12	131
48– 72	117	11	45
72– 96	118	6	22
96–120	117	7	32
>120	123	11	35

Total number: 2611.

It will be seen in Fig. 10.1.1 that mean baseline heart rate decreased from 135 bpm 20–30 min after birth to 111 bpm after 3–4 hours and then remained at that level although there was a tendency to a subsequent increase. Between 96–120 and >120 hours of life this increase was more pronounced.

Comparing the time intervals 0–1 against 3–4 hours after birth the reduction in the mean baseline heart rate of 21 bpm is significant ($t = 13.5$, $n = 752$, $P < 0.001$). The increase of 9 bpm between 24–48 hours and >120 hours is also significant ($t = 4.0$, $n = 166$, $P < 0.001$).

It should be remembered that these baseline heart rate data were only obtained when the infants were quiet. Thus we have established that in agreement with the findings in the literature there is a fall in the mean baseline heart rate during the first three hours after birth followed by a stable period for the rest of the first day of life. Thereafter a tendency to increased heart rate becomes manifest between the fourth and the fifth day of life.

In view of the large number of infants studied these results should be representative of values to be expected in other healthy, quiet infants. Baseline heart rate values outside the limits $\bar{x} \pm 2$ s.d. should be taken as indications of abnormality, i.e. in the second half hour of life values <105 and >160 bpm and from the third hour of life all through the first week values outside <90 and >140 bpm.

10.1.2 Respiratory rate

Fig. 10.1.2 and Table 10.1.2 give the mean respiratory rate for healthy, quiet infants in the first week of life.

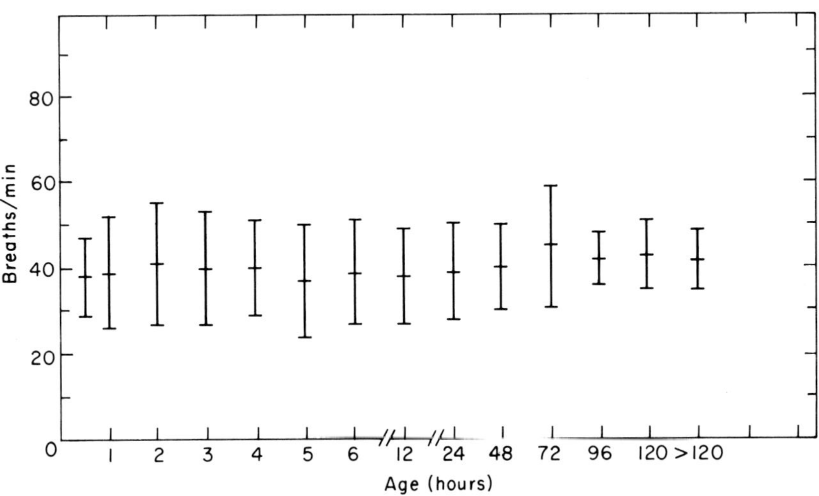

Fig. 10.1.2 Respiratory rate.

We found no tendency to systematic changes in the mean respiratory rate from 20–30 min after birth and all through the first week of life in the infants born after vaginal delivery and with a normal Apgar score. The mean values were close to 40 breaths/min all the time. The decrease in heart rate which was noted from 20 minutes after birth had no equivalent in the respiratory rate.

Table 10.1.2 Respiratory rate (vaginal deliveries, Apgar score ⩾ 7, birth-weight ⩾ 2500 g).

Age in hours	Respiratory rate mean	s.d.	No
20– 30 min	38	9	64
0– 1	39	13	586
1– 2	41	14	152
2– 3	40	13	118
3– 4	40	11	69
4– 5	37	13	87
5– 6	39	12	87
6– 12	38	11	351
12– 24	39	11	555
24– 48	40	10	125
48– 72	45	14	43
72– 96	42	6	22
96–120	43	8	32
>120	42	7	36

Total number: 2327.

Although Fig. 10.1.2 and Table 10.1.2 show very similar mean respiratory rates at the different time periods it should be noted that the variations within each age group are considerable. Because of the large standard deviation and the observation that the distribution is somewhat skewed, the usefulness of the mean values is limited and the data give no clearcut limits for clinical guidance. However, they are in agreement with the clinical experience that a persistent respiratory rate > 60 breaths/min is a warning sign.

As a large part of the variation is due to inter individual variation we have in Chapter 10.6–10.9 studied the changes with time in some individual cases.

10.1.3 tcP_{O_2}

Fig. 10.1.3.1 and Table 10.1.3 give the mean of the highest and the lowest tcP_{O_2} values obtained from each recording as before from healthy, quiet infants. It will be noted that the differences between these two series of mean values are rather constant between 11 and 15 mm Hg (1.5 and 2.0 kPa). In order to stress the fluctuations of tcP_{O_2} even in the quiet infants we have not given the mean tcP_{O_2} value for each recording but rather taken the highest and the lowest tcP_{O_2} observed in each individual infant.

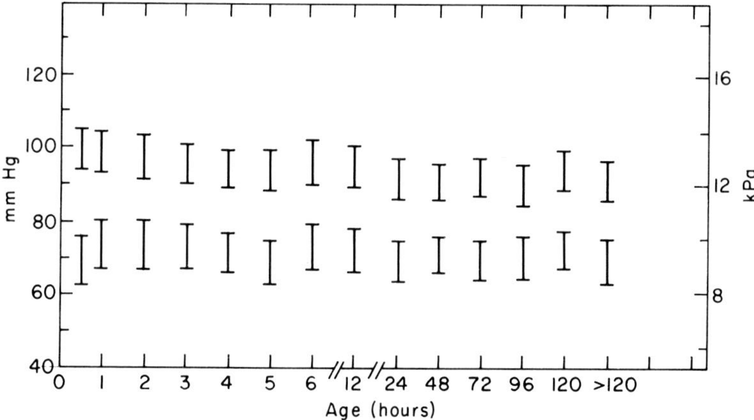

Fig. 10.1.3.1 Highest and lowest tcP_{O_2}.

It will be seen in Fig. 10.1.3.1 that the mean tcP_{O_2} value was highest in the second half hour after birth and that there was a tendency to lower values later. The mean tcP_{O_2} of 93 mm Hg (12.4 kPa) at 0–1 hour after birth was significantly higher than the mean tcP_{O_2} of 86 mm Hg (11.4 kPa) between 12 and 24 hours after birth (t = 11.4, n = 1281, $P < 0.001$).

Table 10.1.3 Highest and lowest tcP_{O_2} (vaginal deliveries, Apgar score ⩾ 7, birthweight ⩾ 2500 g).

Age in hours	Highest tcP_{O_2} mm Hg mean	s.d.	kPa mean	Lowest tcP_{O_2} mm Hg mean	s.d.	kPa mean	No
20– 30 min	94	11	12.5	76	13	10.1	70
0– 1	93	11	12.4	80	13	10.7	666
1– 2	91	12	12.1	80	13	10.7	161
2– 3	90	11	12.0	79	12	10.5	129
3– 4	89	10	11.9	77	11	10.3	75
4– 5	88	11	11.7	75	12	10.0	96
5– 6	90	12	12.0	79	12	10.5	95
6– 12	89	11	11.9	78	12	10.4	382
12– 24	86	11	11.5	75	11	10.0	615
24– 48	86	9	11.5	76	10	10.1	131
48– 72	87	10	11.6	75	11	10.0	44
72– 96	84	11	11.2	76	12	10.1	22
96–120	88	11	11.7	77	10	10.3	30
> 120	86	10	11.5	75	12	10.0	36

Total number: 2552.

The mean of the lowest values observed in the second half of the first hour of life was 80 mm Hg (10.7 kPa) against 75 mm Hg (10.0 kPa) 12–24 hours after birth. This difference is also statistically significant ($t = 7.6$, $n = 1281$, $P < 0.001$).

Thus it appears that during the first hour of life tcP_{O_2} was higher than during the rest of the first week. Comments to this will be given below.

The frequency distributions of all the individual highest and of all the lowest tcP_{O_2} values are shown in Fig. 10.1.3.2. These data are the same as those grouped into time periods in Fig. 10.1.3.1. Both the highest and the lowest tcP_{O_2} values are normally distributed and, as expected from Fig. 10.1.3.1, the frequency distribution for the highest tcP_{O_2} is displaced about 15 mm Hg (2.0 kPa) to the right of that of the lowest tcP_{O_2}.

Fig. 10.1.3.3 illustrates the difference between the highest and the lowest tcP_{O_2} values somewhat differently. Here the individual differences, i.e. the differences between the highest and the lowest tcP_{O_2} values in each case were calculated and the frequency distribution of this is given.

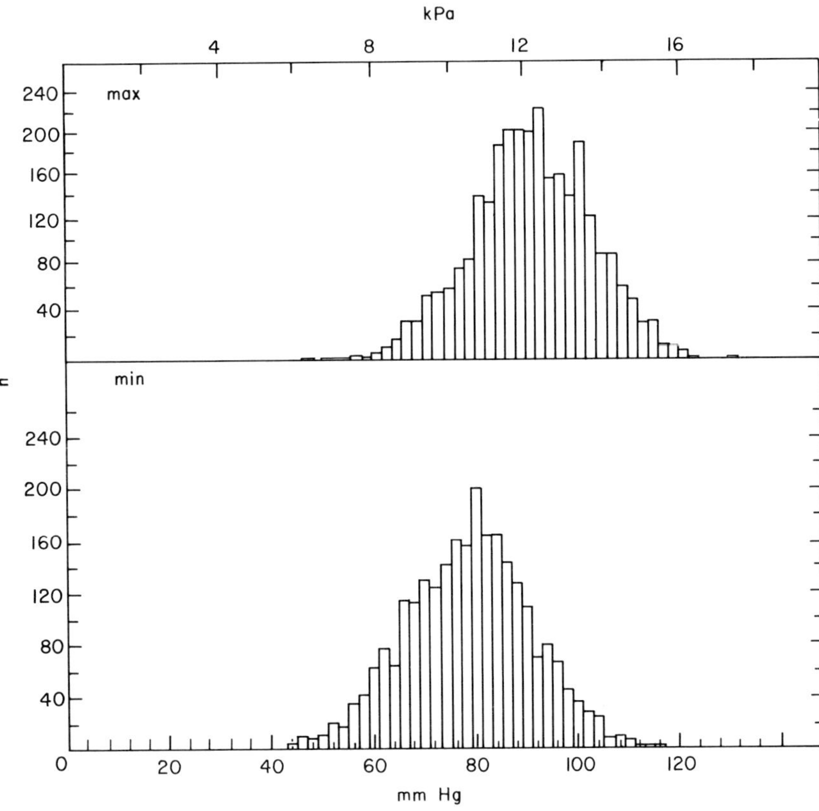

Fig. 10.1.3.2 **Frequency distributions of all the individual highest and lowest tcP_{O_2} values.**

From Figs. 10.1.3.1 and 10.1.3.2 it could be inferred that the mean difference between the highest and the lowest tcP_{O_2} was 15 mm Hg (2.0 kPa). However, the distribution of this difference is skewed as illustrated in Fig. 10.1.3.3. The peak is at 10 mm Hg (1.3 kPa); 92 per cent of the values lie between 0 and 25 mm Hg (0 and 3.3 kPa).

Fig. 10.1.3.3 shows the difference between the highest and the lowest tcP_{O_2} values to be expected in healthy, quiet infants monitored for about one hour during the first week of life. It demonstrates how limited value may be given to any one single P_{O_2} value called 'normal' for healthy infants.

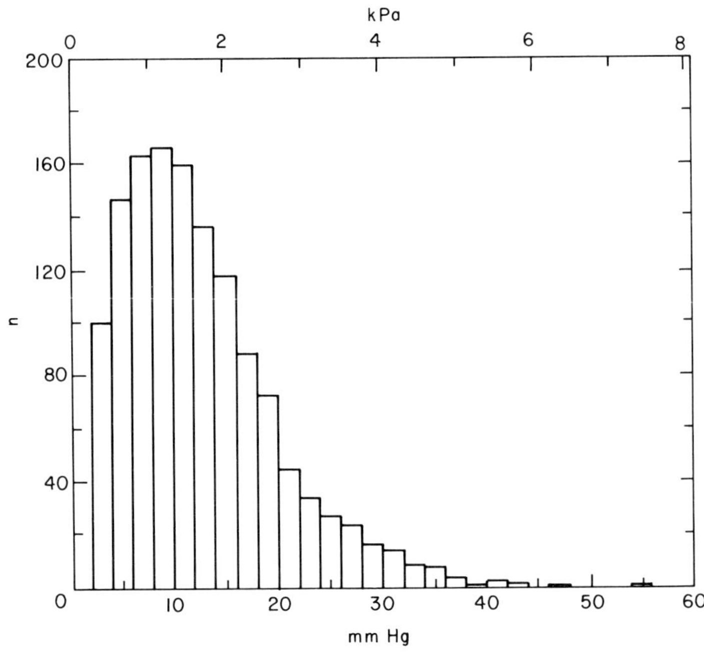

Fig. 10.1.3.3 **Frequency distribution of the differences between the highest and the lowest tcP_{O_2} from each recording.**

Oxygen-cardiorespirograms in Chapter 4.5 have repeatedly shown the tcPo_2 behaviour during crying. Fig. 10.1.3.4 illustrates the distribution of the tcPo_2 changes during crying in healthy newborn infants monitored at different times during the first week of life. As will be seen in this figure 98 per cent of the newborn infants displayed a fall in tcPo_2 during crying, in 0.5 per cent there were no changes, and in only 0.9 per cent did tcPo_2 increase.

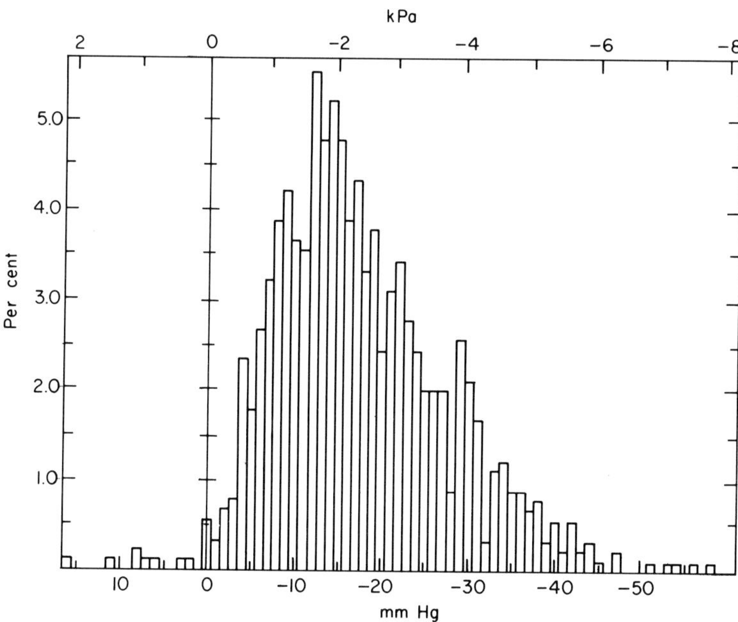

Fig. 10.1.3.4 Frequency distribution of individual tcPo_2 changes during crying.

The oxygen-cardiorespirograms from the healthy infants who demonstrated a decrease in tcP_{O_2} during crying were further analysed. Fig. 10.1.3.5 shows the mean fall in tcP_{O_2} during crying at the different time periods during the first week of life.

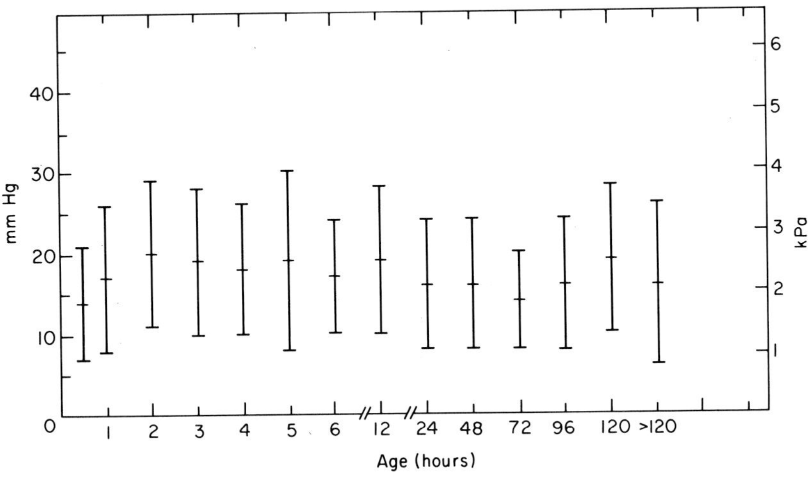

Fig. 10.1.3.5 Fall in tcP_{O_2} during crying.

The corresponding numbers, including the percentage fall in tcP_{O_2} are given in Table 10.1.3.5. The percentage was calculated as relative fall from the previous level when the infant was quiet. It will be seen that the mean fall was about 20 mm Hg (2.7 kPa) with a standard deviation of 10 mm Hg (1.3 kPa). Except for the increase in the level up to 2 hours there are no discernible trends.

Table 10.1.3.5 tcP_{O_2} decrease during crying (vaginal deliveries, Apgar score ⩾ 7, birthweight ⩾ 2500 g).

Age in hours	tcP_{O_2} mm Hg mean	s.d.	kPa mean	per cent	No
20– 30 min	14	7	1.9	16	41
0– 1	17	9	2.3	19	320
1– 2	20	9	2.7	22	89
2– 3	19	9	2.5	21	70
3– 4	18	8	2.4	20	40
4– 5	19	11	2.5	21	43
5– 6	17	7	2.3	20	48
6– 12	19	9	2.5	22	211
12– 24	16	8	2.1	19	280
24– 48	16	8	2.1	19	60
48– 72	14	6	1.9	16	29
72– 96	16	8	2.1	18	18
96–120	19	9	2.5	21	20
> 120	16	10	2.1	17	24

Total number: 1293.

Fig. 10.1.3.6 shows the mean peak tcP_{O_2} levels reached during the oxygen test and the corresponding numbers are given in Table 10.1.3.6. Again the results only refer to healthy, quiet infants. Adequate numbers of measurements were available for the first 48 hours of life. The mean values during this time ranged from 373 to 428 mm Hg (49.7 to 57.1 kPa). With the exception of the fourth hour of life, which was lower, there were no major changes with time. From these mean values a right-to-left shunt of 18–21 per cent was calculated using the formula of Comroe, Forster, DuBois, Briscoe and Carlsen (1962).

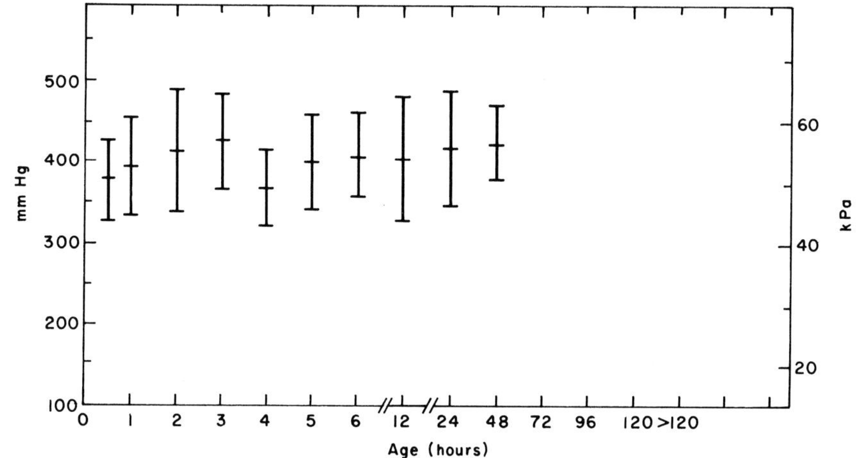

Fig. 10.1.3.6 Peak tcP_{O_2} during the oxygen test.

Table 10.1.3.6 Peak tcP_{O_2} during oxygen test (vaginal deliveries, Apgar score ⩾ 7, birthweight ⩾ 2500 g).

Age in hours	Peak tcP_{O_2} mm Hg mean	s.d.	kPa mean	No
20– 30 min	373	60	49.7	67
0– 1	391	72	52.1	295
1– 2	414	88	55.2	38
2– 3	428	71	57.1	29
3– 4	361	57	48.1	19
4– 5	398	68	53.1	26
5– 6	408	61	54.4	19
6– 12	403	89	53.7	112
12– 24	419	85	55.9	156
24– 48	427	52	56.9	25
48– 72	453	46	60.4	5*
72– 96	427		56.9	3*
96–120	337		44.9	3*
> 120	483		64.4	4*

Total number: 801.

*Not included in Fig. 10.1.3.6.

10.2 Comparisons between vaginal deliveries and Caesarean sections with high and low Apgar scores

10.1 gave the results taken from the oxygen-cardiorespirograms from the vaginal deliveries with Apgar score ⩾7 and birthweight ⩾2500 g. This group of infants will be referred to as A. We will now compare these data with those from the following three populations:

Caesarean section, Apgar score ⩾7, birthweight ⩾2500 g	Group B
Vaginal deliveries, Apgar score ⩽6, birthweight ⩾2500 g	Group C
Caesarean section, Apgar score ⩽6, birthweight ⩾2500 g	Group D

For the groups B, C, and D sufficient data for statistical analysis were obtained in the first hour of life and in the 12–24 hour period.

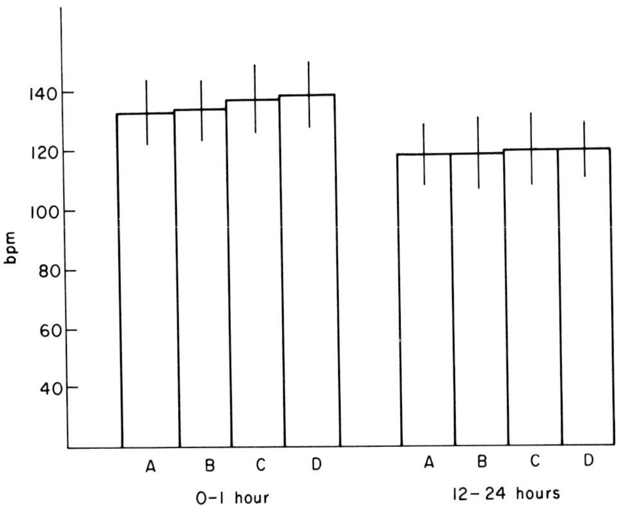

Fig. 10.2.1 Baseline heart rate.

10.2.1 Baseline heart rate

As before baseline heart rate was obtained when the infants were quiet. Fig. 10.2.1 shows the mean baseline heart rate in all the four groups studied in these two time periods. The numbers are given in Table 10.2.1. It will be seen that in the first hour of life there was a stepwise increase in the mean baseline heart rate from group A to group D. At 12–24 hours of life the mean values were almost identical in all the groups.

In the first hour of life, given the same Apgar score group (i.e. ⩽6 or ⩾7) there was no significant difference in the mean baseline heart rate between vaginal deliveries and deliveries by Caesarean section. Mean baseline heart rate in the vaginal deliveries with Apgar score ⩾7 (group A) was 132 bpm against 137 bpm when Apgar score was ⩽6 (group C). This difference is statistically significant ($t = 2.7$, $n = 732$, $P < 0.01$).

Equally statistically significant in the first hour of life was the difference between mean baseline heart rate in the Caesarean deliveries with an Apgar score ⩾7 (group B) which was 133 bpm against 139 bpm when Apgar score was ⩽6 (group D). ($t = 2.4$, $n = 104$, $P < 0.01$.)

The lower mean baseline heart rate at 12–24 hours compared with 0–1 hour is obvious in all four groups.

Table 10.2.1 Baseline heart rate.

		A	B	C	D
0– 1 h	bpm mean	132	133	137	139
	s.d.	13	12	14	13
	n	679	63	53	41
12–24 h	bpm mean	115	115	117	117
	s.d.	12	28	14	11
	n	634	14	25	12

Group A: Vaginal deliveries, Apgar score ⩾7, birthweight ⩾2500 g.
Group B: Caesarean section, Apgar score ⩾7, birthweight ⩾2500 g.
Group C: Vaginal deliveries, Apgar score ⩽6, birthweight ⩾2500 g.
Group D: Caesarean section, Apgar score ⩽6, birthweight ⩾2500 g.

10.2.2 Respiratory rate

Fig. 10.2.2 shows the mean respiratory rate of the quiet infants in groups A–D in the two time periods and the corresponding numbers are given in Table 10.2.2. In the vaginal deliveries (groups A and C), regardless of Apgar scoring, there were no significant changes in mean respiratory rate between the first hour of life and 12–24 hours after birth. In those delivered by Caesarean section with an Apgar score ≤ 6 (group D) there was a decrease in the respiratory rate from the first hour of the 12–24 hours period. This decrease from 42 to 34 breaths/min was statistically significant ($t = 2.5$, $n = 45$, $P < 0.05$).

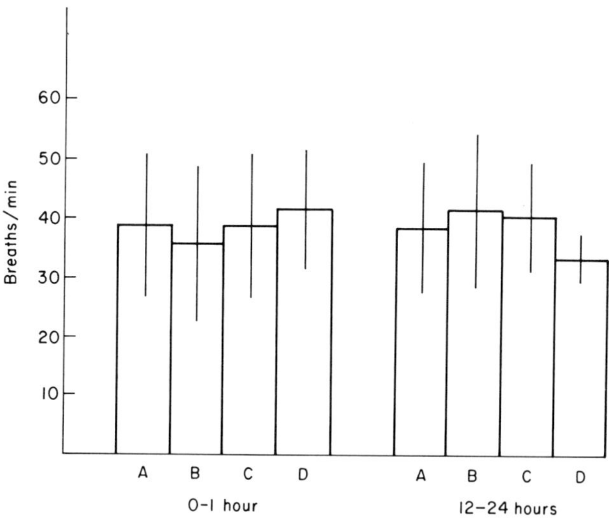

Fig. 10.2.2 Respiratory rate.

Table 10.2.2 Respiratory rate.

		A	B	C	D
0– 1 h breaths/min	mean	39	36	39	42
	s.d.	13	13	12	10
	n	586	54	50	35
12–24 h breaths/min	mean	39	42	41	34
	s.d.	11	13	9	4
	n	555	23	21	10

Group A: Vaginal deliveries, Apgar score ≥ 7, birthweight ≥ 2500 g.
Group B: Caesarean section, Apgar score ≥ 7, birthweight ≥ 2500 g.
Group C: Vaginal deliveries, Apgar score ≤ 6, birthweight ≥ 2500 g.
Group D: Caesarean section, Apgar score ≤ 6, birthweight ≥ 2500 g.

10.2.3 tcPo_2

Fig. 10.2.3.1 shows the mean highest tcPo_2 values from the quiet infants in the groups A–D in the two time periods and the corresponding numbers are given in Table 10.2.3.1.

In all the groups the mean tcPo_2 level at 0–1 hour was higher than at 12–24 hours after birth. Thus, regardless of the type of delivery and regardless of Apgar score, we found the same results as in the uncomplicated vaginal deliveries, i.e. that tcPo_2 was higher at 0–1 hour after birth than later, here at 12–24 hours. For all the groups these differences are significant.

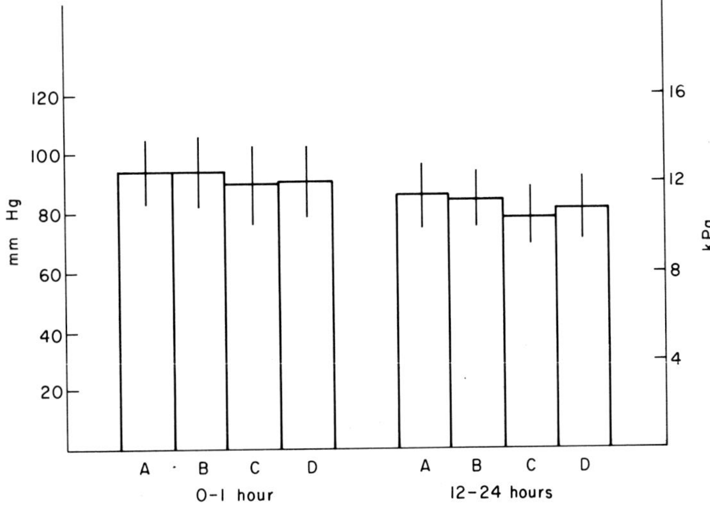

Fig. 10.2.3.1 Highest tcPo_2 values.

There was no difference in the mean of the highest tcPo_2 values seen in the first hour of life comparing vaginal deliveries (A and C) with Caesarean delivery (B and D) provided they were in the same Apgar score group. Pooling the two groups in Table 10.2.3.1, those with Apgar score ≥ 7 (A + B) on the one hand, and those with Apgar score ≤ 6 (C + D) on the other, the mean value of 93 mm Hg (12.4 kPa) in those with the higher Apgar score is statistically different from the 90 mm Hg (12.0 kPa) of those with lower Apgar score ($t = 2.1$, $n = 821$, $P < 0.05$).

The situation was comparable at 12–24 hours in that again the mean values were similar in groups A and B, i.e. in those with normal Apgar score on the one hand, and in those with low Apgar score on the other. The differences between the mean highest tcPo_2 values of 86 mm Hg (11.5 kPa) in the vaginal deliveries with high Apgar score and the mean of 79 mm Hg (10.5 kPa) in those with low Apgar score were more pronounced than in the first hour of life and statistically significant ($t = 3.1$, $n = 640$, $P < 0.01$).

Table 10.2.3.1 Highest tcPo_2 from each recording.

		A	B	C	D
0– 1 h mm Hg	mean	93 (12.4 kPa)	94 (12.5 kPa)	90 (12.0 kPa)	91 (12.1 kPa)
	s.d.	11	14	13	14
	n	666	62	53	40
12–24 h mm Hg	mean	86 (11.5 kPa)	85 (11.3 kPa)	79 (10.5 kPa)	82 (10.9 kPa)
	s.d.	11	10	10	11
	n	615	26	25	12

Group A: Vaginal deliveries, Apgar score ≥ 7, birthweight ≥ 2500 g.
Group B: Caesarean section, Apgar score ≥ 7, birthweight ≥ 2500 g.
Group C: Vaginal deliveries, Apgar score ≤ 6, birthweight ≥ 2500 g.
Group D: Caesarean section, Apgar score ≤ 6, birthweight ≥ 2500 g.

Fig. 10.2.3.2 illustrates the mean lowest tcP_{O_2} values from each recording in the four groups A–D and the corresponding numbers are given in Table 10.2.3.2.

Basically the same differences between the four groups and in the two time periods were found as for the mean of the highest tcP_{O_2} values. Thus the tcP_{O_2} values were always lower at 12–24 hours than in the first hour after birth. Also, at 0–1 hour and at 12–24 hours after birth, mean tcP_{O_2} in the two groups with Apgar score ≤ 6 (C and D) was lower than in the two groups with Apgar score ≥ 7 (A and B).

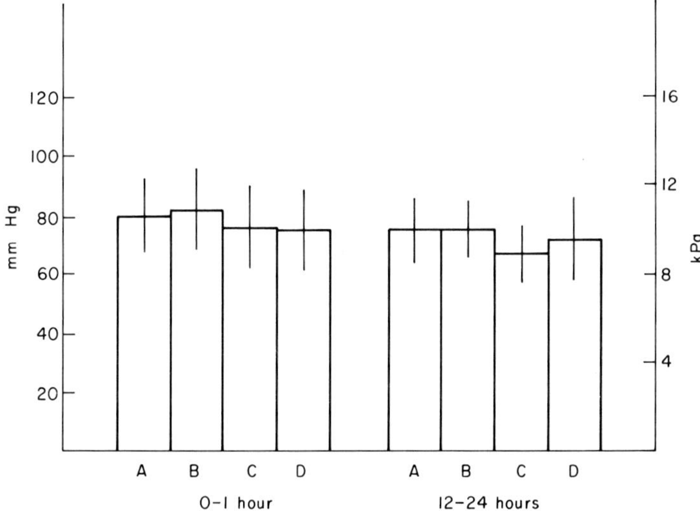

Fig. 10.2.3.2 Lowest tcP_{O_2} values.

Table 10.2.3.2 Lowest tcP_{O_2} from each recording.

		A	B	C	D
0– 1 h mmHg	mean	80 (10.7 kPa)	82 (10.9 kPa)	76 (10.1 kPa)	75 (10.0 kPa)
	s.d.	13	14	14	12
	n	666	62	53	40
12–24 h mmHg	mean	75 (10.0 kPa)	75 (10.0 kPa)	67 (8.9 kPa)	72 (9.6 kPa)
	s.d.	11	10	10	14
	n	615	26	25	12

Group A: Vaginal deliveries, Apgar score ≥ 7, birthweight ≥ 2500 g.
Group B: Caesarean section, Apgar score ≥ 7, birthweight ≥ 2500 g.
Group C: Vaginal deliveries, Apgar score ≤ 6, birthweight ≥ 2500 g.
Group D: Caesarean section, Apgar score ≤ 6, birthweight ≥ 2500 g.

Fig. 10.2.3.3 presents the mean decrease in tcP_{O_2} during crying in the four groups and the two time intervals 0–1 hour and 12–24 hours after birth. The corresponding numbers are given in Table 10.2.3.3. In all groups the mean values are between 15 and 20 mm Hg (2.0 to 2.7 kPa). Because of the large standard deviation statistical significance between the different means will not be attained.

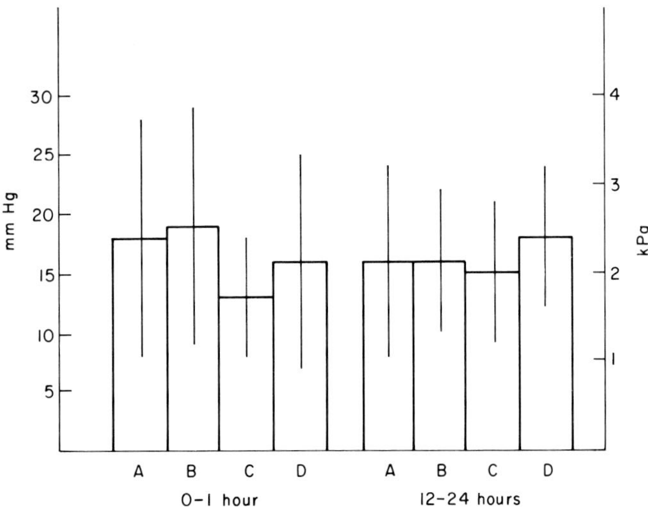

Fig. 10.2.3.3 tcP_{O_2} decrease during crying.

Table 10.2.3.3 tcP_{O_2} decrease during crying.

		A	B	C	D
0– 1 h mm Hg	mean	17 (2.3 kPa)	19 (2.5 kPa)	13 (1.7 kPa)	16 (2.1 kPa)
	s.d.	9	10	5	9
	n	320	35	23	24
12–24 h mm Hg	mean	16 (2.1 kPa)	16 (2.1 kPa)	15 (2.0 kPa)	18 (2.4 kPa)
	s.d.	8	6	6	6
	n	280	13	10	5

Group A: Vaginal deliveries, Apgar score ⩾ 7, birthweight ⩾ 2500 g.
Group B: Caesarean section, Apgar score ⩾ 7, birthweight ⩾ 2500 g.
Group C: Vaginal deliveries, Apgar score ⩽ 6, birthweight ⩾ 2500 g.
Group D: Caesarean section, Apgar score ⩽ 6, birthweight ⩾ 2500 g.

Fig. 10.2.3.4 shows the mean peak values of tcP_{O_2} during the oxygen test at 0 – 1 hour and 12 – 24 hours after birth in the four groups A – D. The corresponding numbers are given in Table 10.2.3.4. In the four groups the peak values attained 12 – 24 hours after birth were 28 to 38 mm Hg (3.7 to 5.1 kPa) higher than at 0 – 1 hour. For the vaginal deliveries with Apgar score ⩾ 7 (group A) this difference was significant (t = 3.7, n = 451, $P < 0.001$).

The mean peak tcP_{O_2} of the vaginal deliveries with normal Apgar score (group A) was 39 and 44 mm Hg (5.2 and 5.9 kPa) higher than for the vaginal deliveries with low Apgar score (group C) in the 0 – 1 and the 12 – 24 hour time period respectively. In the 0 – 1 hour period this difference between groups A and C was statistically significant (t = 2.5, n = 321, $P < 0.01$).

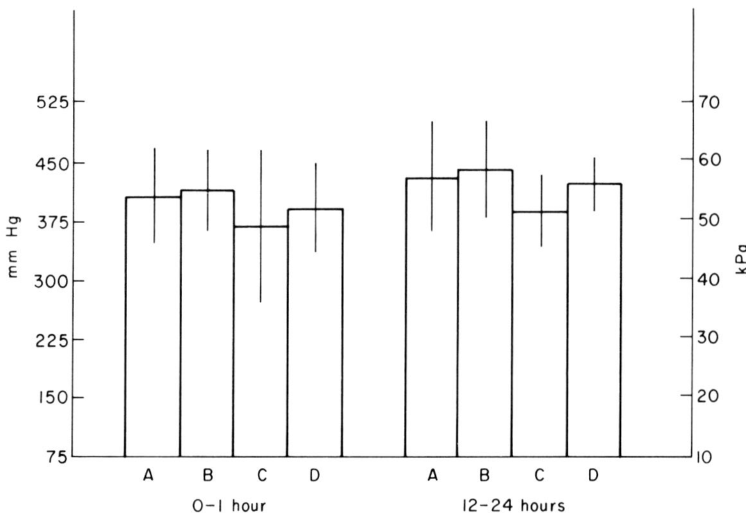

Fig. 10.2.3.4 Peak values of tcP_{O_2} during oxygen test.

Table 10.2.3.4 Peak tcP_{O_2} during oxygen test.

		A	B	C	D
0– 1 h mm Hg	mean	391 (52.1 kPa)	406 (54.1 kPa)	352 (46.9 kPa)	379 (50.5 kPa)
	s.d.	72	61	115	68
	n	295	40	26	30
12–24 h mm Hg	mean	419 (55.9 kPa)	440 (58.7 kPa)	375 (50.0 kPa)	417 (55.6 kPa)
	s.d.	85	73	55	41
	n	156	8	6	2

Group A: Vaginal deliveries, Apgar score ⩾ 7, birthweight ⩾ 2500 g.
Group B: Caesarean section, Apgar score ⩾ 7, birthweight ⩾ 2500 g.
Group C: Vaginal deliveries, Apgar score ⩽ 6, birthweight ⩾ 2500 g.
Group D: Caesarean section, Apgar score ⩽ 6, birthweight ⩾ 2500 g.

Table 10.3 Results from the oxygen-cardiorespirograms in relation to birthweight (vaginal deliveries, Apgar score ≥ 7).

Birthweight (g)	2000–	2250–	2500–	2750–	3000–	3250–	3500–	3750–	4000–	4250–	4500–	4750
Baseline heart rate bpm												
mean	137	139	131	133	135	132	131	129	133	132	139	
s.d.	10	12	14	12	12	13	12	10	12	12	14	
n	8	21	50	107	149	140	119	69	24	8	5	
Respiratory rate breaths/min												
mean	47	39	39	41	39	40	39	36	33	34	47	
s.d.	8	12	9	15	14	13	11	10	12	9	9	
n	7	20	47	92	124	126	107	51	22	7	3	
Highest tcP_{O_2} mm Hg												
mean	94	87	95	95	96	93	92	92	88	89	88	
(kPa)	(12.5)	(11.6)	(12.7)	(12.7)	(12.8)	(12.4)	(12.3)	(12.3)	(11.7)	(11.9)	(11.7)	
s.d.	12	13	11	10	11	9	11	11	12	7	3	
n	8	21	49	104	141	140	117	69	26	8	5	
Lowest tcP_{O_2} mm Hg												
mean	78	74	81	82	81	79	79	78	75	80	69	
(kPa)	(10.4)	(9.9)	(10.8)	(10.9)	(10.8)	(10.5)	(10.5)	(10.4)	(10.0)	(10.7)	(9.2)	
s.d.	12	13	11	14	13	11	12	13	13	7	4	
n	8	21	48	104	143	141	119	69	26	8	5	
tcP_{O_2} decrease during crying mm Hg												
mean	13	12	18	16	15	19	17	17	15	20	22	
(kPa)	(1.7)	(1.6)	(2.4)	(2.1)	(2.0)	(2.5)	(2.3)	(2.3)	(2.0)	(2.7)	(2.9)	
s.d.	1	2	3	2	2	2	2	3	2	1	3	
n	4	12	18	61	72	7	54	35	14	4	3	
Peak tcP_{O_2} during oxygen test mm Hg												
mean	445	354	362	373	383	385	373	391	385	415	325	
(kPa)	(59.3)	(47.2)	(48.3)	(49.7)	(51.1)	(51.3)	(49.7)	(52.1)	(51.3)	(55.3)	(43.3)	
s.d.	74	60	67	72	79	65	76	72	64	53	34	
n	7	17	40	91	135	117	106	64	20	8	5	

10.3 The variables of the oxygen-cardiorespirogram in relation to birthweight

In order to study the effect of birthweight on the different variables of the oxygen-cardiorespirogram we have made up the birthweight groups as shown in Table 10.3. Here, for the first time, are included healthy, quiet infants with a birthweight between 2000 and 2500 g. The analysis is limited to the first hour after birth. As mentioned above this signifies that the recordings were performed in the second half of the first hour of life. Thereby the influence of time after birth was minimized. All were vaginal deliveries with Apgar score ⩾ 7.

The results are summarized in Table 10.3.

10.3.1 Baseline heart rate

Fig. 10.3.1 shows the relation between birthweight and baseline heart rate in the healthy, quiet infants. It suggests a higher mean heart rate in infants with a birthweight < 2500 g than in those with higher birthweights. Comparing the baseline heart rate in the two birthweight groups below 2500 g with the two groups between 2500 and 3000 g the lower birthweight infants have significantly higher rates ($t = 2.4$, $n = 186$, $P < 0.01$).

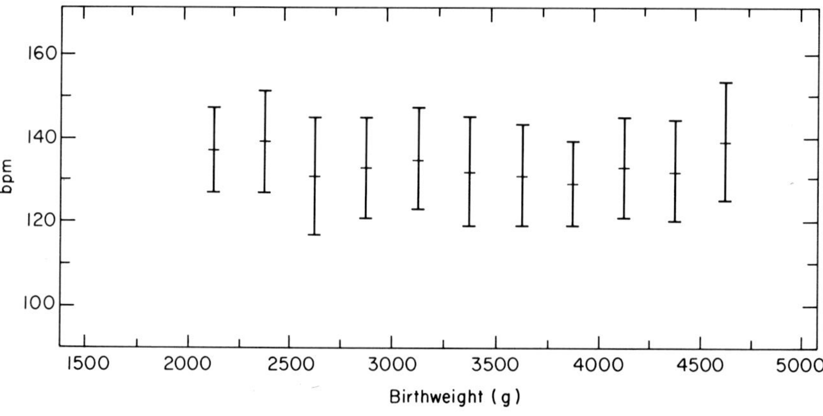

Fig. 10.3.1 Birthweight and baseline heart rate.

10.3.2 Respiratory rate

The mean respiratory rates in the different weight groups are given in Fig. 10.3.2. There is a tendency for respiratory rate to be higher in infants between 2000 and 2250 g (47 breaths/min) compared with the higher weight groups (39 breaths/min) but the difference is not statistically significant ($t = 1.7$, $n = 606$, $P > 0.05$).

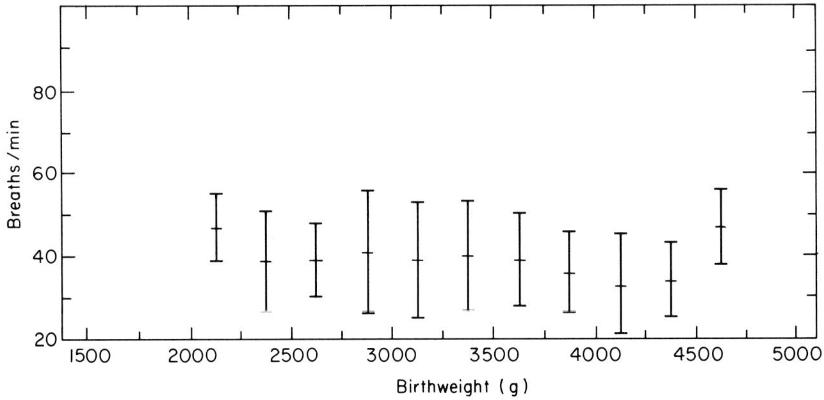

Fig. 10.3.2 Birthweight and respiratory rate.

10.3.3 tcP_{O_2}

Figs. 10.3.3.1 and 10.3.3.2 show the relations between birthweight and the highest and the lowest of the individual tcP_{O_2} values respectively. In both figures tcP_{O_2} is lowest in the weight group 2250–2500 g and compared with the weight group 2500–2750 g the differences are significant. For the highest tcP_{O_2} $t = 2.6$, $n = 70$, $P < 0.01$ and for the lowest tcP_{O_2} $t = 2.3$, $n = 70$, $P < 0.05$.

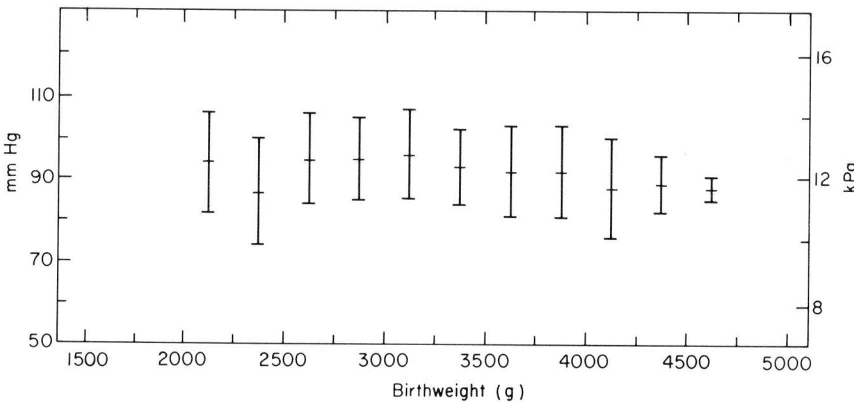

Fig. 10.3.3.1 Birthweight and highest tcP_{O_2} values.

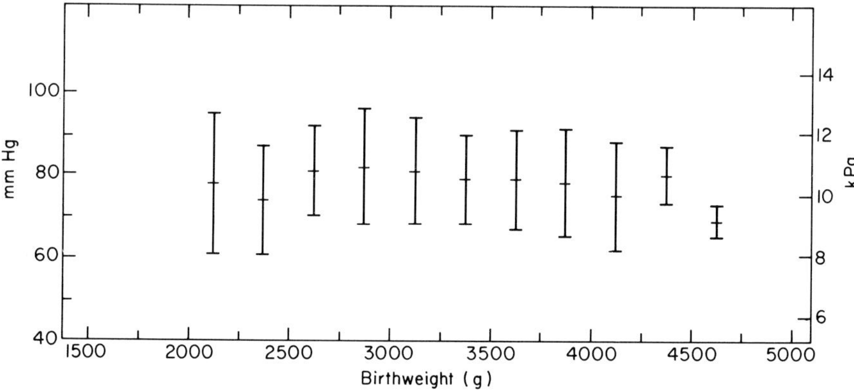

Fig. 10.3.3.2 Birthweight and lowest tcP_{O_2} values.

In Fig. 10.3.3.3 the mean decrease in $tcPo_2$ during crying is illustrated in relation to birthweight. As already pointed out in Chapter 7 when demonstrating the oxygen-cardiorespirograms of the low birthweight infants, the fall in $tcPo_2$ during crying in these infants seemed small. Comparing those with a birthweight $\leqslant 2500$ g with those > 2500 g the difference is statistically significant ($t = 8.2$, $n = 337$, $P < 0.001$).

Fig. 10.3.3.4 gives the mean peak $tcPo_2$ values during the oxygen test in relation to birthweight. It will be seen that those with a birthweight of 2000 to 2250 g reached a peak which was 91 mm Hg (12.1 kPa) higher than those in the next birthweight group. This difference is statistically significant ($t = 3.2$, $n = 24$, $P < 0.01$). Those with a birthweight between 4250 and 4500 g also had higher mean values than the following group 4500 to 4750 g ($t = 3.4$, $n = 13$, $P < 0.01$). In the middle weight ranges the mean values all lie within the 95 per cent confidence intervals of the mean of the largest group.

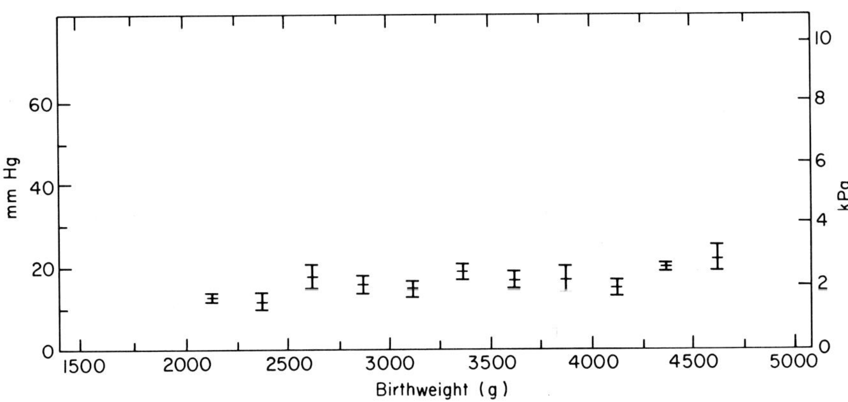

Fig. 10.3.3.3 Decrease in $tcPo_2$ during crying in relation to birthweight.

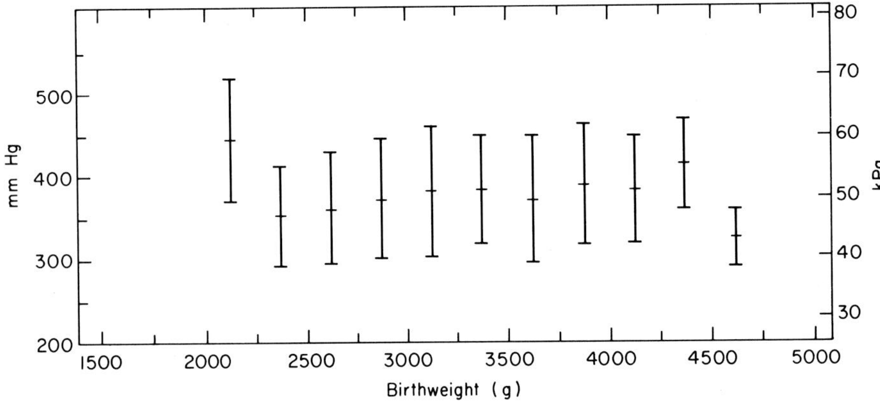

Fig. 10.3.3.4 Peak $tcPo_2$ values during oxygen test in relation to birthweight.

10.4 Baseline heart rate of boys and girls during the first hour of life in relation to birthweight

We have looked at sex differences in baseline heart rate, respiratory rate and tcP_{O_2} and found none except for differences in baseline heart rate between boys and girls when separated into weight groups. As before we have only investigated healthy newborn infants born after vaginal delivery, with Apgar score ⩾7 and birthweight ⩾2000 g and all records were obtained in the second half of the first hour of life when the infants were quiet.

Table 10.4.1 Baseline heart rate of boys and girls in relation to birthweight (vaginal deliveries, Apgar score ⩾7).

Birthweight (g)		2000–	2250–	2500–	2750–	3000–	3250–	3500–	3750–	4000–	4250–	4500–	4750–	5000
	Baseline heart rate bpm													
Boys	mean	143	146	130	130	132	131	129	127	132	125	134	125	
	s.d.	11	10	13	10	12	13	12	9	8	—	12	—	
	n	4	8	27	53	84	78	82	38	9	2	4	2	
Girls	mean	132	135	131	135	138	134	132	130	134	134			
	s.d.	2	14	14	14	10	11	9	10	18	14			
	n	4	13	26	57	71	67	45	33	18	6			

Fig. 10.4.1.1 shows mean baseline heart rate for boys in relation to birthweight and Fig. 10.4.1.2 the corresponding figures for girls. The numbers are listed in Table 10.4.1. It will be noted that there is no trend to different baseline heart rate levels in relation to birthweight in girls, whereas boys with a birthweight below 2500 g have higher baseline heart rate than those with a birthweight above 2500 g. This difference of 15 bpm is statistically significant ($t = 4.4$, $n = 392$, $P < 0.001$). The mean baseline heart rate of boys < 2500 g of 145 bpm is significantly higher than the corresponding mean value of 135 bpm in girls ($t = 2.5$, $n = 30$, $P < 0.01$).

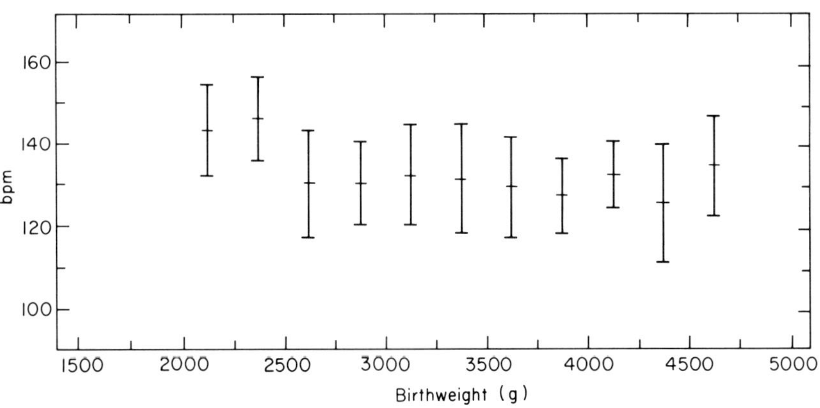

Fig. 10.4.1.1 Baseline heart rate of boys in relation to birthweight.

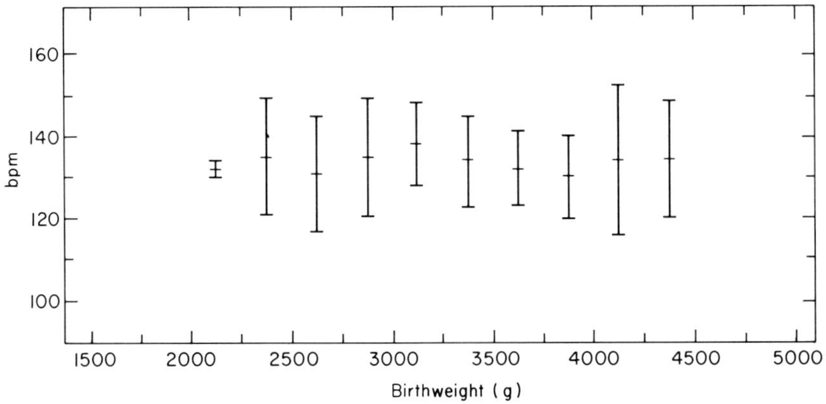

Fig. 10.4.1.2 Baseline heart rate of girls in relation to birthweight.

In Fig. 10.4.1.3 mean baseline heart rate of girls within each weight group is subtracted from that of boys. The Figure illustrates that in birthweight groups < 2500 g mean baseline heart rate is higher in boys than in girls, whereas when birthweight is ⩾ 2500 g girls have higher baseline heart rate than boys. This latter difference is also statistically significant ($t = 4.4$, $n = 704$, $P < 0.001$).

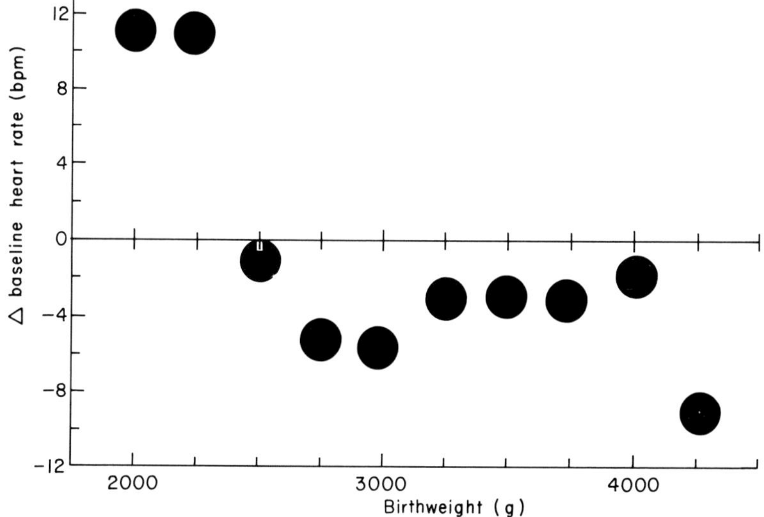

Fig. 10.4.1.3 Difference between mean heart rate of boys and girls in relation to birthweight.

10.5 Comparison between active and quiet sleep

As mentioned in Chapter 3, 500 oxygen-cardiorespirograms were also recorded on tape. This has made additional analysis possible.

In the oxygen-cardiorespirograms shown in Chapters 4–9 it has consistently been emphasized that the different variables behave differently in the various activity states. Before describing some relevant statistical studies we should stress that the activity states described here and seen in clinical practice are often less well defined as to onset and end and as to their distinguishing pattern than the classical activity states described by Prechtl and others. Prechtl observes his infants in specially designed surroundings, maintains fixed intervals between meals, monitors EEG and the ocular movements etc, and only defines the activity state if all his criteria are fulfilled.

In clinical practice such perfection cannot be attained and yet the influence of the activity states cannot be ignored as virtually every figure in Chapters 4–9 has illustrated. With these limitations in mind we have made the following comparisons between different variables in active and in quiet sleep.

10.5.1 Baseline heart rate and amplitude of long-term variability

Table 10.5.1 gives baseline heart rate and amplitude of long-term variability in active and in quiet sleep. Mean baseline heart rate and mean amplitude of long-term variability were obtained from the records during either active or quiet sleep periods. Each recording was only used once. The Table lists the mean of all these individual means. Amplitude of long-term variability was obtained by the computer program described in Chapter 2. It will be remembered that this was devised in order to eliminate decelerations and artifacts (spikes).

Table 10.5.1 Baseline heart rate and amplitude of long-term variability in active and in quiet sleep (vaginal deliveries, Apgar score ⩾ 7, birthweight ⩾ 2500 g).

		Active sleep	Quiet sleep	
Baseline heart rate bpm	mean	123	120	N.S.
	s.d.	13	12	
	n	100	69	
Amplitude of long-term variability bpm	mean	16.2	12.9	$P < 0.01$
	s.d.	7	6	
	n	100	69	

In the two sleep states there was no significant difference in baseline heart rate, partly because of the large standard deviation. However, amplitude of long-term variability was significantly more pronounced in active sleep than during quiet sleep confirming the observations in Chapter 4.3 and 4.4.

10.5.2 Baseline heart rate in different age groups

Fig. 10.1.1 showed that baseline heart rate fell during the first 3–4 hours of life. There the individual mean heart rate had been obtained by inspection of the heart rate tracing. In Fig. 10.5.2 baseline heart rate was obtained in the same way as just described for Table 10.5.1. The five time periods were chosen so that a sufficient number of infants could be included in each group. Both in active sleep and in quiet sleep baseline heart rate was higher 0–3 hours after birth than in the subsequent periods. Furthermore, baseline heart rate was higher in active sleep than in quiet sleep except for the time period 4–6 hours after birth. Thus the figure as well as the table indicate a tendency for mean baseline heart rate to be higher in active sleep than in quiet sleep. The inter individual differences are too high to bring out any statistical significance.

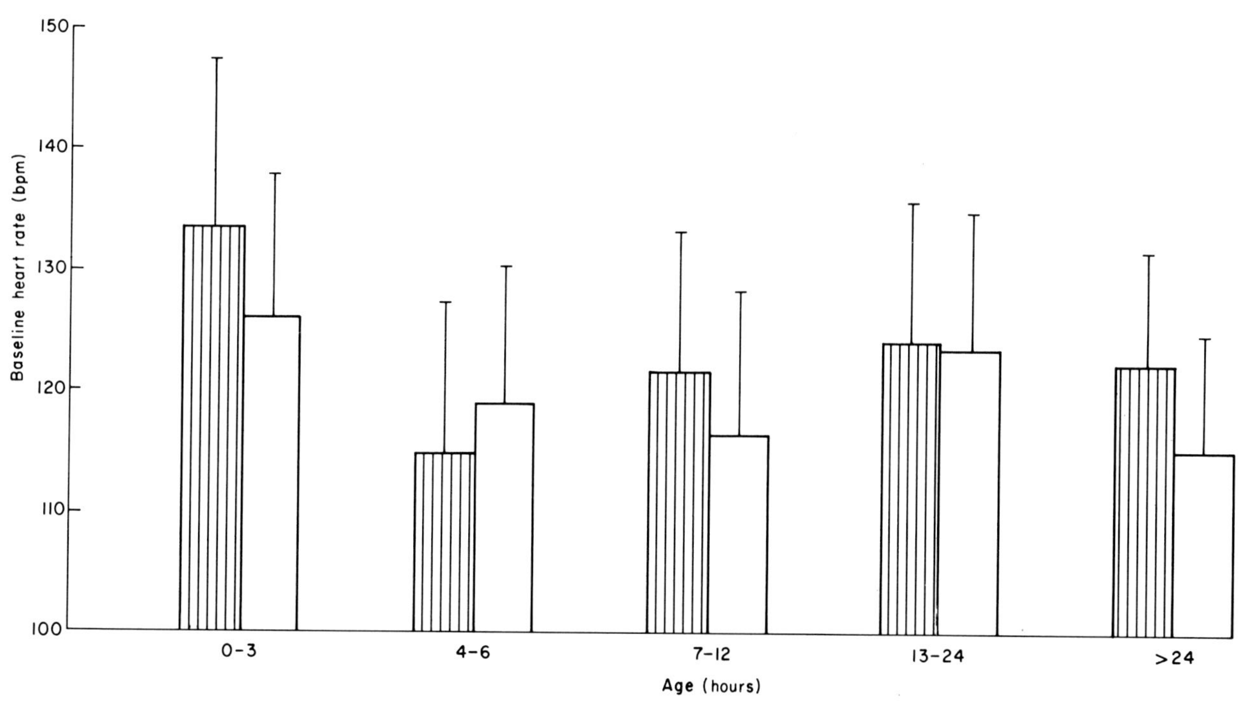

Fig. 10.5.2 Baseline heart rate in active sleep (striped bars) and quiet sleep (open bars) at different time periods.

10.5.3 Amplitude of long-term variability in different age groups

Using the same time periods the amplitude of long-term variability is shown in Fig. 10.5.3. It demonstrates, as did many of the oxygen-cardiorespirograms, that the amplitude of long-term variability is larger in active sleep than in quiet sleep. This difference is constant over the time periods.

Fig. 10.5.3 also illustrates the increase in the amplitude of long-term variability during active sleep within the time span studied. From 0–3 hours after birth to 24–120 hours after birth the mean increase in the amplitude of long-term variability was 11.5 bpm. This is statistically significant ($t = 5.8$, $n = 43$, $P < 0.001$). When the infants were in quiet sleep the mean increase of 7.5 bpm was also statistically significant ($t = 3.3$, $n = 29$, $P < 0.001$).

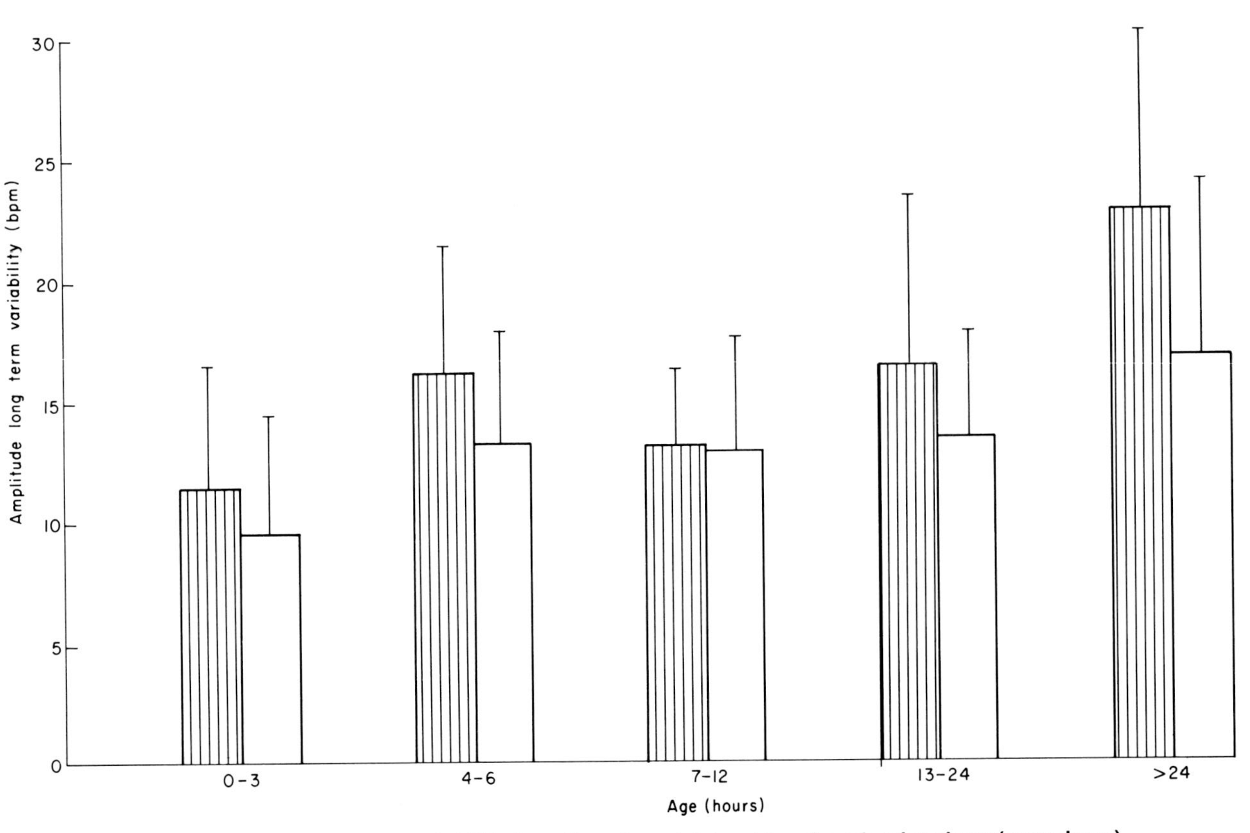

Fig. 10.5.3 Amplitude of long-term variability in active sleep (striped bars) and quiet sleep (open bars) at different time periods.

10.5.4 Correlation between baseline heart rate and amplitude of long-term variability

It is to be expected that with increase in heart rate the amplitude of long-term variability will be reduced. Fig. 10.5.4 demonstrates that in active sleep there is a significant negative correlation between baseline heart rate and the amplitude of long-term variability ($r = -0.30$, $n = 100$, $P < 0.01$). In quiet sleep a similar slope was calculated, but the correlation was not significant ($r = -0.23$, $n = 69$, $P > 0.05$).

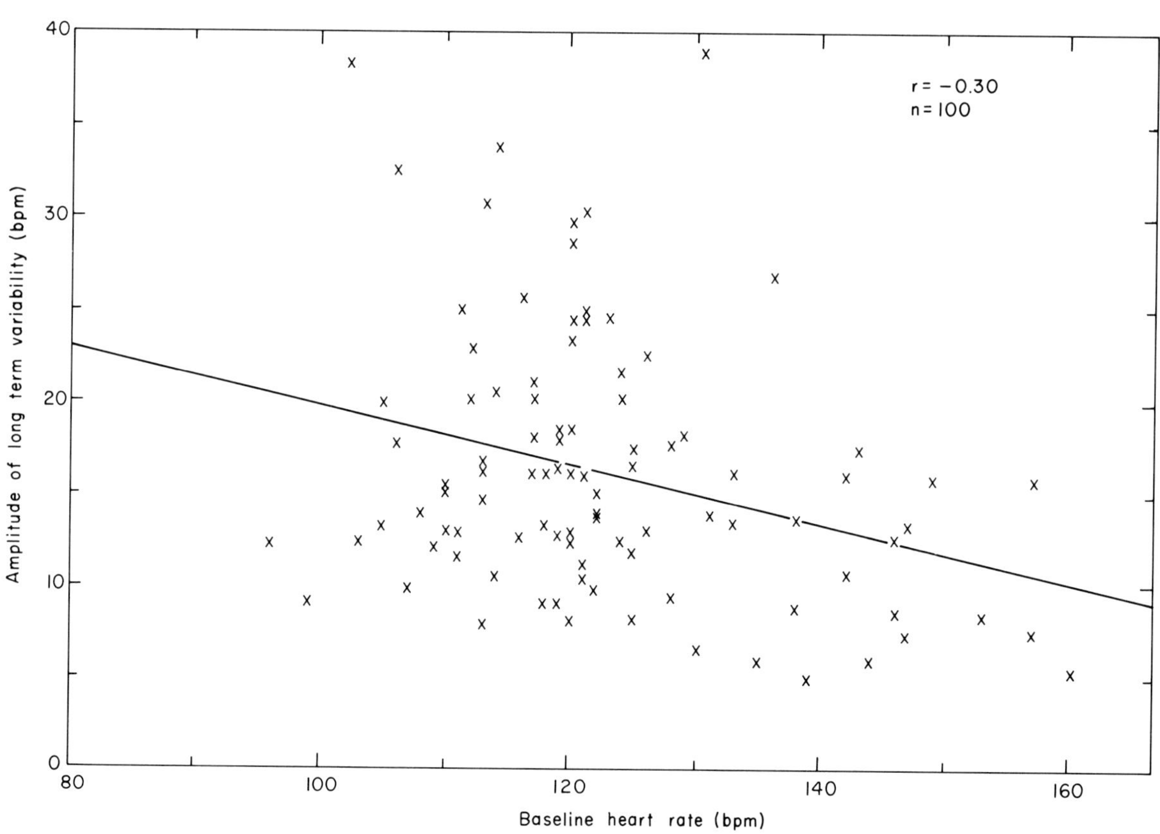

Fig. 10.5.4 Correlation between baseline heart rate and amplitude of long-term variability during active sleep.

10.5.5 Baseline heart rate and amplitude of long-term variability before and during the oxygen test

In the oxygen-cardiorespirograms it was repeatedly illustrated that baseline heart rate fell during oxygen breathing. From the computer-stored records a number of oxygen-cardiorespirograms could be retrieved in which the activity state remained unchanged from before and all through the oxygen test. As Table 10.5.5 shows, the mean fall in baseline heart rate during the oxygen test was 6 bpm in active sleep and 5 bpm in quiet sleep. These changes are statistically significant. By contrast the amplitude of long-term variability was unaffected by the increased oxygen supply.

10.5.6 Respiratory rate before and during the oxygen test

In contrast to heart rate, respiratory rate increases during the oxygen test. Twenty records were randomly chosen when the infants were in active sleep and another 20 when they were in quiet sleep before and during the oxygen test. In active sleep respiratory rate increased in 18 infants and was unchanged in two. In quiet sleep respiratory rate increased in 17 infants, decreased in one and was unchanged in two. See Fig. 10.5.6.1. The mean increase in active sleep was 7 breaths/min and in quiet sleep 9 breaths/min (Table 10.5.6.2). These differences are statistically significant using the paired Student's test.

Table 10.5.6.2 Respiratory rate before and during the oxygen test (vaginal deliveries, Apgar score ⩾ 7, birthweight ⩾ 2500 g).

			In air	In oxygen	
Active sleep	Respiratory rate Breaths/min	mean	38	45	$P < 0.001$
		s.d.	9	9	
		n	20	20	
Quiet sleep	Respiratory rate Breaths/min	mean	36	45	$P < 0.001$
		s.d.	8	10	
		n	20	20	

Table 10.5.5 Baseline heart rate and amplitude of long-term variability before and during the oxygen test (vaginal deliveries, Apgar score ⩾ 7, birthweight ⩾ 2500 g).

			In air	In oxygen	
Active sleep	Baseline heart rate bpm	mean	122	116	$P < 0.01$
		s.d.	14	10	
		n	56	56	
	Amplitude of long-term variability bpm	mean	14.6	14.8	N.S.
		s.d.	6	7	
		n	56	56	
Quiet sleep	Baseline heart rate bpm	mean	119	114	$P < 0.001$
		s.d.	12	12	
		n	33	33	
	Amplitude of long-term variability bpm	mean	14.2	13.1	N.S.
		s.d.	7	6	
		n	33	33	

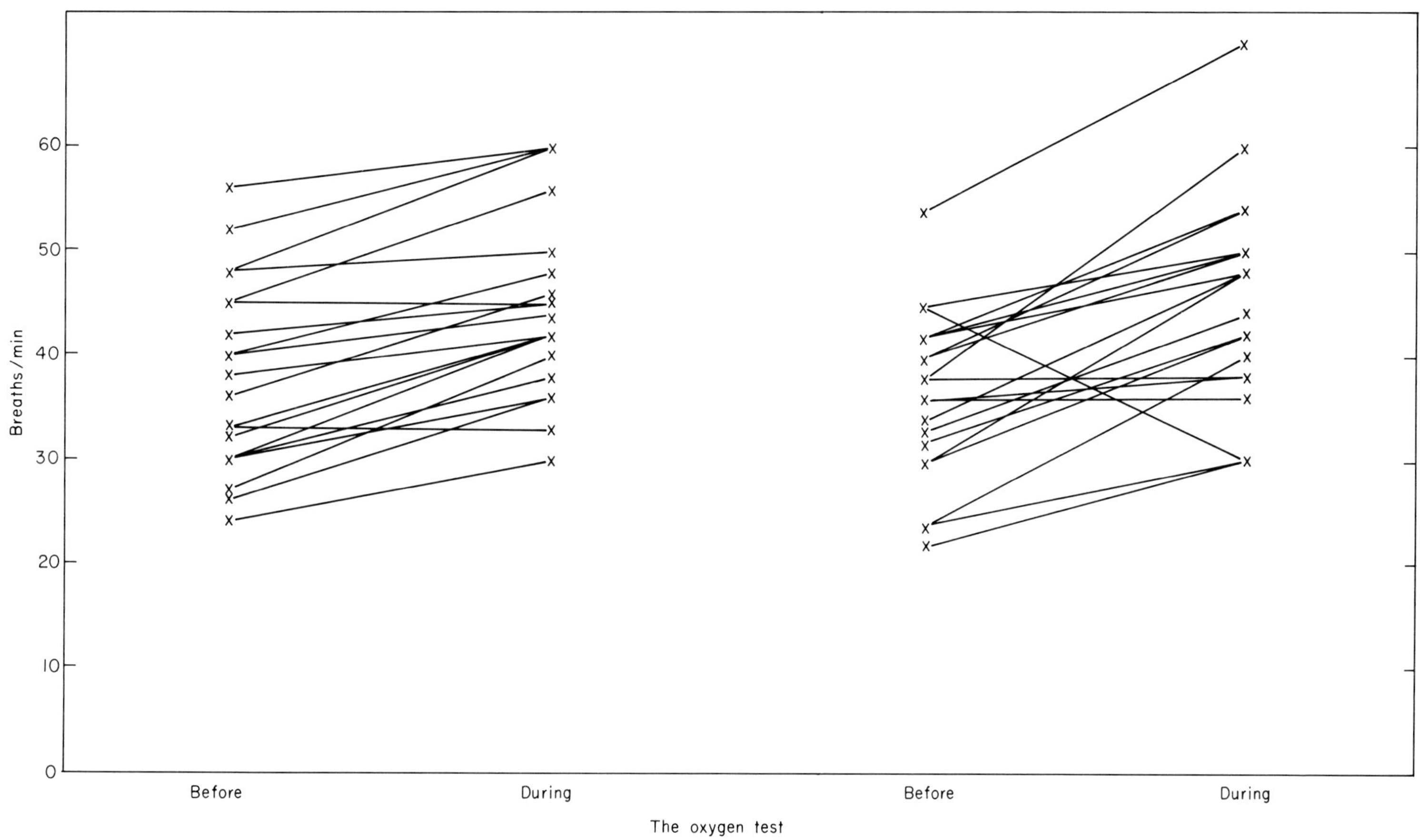

Fig. 10.5.6.1 Individual respiratory rates before and during the oxygen test during active sleep (left) and during quiet sleep (right).

10.5.7 tcPo_2

In Chapter 10.1.3 no mean tcPo_2 values were given in order to stress that tcPo_2 – like arterial Po_2 – varies greatly. However, for comparison between levels in different activity states, mean tcPo_2, as well as the highest and the lowest tcPo_2 observed during active and quiet sleep in the same infant, was obtained. The same computer stored records were used as for Table 10.5.1. The mean values are given in Table 10.5.7. It will be seen that they are virtually identical for both sleep states. We will show below that tcPo_2 is actually higher in quiet sleep than in active sleep, but this is only brought out when the same infant is observed in both sleep states, thereby eliminating the inter individual differences.

Table 10.5.7 Mean tcPo_2, highest tcPo_2 and lowest tcPo_2 in the individual cases in active and in quiet sleep (vaginal deliveries, Apgar score ≥7, birthweight ≥2500 g).

		Active sleep	Quiet sleep	
Mean	tcPo_2 mm Hg			
	mean	77	77	N.S.
	(kPa)	(10.3)	(10.3)	
	s.d.	11	10	
	n	100	69	
Highest	tcPo_2 mm HG			
	mean	83	83	N.S.
	(kPa)	(11.1)	(11.1)	
	s.d.	11	11	
	n	100	69	
Lowest	tcPo_2 mm Hg			
	mean	71	70	N.S.
	(kPa)	(9.5)	(9.3)	
	s.d.	12	11	
	n	100	69	

10.5.8 Rate of increase in tcPo_2 during the oxygen test

It was shown in Chapter 4.7 that when infants were quiet the rate of increase in tcPo_2 was fast during the oxygen test. This rate may be expressed as increase in tcPo_2 in mm Hg/min. As Table 10.5.8 indicates there was no difference in the rate of increase in tcPo_2 comparing the two sleep states.

Table 10.5.8 Rate of increase in tcPo_2 during oxygen test in active and in quiet sleep (vaginal deliveries, Apgar score ≥7, birthweight ≥2500 g).

		Active sleep	**Quiet sleep**	
Rate of increase in tcPo_2	mm Hg/min			
	mean	75	71	N.S.
	(kPa)	(10.0)	(9.5)	
	s.d.	24	24	
	n	51	28	

10.6 Distribution of breath-to-breath respiratory rates in active and in quiet sleep

The series of oxygen-cardiorespirograms illustrated here have shown the great range of values for the different variables even within the same activity state. This has also been documented in the standard deviation in Chapter 10.1–5. One consequence of the inter individual differences is that differences between mean values, for instance obtained in different activity states, may not become significant because of the large standard deviation, the exception being when very large numbers were studied as in 10.1. To supplement this we have chosen some studies demonstrating change with time or with activity state in the same infant.

In Figs. 4.3.1 to 4.3.3 showing quiet sleep and Figs. 4.4.1 to 4.4.2 showing active sleep, it was stressed that in active sleep respiratory rate varied considerably, whereas in quiet sleep respiratory rate was more constant. This is also demonstrated in Fig. 10.6. By the use of the computer respiratory rate was calculated from one breath to another, corresponding to the beat-to-beat heart rate. Three examples of the distribution of the different rates during one 5 minute period of quiet sleep and one 5 minute period of active sleep in the same infant are illustrated. In quiet sleep respiratory rate has a narrow range and a high peak, i.e. most breaths occur within a short frequency range. By contrast, in active sleep the frequencies vary greatly. This is not brought out in the mean respiratory rate. In one of the examples mean respiratory rate was the same in both sleep states although the distributions of the frequencies were very different.

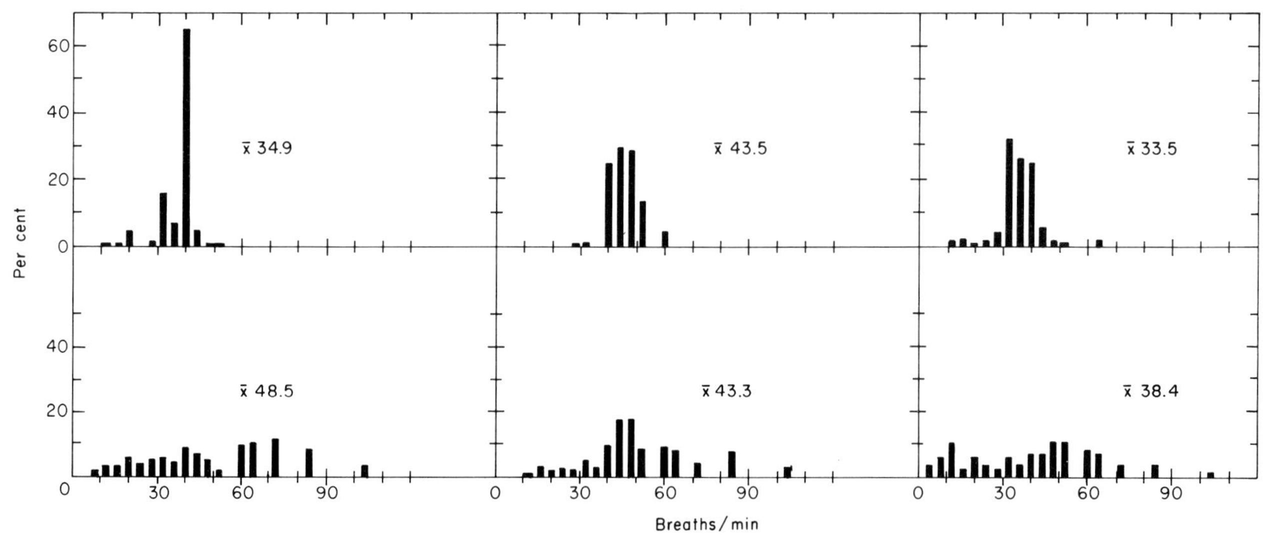

Fig. 10.6 Frequency distribution of respiratory rate (breath-to-breath) in quiet sleep (top level) and in active sleep (bottom level) in three infants.

10.7 Active and quiet sleep in the first and in the 4–6th day of life

From 10 infants with Apgar score $\geqslant 7$, birthweight $\geqslant 2500$ g and born after vaginal delivery oxygen-cardiorespirograms were obtained both from the first day of life and from the 4–6th day. Furthermore, in both time periods active as well as quiet sleep occurred. These recordings were selected from that part of the study in which no tape recording was done. In spite of the small number of case studies some differences between the two sleep states become manifest once, as here, the inter individual differences are eliminated. Table 10.7 summarizes the results. The statistical significances refer to the differences between active and quiet sleep.

Baseline heart rate was higher in active sleep than in quiet sleep but only on the 4–6th day of life was this difference statistically significant.

The amplitude of long-term variability of the heart rate was significantly larger in active than in quiet sleep in both time periods.

Decelerations were more frequent in active than in quiet sleep.

There were no significant differences in respiratory rate.

Both on the first day of life and on the 4–6th day $tcPo_2$ was higher during quiet sleep than during active sleep.

The data also allow for individual comparison in the same sleep states on the first and on the 4–6th day of life. As in Table 10.7 the paired t-test was used except when in all the 10 infants the direction of the changes were the same. In that case the sign test was utilized giving a P value of 1/1024.

Baseline heart rate was higher on the first day of life in agreement with Fig. 10.1.1 but this was only significant in quiet sleep ($t = 2.5$, $n = 10$, $P < 0.05$).

The amplitude of long-term variability of the heart rate increased with time but this too was only significant in quiet sleep ($t = 3.4$, $n = 10$, $P < 0.01$).

Decelerations became more frequent with time in both sleep states ($t = 2.4$, $n = 10$, $P < 0.05$ in active sleep; $t = 3.2$, $n = 10$, $P < 0.05$ in quiet sleep).

As before there were no significant changes in respiratory rate. Although $tcPo_2$ tended to be higher on the first day of life in both sleep states these differences were not significant.

Table 10.7 Several observations from the oxygen-cardiorespirograms of 10 infants in active and in quiet sleep obtained in the first and in the 4–6th day of life (vaginal deliveries, Apgar score $\geqslant 7$, birthweight $\geqslant 2500$ g).

		1st day of life			4–6th day of life		
		Active sleep	Quiet sleep		Active sleep	Quiet sleep	
Baseline heart rate bpm	mean	122	118	N.S.	119	111	$P < 0.01$
	s.d.	7	8		11	12	
Amplitude of long-term variability bpm	mean	17.2	8.9	$P < 0.001$	20.1	12.1	$P < 0.001$
	s.d.	4.1	2.5		2.7	2.2	
Decelerations per min	mean	0.6	0.2	$P < 0.01$	1.0	0.7	$P < 0.05$
	s.d.	0.3	0.3		0.5	0.5	
Respiratory rate Breaths/min	mean	37	40	N.S.	41	43	N.S.
	s.d.	7	8		7	9	
$tcPo_2$ mm Hg	mean	76	82	$P < 0.01$	73	79	$P < 0.05$
	(kPa)	(10.1)	(10.9)		(9.7)	(10.5)	
	s.d.	13	11		7	8	

10.8 Active and quiet sleep in the same recording

Among the oxygen-cardiorespirograms recorded on tape 16 demonstrated distinct periods of both active and quiet sleep. The main results are shown in Table 10.8.1. Again the paired *t*-test was used to calculate a statistical significance.

Heart rate was significantly higher in active sleep than in quiet sleep.

Amplitude of the long-term variability was also higher in active sleep than in quiet sleep.

Neither here nor in the previous series was there any significant change in respiratory rate.

As in 10.7 tc$P$O$_2$ was significantly higher in quiet sleep than in active sleep. This is also illustrated in Fig. 10.8.2 which shows that in 15 of these 16 infants tc$P$O$_2$ was higher in quiet sleep than in active sleep. Using the sign test this difference is significant.

We also tried to evaluate whether tc$P$O$_2$ varied differently in the two sleep states. To achieve this the highest and the lowest tc$P$O$_2$ values were noted in a one minute window which overlapped the previous window by 30 seconds. The differences were generated. The mean values for the active and for the quiet sleep periods were calculated. As Table 10.8.1 demonstrates tc$P$O$_2$ varied significantly less in quiet sleep than in active sleep.

Table 10.8.1 Several observations from the oxygen-cardiorespirograms of 16 infants in active and in quiet sleep (vaginal deliveries, Apgar score ⩾ 7, birthweight ⩾ 2500 g).

		Active sleep	Quiet sleep	
Baseline heart rate bpm	mean	121	115	$P < 0.01$
	s.d.	11	14	
Amplitude of long-term variability bpm	mean	16.2	12.5	$P < 0.001$
	s.d.	5.6	5.6	
Respiratory rate Breaths/min	mean	41	39	N.S.
	s.d.	7	10	
tc$P$O$_2$ mm Hg	mean	71	78	$P < 0.001$
	(kPa)	(9.5)	(10.4)	
	s.d.	10	11	
tc$P$O$_2$ variability mm Hg	mean	3.4	2.1	$P < 0.05$
	(kPa)	(0.5)	(0.3)	
	s.d.	1.1	1.0	

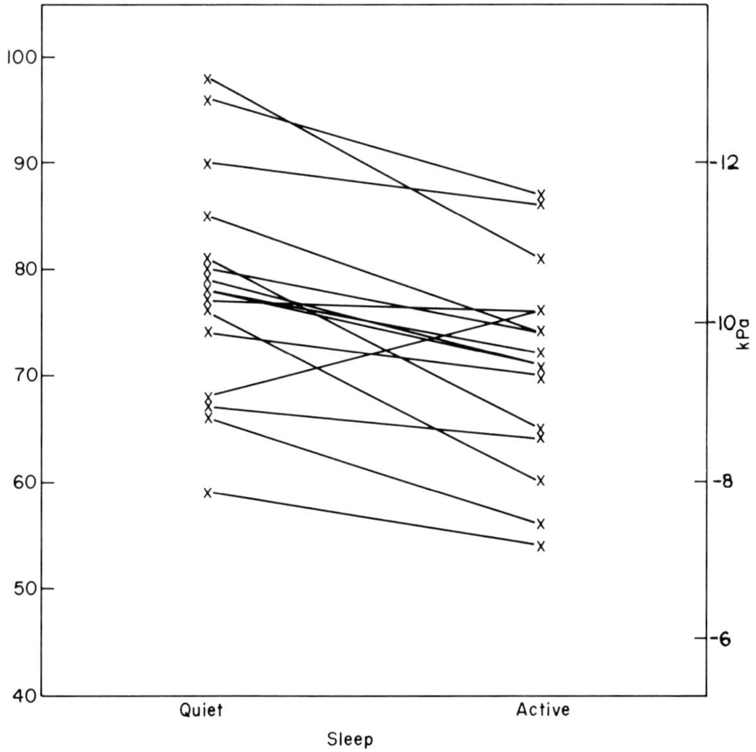

Fig. 10.8.2 Individual tc$P$O$_2$ changes in 16 newborn infants from quiet to active sleep.

10.9 Respiratory rate at 30 min and at one hour of life

In order to test if respiratory rate decreased during the first hour of life we compared respiratory rate twice from the same recording in 21 infants.

Table 10.9 shows that respiratory rate fell from a mean value of 45 breaths/min to 39 breaths/min during the second half hour of life. Using the paired *t*-test this decrease was statistically significant.

Table 10.9 Respiratory rate at two time periods (vaginal deliveries, Apgar score ≥ 7, birthweight ≥ 2500 g).

		Age at first observation (min)	Age at second observation (min)	
		30 ± 5.5	67 ± 11.5	
Respiratory rate				
Breaths/min	mean	45	39	$P < 0.05$
	s.d.	16	12	
	($n = 21$)			

11 Comments

11.1 The activity states

Reviewing the oxygen-cardiorespirograms in Chapters 4–9 it is clear that whatever may influence the pattern, such as birthweight, age, and so on, the most dominant factor is the activity state. In spite of the large variations in the individual variables the patterns for the activity states can be identified.

Both in the awake quiet and awake unquiet state there are changes in respiratory rate, transthoracic impedance, heart rate and usually also in tcP_{O_2}. The main differences between the quiet and the unquiet states are that respiratory excursions and heart rate are more constant in the quiet state and that tcP_{O_2} tends to increase in the quiet state.

In quiet sleep the pattern is very distinct and recognizable. The respiratory excursions are regular, heart rate is stable and the amplitude of long-term variability is small. At irregular intervals this picture is interrupted by 'startles', deep signs, heart rate accelerations and increases in 'flow'.

In active sleep respiratory rate changes all the time, and the transthoracic impedance curve shows, alternately, large and small excursions. Although baseline heart rate may be about the same as in quiet sleep the amplitude of long-term variability is often marked in active sleep in contrast to quiet sleep when it may be < 5 bpm. Using fetal terminology this would be considered pathologically reduced. However, it could be that in the neonate this amplitude is within the normal limits seen during quiet sleep.

In quiet sleep tcP_{O_2} tends to be higher than in active sleep. In quiet sleep there is often a gradual increase in tcP_{O_2} whereas, if anything, in active sleep tcP_{O_2} falls.

Crying also shows a distinct pattern. The transthoracic excursions increase in size and in variation, respiratory rate changes and may be very high. Breath-to-breath recording will show marked variations. Heart rate accelerates parallel to the crying periods or remains at a high level if crying continues. There is a fall in tcP_{O_2} in most cases.

A few other patterns also are easily distinguished. During suckling or drinking there are cyclic waves in heart rate and 'flow'. During the oxygen test, tcP_{O_2} increases, heart rate decreases and respiratory rate usually increases. When maternal pethidine is given the amplitude of the long-term variability of the fetus is reduced. Also there are correlations between fetal heart rate pattern and low pH and low Apgar score. No similar patterns could be identified in the oxygen-cardiorespirogram of the neonate. This, however, does not imply that maternal pethidine administration has no effect on the neonate. A separate study (Rooth, Lysikiewicz, Huch and Huch, 1982) demonstrated that infants whose mothers were given pethidine spent significantly less time crying, had higher baseline heart rate, higher neonatal arterial P_{CO_2} and lower pH than control infants.

It is not the aim of the present Atlas to describe the range of possible patterns in disease. However, the examples in Chapters 8 and 9 help to demonstrate that the diagnostic possibilities are greatly increased by monitoring several variables at one time. To cite two examples. If in Fig. 8.2.3 showing the tachycardia only a heart rate monitor had been used the infant would probably have been suspected of having hypoxia or other disturbance. However, the normal tcP_{O_2} was reassuring. In Fig. 9.2.1 neither respiratory rate nor heart rate was abnormal, whereas a tcP_{O_2} value of 35 mm Hg (4.6 kPa) is pathological and indicated a congenital heart disease as there were no clinical signs of respiratory distress.

11.2 The statistical analyses

11.2.1 Heart rate

Heart rate is labile and greatly affected by movements, and so on. A prerequisite for comparing baseline heart rate levels in different groups of infants is that activity is standardized. All statistics therefore only refer to baseline heart rate when the infants were quiet.

Fig. 10.1.1 showed that mean baseline heart rate about 20–30 minutes after birth was 135 bpm falling to 111 bpm 3–4 hours after birth. During this time the infant gradually settles down. Immediately after birth the healthy newborn infant has a heart rate between 170 and 200 bpm. At this time the infant is restless and the baseline heart rate of a quiet infant cannot be evaluated. After the long period of sensory deprivation (Reynolds, 1962) *in utero* the infant is chilled by the environment, gets tactile and acoustic influences, has a peak catecholamine level contributing to a high oxygen consumption etc, all this necessitating a high heart rate. Gradually the immediate adaptation phase is over and the infant becomes quieter. To judge from heart rate this takes some 3 to 4 hours.

After this initial fall in mean baseline heart rate there is a tendency to a gradual increase which becomes statistically significant at the end of the first week. These results agree with those of the literature (Välimäki and Tarlo, 1971; Smith and Nelson, 1976), but little seems to be known – or even discussed – about the nature of this increase. Mean blood pressure shows similar time related changes as baseline heart rate (Contis and Lind, 1963). The gradual increase in baseline heart rate continues for 1–3 months and has been attributed to the physiological anaemia of the newborn, which begins in the first week of life (Betke, 1958). Whether this early rise is the first manifestation of a slow adaptation to tissue oxygen requirements is as yet uncertain.

Over and above the main group of healthy newborn infants with Apgar score ⩾7 and birthweight ⩾2500 g, mean baseline heart rate was studied in three other groups. They comprise infants with birthweight ⩾2500 g and Caesarean section, Apgar score ⩾7; vaginal deliveries, Apgar score ⩽6; Caesarean section, Apgar score ⩽6. There was a stepwise, albeit small, increase in mean baseline in these heart rate groups in the first hour of life, but none at 12–24 hours after birth. Similar results were seen by Fournier, Burgun and Renaud (1977) and Klöck, Closs, Austermann, Lamberti and Schwenzel (1972). By contrast Cordero (1972) found lower mean baseline heart rates when Apgar score was ⩽6 than in a group of infants with Apgar score ⩾7. The published series are small and the differences, as in our series, also small. In the individual case baseline heart rate therefore cannot be used for diagnostic purposes although values outside the limits <105 and >160 bpm at one hour after birth and < 90 and >140 bpm subsequently during the first 1–4 days of life should motivate a further study of the health of the infant.

The influence of birthweight was studied in infants with Apgar score ⩾7. In order to eliminate the effect of time as just discussed only data obtained during the second half of the first hour of life were included. On the whole birthweight did not seem to have much influence on baseline heart rate. Only in the two birthweight groups between 2000 and 2500 g was mean baseline heart rate significantly higher than in the two groups between 2500 and 3000 g.

When studying the effect of sex and birthweight together in the infants with Apgar score ⩾7 and during the first hour of life we found that boys with a birthweight < 2500 g had significantly higher baseline heart rate than girls weighing less than 2500 g. In the weight groups above 3000 g mean baseline heart rate was always higher in girls than in boys. Watson and Lowrey (1967) state that heart rate is slightly higher in girls than in boys without commenting why this is so. Iliff and Lee (1952) described the higher heart rate in boys at one year of age. At 10 to 15 years of age heart rate of boys is lower than that of girls. This higher mean value in low birthweight boys does not seem to have been observed before.

The increased baseline heart rate in the low birthweight boys compared with girls may perhaps be seen as one sign that such boys are more stressed than girls, even when healthy. When sick with respiratory distress or other diseases, the boys have a reduced survival rate. It is well known that perinatal mortality is higher in boys than in girls. However, this difference is not the same in all weight groups. The relative risk of boys dying in the perinatal period is most pronounced in the weight groups 2000 to 3000 g. Below 1000 g and above 3500 g there are no sex differences (WHO, 1978). Perhaps the higher baseline heart rate in the low birthweight boys may be seen in the same context.

In the studies so far commented upon baseline heart rate was evaluated visually from the tracings and computer analysis was only used for the subsequent handling of the data. In one part of all the infants monitored the physiological variables were recorded on tape as well and computer calculation of mean baseline heart rate and mean amplitude of long-term variability could be done.

Comparisons were then made between active and quiet sleep. Studying mean values of different infants in either sleep state we found no difference in baseline heart rate level, whereas the amplitude of long-term variability was larger in active sleep than in quiet sleep as was already evident from the oxygen-cardiorespirograms. In both states the amplitude of long-term variability increased gradually from 1–3 hours after birth to 24–120 hours after birth. A similar increase in the amplitude of long-term variability during the first week of life was noted by Cabal, Siassi, Zanini, Hodgman and Hon (1980). Eliminating the inter individual variations in healthy preterm infants by studying individual cases (10.7 and 10.8.1) it was possible to demonstrate that mean baseline heart rate was higher during active sleep than during quiet sleep. Ashton and Connolly (1971), eliminating the inter individual differences by two-way analysis of variance, and Theorell, Prechtl and Vos (1974) as well as deHaan, Patrick, Chess and Jaco (1977), by studying the same infant at different times, also found higher baseline heart rate during active sleep than during quiet sleep.

During oxygen breathing as in the oxygen test, mean baseline heart rate decreased in the newborn infants as originally described by Brady, Cotton, and Tooley (1964). In quiet sleep the mean decrease was 6 bpm and in active sleep 5 bpm (10.5.6.2) but no changes were seen in the amplitude of long-term variability. This fall in heart rate during oxygen breathing is not confined to neonates. A drop of similar magnitude was found in women during labour and in their fetuses (Huch, Huch, Schneider and Rooth, 1977) when supplementary oxygen was given to the mothers.

11.2.2 Respiratory rate

Before commenting upon the results a discussion of the validity of respiratory rate is needed. It will be remembered from Chapter 2 that the transthoracic impedance, Monitor I, mostly used in the present study had a time constant of 3 seconds for respiratory rate, whereas Monitor II had a time constant of 20 seconds. As nurses often count respiratory rate by observing the infants for 15 seconds, the figures obtained from direct observation and from Monitor II should agree fairly well. By contrast, Monitor I gives figures that vary so often that no reasonable mean respiratory rate may be obtained from the instantaneous figures for respiratory rate. However, from a tracing, as in the oxygen-cardio-respirograms, both the changes and the mean levels may be read off by visual estimation. We have checked these visually assessed mean respiratory rates both with computer calculated mean values and mean values obtained from counting each single breath. There has been a very close agreement between the results gathered by these three different techniques. So, however respiratory rate has been obtained, it has not significantly influenced the results.

The transthoracic impedance equipment will fail to give respiratory rate entirely, or partially, if the triggering is improperly set (see Chapter 2.6.1). Some examples of this are demonstrated in the oxygen-cardio-respirograms. As the monitoring of the newborn infants was done by experienced technicians or doctors and with continuous supervision the triggering has only been erroneous in a small percentage of the records. In clinical practice the risk cannot be ignored and an intermittent checking of the triggering is recommended.

Fig. 10.1.2 indicated that only small changes occur in mean respiratory rate during the first week of life. It is somewhat surprising that the mean values during all the time periods in Fig. 10.1.2 are so close to 40 breaths/min in spite of the large standard deviation and the difference in the number of observations in the time groups. With large numbers similar means are expected – if they are similar – but in some of the time groups the number of observations was limited, but still the same mean values were found.

All the published reports show a wide range of values (for an extensive review see Schwartze and Schwartze, 1977). Most authors have studied a small number of patients. Their mean values are between 33 and 68 breaths/min. The different 'normal' values found may partly be due to different techniques and to variable attention to the activity states of the infants, but other factors are also of importance. Oh, Lind and Gessner (1966) found that after late clamping of the cord neonatal respiratory rate was higher, 59 breaths/min, than after early clamping of the cord, 48 breaths/min. This could explain the mean respiratory rates of 74–85 breaths/min 30–45 minutes after birth in the three series of 15 infants reported by Bratteby, Andersson and Swanström (1978).

All authors agree on the frequently large range in respiratory rate even in quiet infants and the difficulty of distinguishing between normal and abnormal respiratory rate.

Within the first hour of life respiratory rate changes in the individual infant as more detailed studies within this time period have shown. In 21 infants monitored from 30 minutes after birth and onwards we found a significant decrease in the individual respiratory rate from 45 breaths/min at 30 minutes to 30 breaths/min by 67 minutes after birth. Oh, Lind and Gessner (1966) found a fall in mean respiratory rate from 55 to 48 breaths/min in the same time periods. They attributed the higher earlier respiratory rate to a mild degree of pulmonary oedema as judged from their studies of haematocrit. Another, perhaps more important, factor may be the decrease in respiratory work occurring early in life. Karlberg and Koch (1962) found that respiratory work decreased to about half from 15 minutes after birth to 3 hours after birth. Moreover, even if respiratory rate was always obtained when the infants were quiet they were more quiet and more often quiet at one hour after birth than at 30 minutes. Thus several factors probably contribute to a modest fall in respiratory rate during the first hour of life. Thereafter mean respiratory rate stays very close to 40 breaths/min all through the first week of life.

We found some significant differences in mean respiratory rate between infants delivered by Caesarean section. Those with Apgar score ⩾7 decreased their respiratory rate between 1 and 12–24 hours of life, whereas those with Apgar score ⩽6 increased their respiratory rate during this time. The physiological background for this is uncertain, but it may be that the low Apgar score after Caesarean section is to some extent a result of maternal anaesthesia and that this effect wears off between 12 and 24 hours after birth.

The influence of birthweight was studied in the second half of the first hour of life but mean respiratory rate was the same in all weight groups.

The different information obtained from breath-to-breath monitoring compared with mean respiratory rate was illustrated in Fig. 10.6. Mean respiratory rate was similar, whereas the distribution of the respiratory rates over a certain time period gave different pictures in active sleep compared with quiet sleep. In the latter case a few frequencies dominate while in active sleep respiratory rate varies greatly. During activity, including crying, respiratory rate also varies markedly.

Curzi-Dascalova, Gaudebout and Dreyfus-Brisac (1980), studying 22 full-term, healthy infants and 35 2–18 week old infants, found respiratory rate between 33 and 90 breaths/min. However, with each infant respiratory rate remained at similar levels in spite of differences between active and quiet sleep. Thus they found a significant correlation between respiratory rate at different time periods in the same infant. Similar results were noted in the present study. The correlation coefficient between the respiratory rate at 30 and 67 minutes of life in the 21 infants was 0.58. Thus different infants, for reasons which do not as yet seem to have been studied, have different levels of respiratory rate. It follows that more detailed information about changes or abnormalities in respiratory rate will best be obtained in studies which eliminate the inter individual differences.

We found no difference in mean respiratory rate between active or quiet sleep either in the first day of life or during the 4–6th day of life even when studying the individual infant (10.7). There was a tendency for higher respiratory rate in active sleep and with larger numbers we might have found a significant difference as did Brooks, Schlueter, Navelet and Tooley (1978) and Curzi-Dascalova, Gaudebout and Dreyfus-Brisac (1980). However, when different infants were observed even larger numbers did not bring out any differences (10.8).

It has already been shown that heart rate decreases during oxygen breathing, and reasons were given for considering this a true oxygen effect. By contrast respiratory rate increases often quite markedly during the oxygen test (10.5.7). Brady, Cotton and Tooley (1964) observed a fall both in heart rate and respiratory rate during oxygen breathing. Failing further studies we can only speculate on this discrepancy. One possibility is that in our study the oxygen was given in a small hood over the head of the infants and that the increased air flow over the face stimulated respiration.

11.2.3 tcP_{O_2}

Figs. 10.1.3.1 and 10.1.3.2 show that the tcP_{O_2} level of the newborn infant is high in the first week of life. Moreover, the level is highest in the first hour after birth. The figures also reconfirm previous experience with transcutaneous and intra-arterial continuous P_{O_2} monitoring, demonstrating that P_{O_2} varies greatly and that this is a physiological reaction.

Thus these non-invasive measurements of tcP_{O_2} in newborn infants have partly changed the previous conception about the gradual increase in P_{aO_2} during the first day or even during the first week of life. Earlier studies were based on intermittent arterial blood sampling almost always obtained from below the ductus arteriosus (Oliver, Demis and Bates, 1961; Wulff, 1966; Koch and Wendel, 1967; Berg and Dörrler, 1969). Previous results including our own indicated that the main postnatal cardiopulmonary adaptation takes place within minutes after birth (Rooth, Fall, Schachinger, Huch and Huch, 1979). The present study found mean highest tcP_{O_2}, in quiet infants, during the first hour of life, to be 93 mm Hg (12.4 kPa) and the corresponding mean lowest level was 80 mm Hg (10.6 kPa). After 3 – 4 hours a lower plateau was reached. The mean highest tcP_{O_2} was 85 mm Hg (11.3 kPa) and the mean lowest level was 75 mm Hg (10.0 kPa).

In considering the absolute values it must be remembered that the transcutaneous P_{O_2} figures are about 10 per cent higher than those from arterial blood. This is mainly because of the effect of local heating on the oxygen dissociation curve of haemoglobin. By constant oxygen saturation P_{O_2} increases. The correlation between the individual P_{aO_2} and tcP_{O_2} measurements in the present study (Fig. 2.2.3.2) confirms that tcP_{O_2} is about 10 per cent higher than P_{aO_2}.

A second and important reason why the present tcP_{O_2} values are high by published standards is that all measurements were performed in skin areas supplied by praeductal vessels. The otherwise well established difference in prae- and postductal P_{aO_2} during the first week of life has not been adequately taken into account when giving normal values for P_{O_2}. Most 'normal' values in the literature concerning P_{O_2} in the first week of life refer to measurements from postductal areas and are between 60 and 65 mm Hg (8.0 to 8.7 kPa). In the few studies based on blood sampling from praeductal vessels as high P_{O_2} values as in our study were found (Reardon, Baumann and Haddad, 1960, temporal arteries; Oh, Arcilla, Lind and Gessner, 1966, left atrium; Engström, Karlberg, Rooth and Tunell, 1966, arcus aortae or left atrium).

A third reason for high P_{O_2} values is that only phases when the infants were quiet were studied. This is difficult to achieve during intermittent blood sampling. The fall in tcP_{O_2} during crying will be discussed below.

It was both unexpected and surprising to find higher tcP_{O_2} levels during the first hour after birth than subsequently in the first week of life. This observation was made both in those with vaginal deliveries, Apgar score $\geqslant 7$ and in those with Apgar score $\leqslant 6$. The same held true for those born after Caesarean deliveries, again regardless of Apgar score.

Only two causes for this high P_{O_2} value in the first hour of life need to be considered; hyperventilation or a gradual reduction in the right-to-left shunting. The studies during hyperoxia, i.e. the oxygen test (Fig. 10.1.3.6), show that the right-to-left shunt remains rather constant during the first week of life and thereby excludes such an explanation. Thus only hyperventilation remains as the probable cause for the particularly high values during the first hour of life. Actually an alveolar hyperventilation is needed after birth to eliminate a hypercapnia and a metabolic acidosis.

The technique used for monitoring respiration in the present study, i.e. transthoracic impedance, gives no quantitative information about the gas exchange but the reduction in respiratory rate at one hour of life compared with 30 minutes after birth (Table 10.9) supports the hyperventilation theory.

To those used to intermittent blood sampling the rapid changes in tcP_{O_2} must be surprising. These are present even when the infants are quiet. If rapid changes occur in P_{aO_2} these are only partially reflected in tcP_{O_2} because of the damping effect of the skin etc. Thus it may be inferred that the actual P_{aO_2} changes are even larger and faster than those illustrated in the oxygen-cardiorespirograms.

One characteristic feature of the oxygen-cardiorespirograms during crying is a fall in tcP_{O_2}. This was observed in 98 per cent of the crying periods studied. The mean fall in tcP_{O_2} was 20 mm Hg (2.7 kPa). A similar fall in arterial blood P_{O_2} was earlier demonstrated by intermittent blood sampling (Versmold, Onken, Höpner and Riegel, 1976, and Dinwiddie, Pitcher-Wilmott, Schwartz, Shaffer and Fox, 1979). This P_{O_2} drop may be caused by increased venous admixture in the heart and/or in the lung or a change in the ventilation/perfusion ratio. Such P_{O_2} drops are seen during the Valsalva manoeuvre and to some extent crying can be considered such a manoeuvre. If the P_{O_2} fall is due to a shunt then it is a praeductal one as all the present measurements were praeductal. During the first week of life, covered by the present study, the tcP_{O_2} fall during crying remained of the same order of magnitude.

The praeductal anatomical right-to-left shunt was evaluated by the use of the oxygen test. The physiological shunts caused by alveolar hypoventilation, restriction in diffusion, or uneven ventilation/perfusion become negligible during inhalation of 100 per cent oxygen and any reduction in $P\text{O}_2$ is due to a right-to-left flow of venous blood which, bypassing ventilated alveoli, flows directly into the arterial circulation. Fig. 10.1.3.6 showed mean peak tc$P\text{O}_2$ levels during the oxygen test in the first 48 hours of life in quiet, healthy infants. There was no tendency for a change in the size of the shunt which was calculated as 18–21 per cent. However, comparing in Fig. 10.2.3.2 and Table 10.2.3.2 four different clinical groups in the first hour of life and at 12–24 hours after birth, the mean value was lower in all the four groups in the later time period, indicating some reduction in the shunt.

Our results differ from those of Ulrich (1969) and Koch (1968) regarding the size of the shunt and its temporal changes. Thus Koch (1968) reports a significant reduction in the size of the shunt by 24 per cent in the first 5 hours of life. At that time he finds it to be 10 per cent and explains this change by the closure of the ductus arteriosus. Nelson, Prod'hom, Cherry, Lipsitz and Smith (1963) and Prod'hom, Levison, Cherry, Drorbaugh, Hubbell and Smith (1964) also found shunts of about 20 per cent and observed no changes with time during the first 58 hours of life. But comparison with these studies is difficult, as they all measured $P\text{O}_2$ in blood taken from postductal vascular regions.

Whether the shunt is calculated from arterial blood $P\text{O}_2$ measurements or from transcutaneous monitoring, the formula for the calculation uses several assumptions. Consequently only approximate values are obtained. The largest error lies in the assumption of a constant arterio-venous difference. In the present study there was a risk that the shunt was calculated from a tc$P\text{O}_2$ value taken before the true peak was obtained. Fortunately this only leads to a small error.

It has repeatedly been reported that newborn infants with fetal asphyxia, low Apgar score and/or low umbilical blood pH have cardio-pulmonary adaptation problems. The comparison of the four different clinical groups, vaginal or Caesarean deliveries, high or low Apgar score, also substantiates this opinion. When Apgar score was $\leqslant 6$ tc$P\text{O}_2$ was significantly lower than when Apgar score was $\geqslant 7$. No influence from Caesarean section *per se* was revealed.

We found that tc$P\text{O}_2$ was higher and the tc$P\text{O}_2$ variability smaller in quiet sleep than in active sleep. This was only revealed when oxygen-cardiorespirograms from the same infant in the two sleep states were compared. Similar observations were made by Martin, Okken and Rubin (1979), Friis-Hansen, Lou, Marstrand-Christiansen and Scheibel (1979) and Gabriel, Helmin and Albani (1980) and may be explained by the differences in chest and abdominal breathing during the sleep states. Moreover, in comparison with quiet sleep, active sleep is characterized by irregular and reduced ventilation.

11.3 Summary

1 The Atlas describes the principle, the technical equipment, and the clinical application of the oxygen-cardiorespirogram, i.e. the simultaneous, continuous, non-invasive recording of transthoracic impedance, heart rate, transcutaneous PO_2 and skin blood flow.

2 The oxygen-cardiorespirograms of 3000 newborn infants were obtained in order to define the limits of variability in vital signs of the healthy infant during the first week of life in relation to time and different clinical and physiological situations.

3 Excerpts from 115 oxygen-cardiorespirograms are shown in Chapters 4–9 in order to describe the influence of the activity state of the infants, time after birth, type of birth, Apgar score, cord blood gases, maternal anaesthesia and analgesia, and birthweight. Emphasis is placed on the covariability of the different variables.

Chapter 10 contains statistical analyses of healthy newborn infants with a birthweight ⩾2500 g and Apgar score ⩾7. The descriptive and statistical studies are summarized as follows:

4 The pattern of the different variables is dominated by the activity states of the infants.

5 Baseline heart rate changes characteristically in quiet, healthy newborn infants ⩾2500 g, Apgar score ⩾7; 20–30 min after birth the mean was 135 bpm falling to 111 bpm 3–4 hours after birth. An increase then occurred >120 hours after birth. Thus values during the second half hour of life <105 and >160 bpm and subsequently in the first week of life <90 and >140 bpm should raise suspicion of some disturbance.

6 During the first week of life there is no tendency to systematic changes in mean respiratory rate in quiet, healthy newborn infants ⩾2500 g, Apgar score ⩾7. During this time the mean values all are close to 40 breaths/min with considerable variations from child to child. Infants with persistent respiratory rate >60 breaths/min should be investigated for disease.

7 Transcutaneous PO_2 varies greatly in healthy newborn infants. The mean level of 93 mm Hg (12.4 kPa) at 1 hour after birth was higher than at 12–24 hours after birth when it was 86 mm Hg (11.4 kPa).

8 During crying tcPO_2 fell in 98 per cent of the infants. The mean fall was about 20 mm Hg (2.7 kPa) and was not affected by the time after birth.

9 During the oxygen test the peak values were between 373 and 428 mm Hg (49.7–57.1 kPa) in the first 48 hours of life. This corresponds to a right-to-left shunt of 18–21 per cent.

10 The results from the healthy newborn infants delivered vaginally, with birthweight ⩾2500 g and Apgar score ⩾7, Group A, were compared with three other groups:
Group B, Caesarean section, birthweight ⩾2500 g,
Apgar score ⩾7
Group C, vaginal deliveries, birthweight ⩾2500 g,
Apgar score ⩽6
Group D, Caesarean section, birthweight ⩾2500 g,
Apgar score ⩽6.

11 At one hour after birth mean baseline heart rate levels increased stepwise from A to D, but at 12–24 hours no differences were found.

12 Provided the Apgar score grouping is the same there were no differences in the mean baseline heart rate between vaginal deliveries and Caesarean sections.

13 In all the four groups mean tcPO_2 was higher in the first hour after birth than 12–24 hours after birth.

14 As with baseline heart rate there were no significant tcPO_2 differences during the first hour after birth between vaginal deliveries and Caesarean section provided the Apgar grouping was the same. When Apgar score ⩾7 mean tcPO_2 was 93 mm Hg (12.4 kPa) against 90 mm Hg (12.0 kPa) when Apgar ⩽6. A similar situation was found 12–24 hours after birth.

15 In all the four groups mean tcPO_2 decrease during crying was between 15 and 20 mm Hg (2.0–2.7 kPa).

16 In all four groups the peak values during the oxygen test were 28–38 mm Hg (3.7–5.1 kPa) higher 12–24 hours after birth than 1 hour after birth. In both time periods, the peak values of infants delivered vaginally with Apgar score ⩽6 (Group C) were lower than in corresponding infants with Apgar score ⩾7 (Group A).

17 Studying the influence of birthweight we found that mean baseline heart rate was significantly higher in infants with a birthweight < 2500 g compared with those with a birthweight between 2500 and 3000 g.

18 Mean tcP_{O_2} was lower in the birthweight groups 2000–2500 g than in those weighing between 2500 and 2750 g.

19 Mean tcP_{O_2} fell less during crying in infants with a birthweight below 2500 g than in those with a birthweight above 2500 g.

20 Studying the influence of sex we found that in boys with a birthweight < 2500 g mean baseline heart rate was significantly higher than in higher weight groups. Mean baseline heart rate in boys weighing < 2500 g was 145 bpm which was significantly higher than the corresponding value of 135 bpm in girls in the same weight group.

21 Several comparisons were made between the variables in active sleep and in quiet sleep. We found no significant differences in mean baseline heart rate whereas there were significant differences in the amplitude of long-term variability.

22 Furthermore we found that, in both sleep states, the amplitude of long-term variability increased with time after birth.

23 During the oxygen test mean baseline heart rate fell significantly by 6 bpm in active sleep and by 5 bpm in quiet sleep.

24 By contrast, respiratory rate increased significantly in both sleep states during the oxygen test.

25 tcP_{O_2} was significantly higher during quiet sleep than during active sleep in any one infant.

26 The range of the breath-to-breath respiratory rates was much greater in active sleep than in quiet sleep.

27 Differences in the variables become more distinct or only become manifest when the inter individual differences are eliminated. Therefore significant differences, for instance between active and quiet sleep, may not become apparent even in large series.

28 Studying one particular infant in the same activity state first at about 30 min after birth and then some 60 minutes after birth we found a significant fall in respiratory rate.

Bibliography

Ashton, R. and Connolly, K. (1971) The relation of respiration rate and heart rate to sleep states in the human newborn. *Develop. Med. Child Neurol.* **13**, 180–187.

Avery, M.E. (1964) The lung and its disorders in the newborn infant. In *Major Problems in Clinical Pediatrics* (Schaffer, A., ed). Philadelphia: W.B. Saunders.

Berg, D. and Dörrler, J. (1969) Das Verhalten des Säure-Basen-Haushalts am ersten Lebenstag unter besonderer Berücksichtigung der ersten Lebensminuten. *Geburtsh.u.Frauenheilk.* **29**, 980–994.

Betke, K. (1958) Hämatologie der ersten Lebenszeit. In *Ergebnisse der Inneren Medizin und Kinderheilkunde.* (Heilmeyer, L., Schoen, R., Glanzmann, E. and de Rudder, B., eds), p. 9. Berlin-Göttingen-Heidelberg: Springer.

Brady, J.P., Cotton, E.C. and Tooley, W.H. (1964) Chemoreflexes in the newborn infant: effects of 100% oxygen on heart rate and ventilation. *J. Physiol.* **172**, 332–341.

Brady, J. and James, L.S. (1962) Heart rate changes in the fetus and newborn infants during labour, delivery and the immediate neonatal period. *Am. J. Obstet. Gynecol.* **84**, 1–12.

Bratteby, L.-E., Andersson, L. and Swanström, S. (1979) Effect of obstetric regional analgesia on the change in respiratory frequency in the newborn. *Br. J. Anaesth.* **51**, 41S–45S.

Brooks, J.G., Schlueter, M.A., Navelet, Y. and Tooley, W.H. (1978) Sleep state and arterial blood gases and pH, in human newborn and young infants. *J. Perinat. Med.* **6**, 280–286.

Bryan, A.C. and Bryan, M.H. (1975) Respiratory control in newborn infants. In *Perinatale Medizin VI.* (Dudenhausen, J.W., Saling, E. and Schmidt, E., eds), p. 299. Stuttgart: Georg Thieme Verlag.

Cabal, L.A., Siassi, B., Zanini, B., Hodgman, J.E. and Hon, E.E. (1980) Factors affecting heart rate variability in preterm infants. *Pediatrics.* **65**, 50–56.

Chernick, V. (1977) Onset and control of fetal and neonatal respiration. *Seminar in Perinatology.* **1**, 321–392.

Comroe, J.H., Jr, Forster, R.E., DuBois, A.B., Briscoe, W.A. and Carlsen, E. (1962) *The Lung*, 2nd edn. Chicago: Year Book Publishers.

Clark, L.C. Jr. (1956) Monitor and control of blood and tissue oxygen tension. *Trans. Am. Soc. for Art. Int. Org.* **2**, 41.

Contis, G. and Lind, J. (1963) Study of systolic blood pressure, heart rate, body temperature of normal newborn infants through the first week of life. *Acta Paediatrica.* **146**, 41–47.

Cordero, L. (1972) Heart rate changes during the first hour of life. *Biol. Neonat.* **20**, 270–286.

Cross, K.W. (1949) The respiratory rate and ventilation in the newborn baby. *J. Physiol.* **109**, 459–474.

Curzi-Dascalova, L., Gaudebout, C., Dreyfus-Brisac, C. (1981) Respiratory frequencies of sleeping infants during the first months of life: correlations between values of different sleep states. *Early Human Development.* **5**, 39–54.

Desmond, M.M., Franklin, R.R., Vallbona, C. *et al.* (1963) The clinical behavior of the newly born. *J. Pediat.* **62**, 306–325.

Dinwiddie, R., Pitcher-Wilmott, R., Schwartz, J.G., Shaffer, T.H. and Fox, W.W. (1979) Cardiopulmonary changes in the crying neonate. *Pediat. Res.* **13**, 900–903.

Engström, L., Karlberg, P., Rooth, G. and Tunel, R. (1966) *The Onset of Respiration.* Association for the Aid of Crippled Children, New York.

Fournier, J.C., Burgun, P. and Renaud, R. (1977) Le rythme cardiaque instantané au cours de la première heure de vie chez les prématurés, les enfants en état d'acidose, les enfants nés per césarienne. In *1er Symposium Européen de cardiorespirographie néonatale,* pp. 27–45. Hewlett Packard, France.

Friis-Hansen, B., Lou, H.C., Marstrand-Christiansen, P. and Scheibel, E. (1979) The influence of apnoea and physical activity on arterial blood pressure and transcutaneous oxygen tension in the newborn. In *Continuous Transcutaneous Blood Gas Monitoring* (Huch, A., Huch, R. and Lucey, J.F., eds), pp. 461–468. Original Article Series – Birth Defects – The National Foundation March of Dimes, New York: Liss AR.

Gabriel, M., Helmin, U. and Albani, M. (1980) Sleep induced Po_2 – changes in preterm infants. *Eur. J. Pediat.* **134**, 153–154.

De Haan, R., Patrick, J., Chess, G.F. and Jaco, N.T. (1977) Definition of sleep state in the newborn infant by heart rate analysis. *Am. J. Obstet. Gynecol.* **127**, 753–757.

Hartreiter, A.R. and Abella, J.B. (1971) The electrocardiogram in the newborn period. I The normal infant. *J. Pediat.* **78**, 146–153.

Hathorn, M.K.S. (1974) The rate and depth of breathing in newborn infants in different sleep states. *J. Physiol.* **243**, 101–113.

Huch, R. and Huch, A. (1981) Transcutane Po_2 – Messung (tcPo_2 – Messung) beim Neugeborenen. In *Kardiotokographie* (Fischer W.M., ed), pp. 580–591. Stuttgart-New York: Georg Thieme Verlag.

Huch, R., Huch, A. and Lübbers, D.W. (1981) *Transcutaneous Po_2.* New York: Thieme-Stratton Inc.

Huch, A., Huch, R., Schneider, H. and Rooth, G. (1977) Continuous transcutaneous monitoring of fetal oxygen tension during labour. *Br. J. Obstet. Gynaec.* **84**, suppl. 1, 1–39.

Huch, R., Schneider, H. and Huch, A. (1978) Einfluss der mütterlichen O_2 – Atmung auf Herzfrequenz und tcPo_2 bei Mutter und Fet. In *Perinatale Medizin VII* (Schmidt, E., Dudenhausen, J.W. and Saling, E., eds), pp. 211–214. Stuttgart: Georg Thieme Verlag.

Iliff, A. and Lee, V.A. (1952) Pulse rate, respiratory rate, and temperature of children between two months and eighteen years of age. *Child Develop.* **23**, 237–245.

Junge, H.D. (1979) Behavioral states and state related heart rate and motor activity patterns in the newborn infants and the fetus ante partum. A comparative study II. Computer analysis of state related heart rate baseline and macro-fluctuation patterns. *J. Perinat. Med.* **7**, 134–148.

Karlberg, P. and Koch, G. (1962) Respiratory studies in newborn infants III. Development of mechanics of breathing during the first week of life. A longitudinal study. *Acta Paediatrica.* Suppl. 135, 121–129.

Kerpel-Fronius, E., Vegheleyi, P.V. and Rosta, J. (1978) *Perinatal Medicine.* Budapest: Akademiai Kiado.

Klöck, F.K., Closs, H.P., Austermann, R., Lamberti, G. and Schwenzel, W.(1972) Das Kardio-Respirogramm. Eine Erweiterung der postpartalen Zustands-diagnostik des Neugeborenen. *Z. Geburtsh. Perinat.* **176**, 266–274.

Koch, G. (1968) Venous admixture due to true anatomic shunt in the newborn infant during the first week of life. *Pädiatrie und Pädologie.* **4**, 211–224.

Koch, G. and Wendel, H. (1968) Adjustment of arterial blood gases and acid base balance in the normal newborn infant during the first week of life. *Biol. Neonat.* **12**, 136–161.

Martin, R.J., Okken, A. and Rubin, D. (1979) Changes in arterial oxygen tension during active and quiet sleep in the neonate. In *Continuous Transcutaneous Blood Gas Monitoring* (Huch, A., Huch, R. and Lucey, J.F., eds), pp. 493–494. Original Article Series – Births Defects – The National Foundation March of Dimes, New York: Liss AR Inc.

Nelson, N.M., Prod'hom, L.S., Cherry, R.B., Lipsitz, P.J. and Smith, C.A. (1963) Pulmonary function in the newborn infant: the alveolar-arterial oxygen gradient. *J. Appl. Physiol.* **18**, 534–542.

Oh, W., Arcilla, R.A., Lind, J. and Gessner, I.H. (1966) Arterial blood gas and acid base balance in the newborn infant: effects of cord clamping at birth. *Acta Paediatrica Scandinavica.* **55**, 593–599.

Oh, W., Lind, J. and Gessner, I.H. (1966) The circulatory and respiratory adaptation to early and late cord clamping in newborn infants. *Acta Paediatrica Scandinavica.* **55**, 17–25.

Oliver, T.K., Demis, J.A. and Bates, G.D. (1961) Serial blood-gas tensions and acid–base balance during the first hour of life in human infants. *Acta Paediatrica.* **50**, 346–360.

Parmelee, A.H., Schulz, H.R. and Disbrow, M.A. (1961) Sleep patterns of the newborn. *J. Pediat.* **58**, 241–250.

Peabody, J.L., Gregory, G.A., Willis, A.M. and Tooley, W.H. (1978) Transcutaneous oxygen tension in sick infants. *Amer. Rev. Resp. Dis.* **118**, 83.

Prechtl, H.F.R. (1968) Polygraphic studies of the full-term newborn: II computer analysis of recorded data. In *Studies in Infancy, Clinics in Developmental Medicine, 27* (Bax, M. and MacKeith, R.C., eds), pp. 26–40. London: Heinemann.

Prechtl, H.F.R. (1974) The behavioural states of the newborn infant. *Brain Research.* **76**, 185–212.

Prechtl, H.F.R. and Beintema, D. (1964) The neurological examination of the full-term newborn infant. In *Little Club Clinics in Developmental Medicine,* p. 74. London: Heinemann.

Prechtl, H.F.R., O'Brien, M.J. and Van Eykern, L.A. (1979) Neonatal breathing in different states of sleep and wakefulness. In *Central Nervous Control Mechanisms in Breathing* (Euler, C. and Lagercrantz, H., eds). Oxford and New York: Pergamon Press, 443–455.

Prod'hom, L.S., Levison, H. Cherry, R.B., Drorbaugh, J.E., Hubbell, J.P. and Smith, C.A. (1964) Adjustment of ventilation, intrapulmonary gas exchange and acid–base balance during the first day of life. Normal values in well infants of diabetic mothers. *Pediatrics.* **33**, 682–693.

Reardon, H.S., Baumann, M.L. and Haddad, E.J. (1960) Chemical stimuli of respiration in the early neonatal period. *J.Pediat.* **57**, 151–169.

Reynolds, S.R.M. (1962) Nature of fetal adaptation to the uterine environment: a problem of sensory deprivation. *Am. J. Obstet. Gynecol.* **83**, 800–808.

Rooth, G., Fall, O., Schachinger, H., Huch, A. and Huch, R. (1980) Continuous transcutaneous P_{O_2} measurement in the newborn immediately after delivery. In *Gynecology and Obstetrics – International Congress Series No. 512* (Sakamoto, S. and Tojo, S., eds), Proceedings of the IX World Congress of Gynecology and Obstetrics, pp. 419–422 Amsterdam: Excerpta Medica.

Rooth, G., Lysikiewicz, A., Huch, A. and Huch, R. (1982) Some effects of maternal pethidine administration on the newborn infant. *Br. J. Obstet. Gynaec.* In press.

Schachinger, H. (1980) Nicht-Invasive Messmethoden zur Ueberwachung der postpartalen Anpassung Neugeboner (Non-Invasive Monitoring of the Postnatal Adaptation of Newborn Infants). Thesis. Berlin FRG.
Scholten, C.A. and Vos, J.E. (1981) Descriptors of the rhythmicity in respiration and heart beat of newborn infants. *Med. & Bio. Eng. & Comp.* **19**, 83–90.
Schulte, F.J. (1975) Polygraphische Kontrolle von Apnoen. In *Perinatale Medizin VI* (Dudenhausen, J.W., Saling, E. and Schmidt, E., eds), p. 298. Stuttgart: Georg Thieme-Verlag.
Schwartze, H. and Schwartze, P. (1977) *Physiologie des Foetal-, Neugeborenen und Kindesalters.* Stuttgart-New York: G. Fischer.
Smith, C.A. and Nelson, N.M. (1976) *The Physiology of the Newborn Infant*, Springfield: Thomas C.C. Publishers.
Theorell, K., Prechtl, H.F.R. and Vos, J.E. (1974) A polygraphic study of normal and abnormal newborn infants. *Neuropädiatre.* **5**, 279–317.
Ulrich, U. (1969) Bestimmungen der arteriellen Blutgase unter Normoxie und Hyperoxie bei gesunden Säuglingen. Thesis, University Tübingen.
Välimäki, I. and Tarlo, P.A. (1971) Heart rate pattern and apnea in newborn infants. *Am. J. Obstet. Gynecol.* **110**, 343–349.
Vallbona, C., Desmond, M.M. and Rudolph, A.J. *et al* (1963) Cardiodynamic studies in the newborn. *Biol. Neonat.* **5**, 159–199.
Versmold, H.T., Onken, D., Höpner, F. and Riegel, K.P. (1976) Transcutaneous monitoring of Po_2 in the sick newborn. In *Intensive Care in the Newborn* (Stern, L., Friis-Hansen, B. and Kildeberg, P., eds), pp. 269–277. New York: Masson Publishing U.S.A.
Walsh, S.Z. and Lind, J. (1978) The fetal circulation and its alteration at birth. In *Perinatal Physiology* (Stawe, U., ed), pp. 129–181. New York: Plenum Medical Book.
Watson, E.H. and Lowrey, G.H. (1967) *Growth and Development of Children.* Chicago: Year Book Medical Publishers.
Willard, D. and Ott, W. (1978) La surveillance cardiorespirographique chez le nouveau-né. *Le médecine infantile.* **85**, 565–567.
World Health Organisation (1978) *A WHO Report on Social and Biological Effects on Perinatal Mortality.* Geneva.
Wulf, H. (1966) Die arterielle Sauerstoffspannung in der Neugeborenenzeit. Geburtsh. und Frauenheilk. **26**, 833–836.